Macular Diseases - An Update

Edited by Sara Crespo Millas and Salvatore Di Lauro

Published in London, United Kingdom

Macular Diseases - An Update
http://dx.doi.org/10.5772/intechopen.111271
Edited by Sara Crespo Millas and Salvatore Di Lauro

Contributors
Alessia Amato, Ali A. Hussain, Andrea Tamine Hoyos Dumar, Andrew Lamborn, Anselmo Feliciano Sánchez, Binita Patel, Brijesh Gelat, Chineze Thelma Agweye, Erick A. Quiroz-Gonzalez, Haroon Tayyab, Juan Carlos Lugo Prada, Kaid Johar, Krupali Trivedi, Laura Fernández García, Lesley Everett, Mark E. Pennesi, Miguel A. Quiroz-Reyes, Natalia Lobanovskaya, Nida Wongchaisuwat, Ogugua Ndubuisi Okonkwo, Paula Boned-Fustel, Paul Yang, Pooja Malaviya, Pooja Rathaur, Rahul Gelat, Romana García Gil, Tina Guanting Qiu, Toyin Akanbi, Utam Ashibel Utam, Yunhee Lee

First published in London, United Kingdom, 2024 by IntechOpen
IntechOpen is the global imprint of INTECHOPEN LIMITED, registered in England and Wales, registration number: 11086078, 167-169 Great Portland Street, London, W1W 5PF, United Kingdom

British Library Cataloguing-in-Publication Data
A catalogue record for this book is available from the British Library

Additional hard and PDF copies can be obtained from orders@intechopen.com

Macular Diseases - An Update
Edited by Sara Crespo Millas and Salvatore Di Lauro
p. cm.
Print ISBN 978-0-85466-455-9
Online ISBN 978-0-85466-454-2
eBook (PDF) ISBN 978-0-85466-456-6

Meet the editors

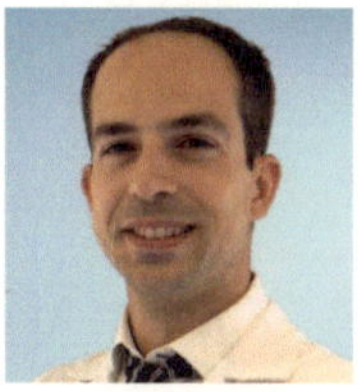

Salvatore Di Lauro graduated in medicine and surgery from the University of Naples "Federico II" (Italy) in 2009. He obtained a master's degree in vitreo-retina from the University of Valladolid (Spain), becoming a specialist in ophthalmology. He is a fellow of the European Board of Ophthalmology and has been an honorific collaborator of the University of Valladolid. He is an active researcher in retinal and ocular surface diseases, participating as investigator and study coordinator in numerous clinical trials, and has published several papers and book chapters. He is part of the REPRISE (database of expert reviewers created by the Italian Ministry of Education, Universities and Research).

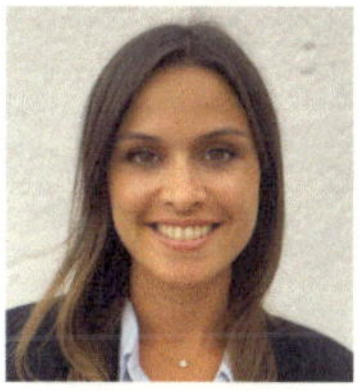

Sara Crespo Millas graduated in medicine and surgery from the Autonomous University of Madrid (Spain), receiving a master's degree in vitreo-retina from the University of Valladolid (Spain) and the title of specialist in ophthalmology. She is a researcher in retinal and ocular surface diseases, participating as an investigator in various clinical trials, and has presented at several recent international congresses.

Contents

Preface

Ophthalmology is continuously evolving, with new imaging techniques, diagnostic tools, and therapeutic options. In this sense, retinal diseases have experienced huge advances in the last few years. Optic coherence tomography (OCT) has revolutionized the classification, diagnosis, follow-up, and treatment of many macular diseases, especially age-related macular degeneration (AMD) and diabetic macular edema (DME).

New therapies are now available for AMD and DME, changing therapeutic intervals and maybe improving anatomical and functional results.

Furthermore, surgical techniques and technologies have improved for the treatment of epiretinal membranes and macular holes.

The reader will find in this book a combination of review chapters from international experts and original research chapters, including recent innovations in macular diseases.

Salvatore Di Lauro, MD, FEBO and Sara Crespo Millas, MD
Department of Ophthalmology,
Hospital Clinico Universitario de Valladolid,
Valladolid, Spain

Retina-Vitreous Department,
Instituto Oftalmologico Recoletas,
Valladolid, Spain

Section 1

Medical Retina

Chapter 1

A New Therapeutic Option for Reversing the Deficits in Dark Adaptation Associated with Age-Related Macular Degeneration (AMD)

Yunhee Lee and Ali A. Hussain

Abstract

The earliest functional marker in age-related macular degeneration (AMD) is the delayed recovery of rod photoreceptor sensitivity following a bright flash. Underlying mechanism is thought to be reduced levels of retinoids in the retinal pigment epithelium (RPE) compromising the rate of transfer of 11-cis retinal to the photoreceptor for rhodopsin regeneration. Normally, retinoids are lost due to photo-oxidation in the photoreceptor cell and inefficient processing of outer segment discs by the RPE but this loss is compensated for by delivery of plasma retinol across Bruch's membrane. Ageing of Bruch's membrane is associated with a 10-fold decrease in capacity for transport that is further exaggerated in AMD. We had previously shown that saponins can remove deposits from Bruch's membrane resulting in improved transport. As a proof-of-principle we have undertaken a pilot study with six AMD patients on oral saponin supplementation for 2 months (200 mg saponins/day) to assess the possibility of improving the transport across Bruch's membrane. Saponin supplementation improved the rate of recovery in rod sensitivity following a bright flash in all AMD subjects ($p < 0.005$, paired t-test), indicative of improved delivery of retinol across Bruch's membrane. The saponin intervention provides a new approach to slow, halt, or reverse the progression of AMD.

Keywords: macular degeneration, dark adaptation, vitamin A, Bruch's membrane, saponins

1. Introduction

Age-related macular degeneration (AMD) is the single largest cause of untreatable blindness in the elderly population [1]. In the European Union (EU), the number of affected individuals has been estimated as 67 million, with the figure predicted to increase to 77 million by 2050 [2].

Clinically, AMD is divided into early, intermediate, and late stages. Early AMD is characterised by the presence of drusen and pigmentary abnormalities of the fundus such as hypo- or hyperpigmentation. Although the presence of drusen remains a hallmark of AMD, it is important to realise that they are also present in normal elderly eyes. It is the size, number, and degree of confluency of druse that determines the risk for AMD pathology [3]. Progression to the late form results in geographic atrophy of the RPE followed by photoreceptor degeneration, also known as 'dry' AMD. The late phase is also associated with secondary complications of pigment epithelial detachments (PEDs, accounting for 12–20% of patients) and neovascular episodes (comprising 10–20% patients), the latter being designated as 'wet' AMD.

Epidemiological studies have shown AMD to be a highly complex, multi-factorial disease that has both a genetic disposition and considerable gene-environmental interactions [4, 5]. The diverse genetic associations with AMD best reflect the complex nature of the disease process. These genetic variations include several members of the complement pathway, components in lipid metabolism (cholesterylester transfer protein (CETP), hepatic lipase (LIPC), apolipoprotein E), and heat shock serine protease (Htra1), amongst others [6–9]). This complexity is further enlarged by the additional association of dietary, environmental, and cardiovascular risk factors.

The complexity of underlying mechanisms involved makes it very difficult to nominate suitable targets for intervention. Current efforts at intervention have addressed the late-stage complications of inflammatory and neovascular processes with some degree of short-time success but since the underlying instigators have not been targeted, the underlying degenerative phase will continue, leading to the death of RPE and photoreceptors.

We have adopted an alternative approach for understanding the causative mechanisms in AMD. Since age is the highest risk factor in AMD, it would appear that some component of the normal ageing process is accelerated in this disease leading to the pathological outcomes. Based on an assessment of the earliest functional alteration in AMD (namely, slowed rod dark-adaptation), we have nominated the transport system in Bruch's membrane as a specific target for intervention and the reasoning for this approach is discussed below.

2. Delayed recovery of rod sensitivity following a bright flash

The earliest functional marker in AMD is the delayed recovery of rod photoreceptor sensitivity following a bright flash [10–12]. Briefly, when a subject is dark-adapted for about 30 min, their retinal sensitivity to light is very high, given as the dark-adapted threshold (**Figure 1**, point A). Following a bright light flash that bleaches 95–100% rhodopsin, their retinal sensitivity is reduced, denoted by point B (**Figure 1**). Recovery in sensitivity begins with cones reaching a plateau in about 12–20 min. This is followed by recovery of rod sensitivity reaching the dark-adapted threshold in 30–40 min. The switch from cone to rod recovery is known as the cone-rod break (CRB). The initial rate of rod recovery is known as the S2 gradient and in this 30-year-old subject, it was determined as 2.0 dB/min. In AMD subjects, the S2 gradients are much lower, reaching dark-adapted thresholds much later (curve C, **Figure 1**) [13, 14]. In some AMD patients, the rod component is absent within the period of experimentation and may require hours to days to reach the dark-adapted threshold (curve D, **Figure 1**) [15, 16].

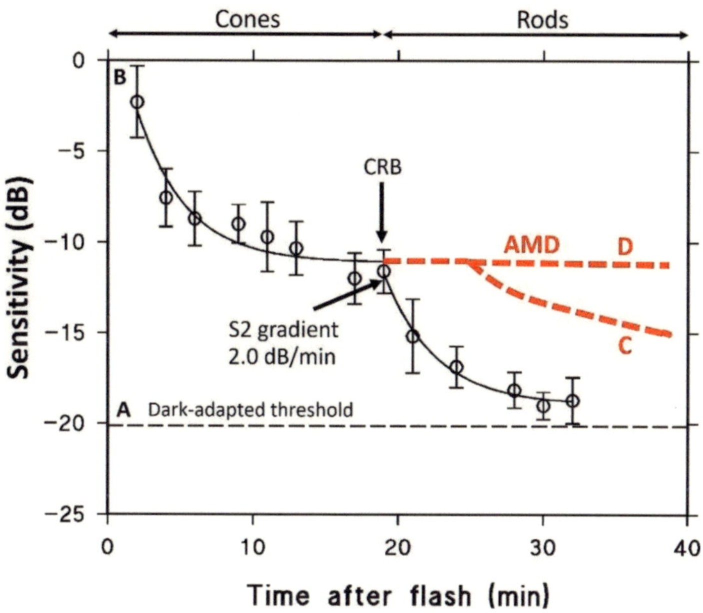

Figure 1.
Representative dark-adaptation curves for control and patients with AMD. In control subjects, there is an early recovery in cone sensitivity followed by recovery in rod sensitivity, reaching the dark-adapted threshold in about 30 min. In AMD, the cone-rod break (CRB) is usually delayed with slowed recovery in sensitivity (C). In some AMD patients, rod recovery may be absent within the period of observation (D).

Molecular mechanisms underlying the recovery in rod sensitivity are described briefly (**Figure 2**). Following a light flash, rhodopsin is converted to the apoprotein opsin and all-trans retinal (AT-RL), with retinal sensitivities falling from threshold A to B. Because of the toxic nature of AT-RL, it is converted to all-trans retinol and transported to the RPE to enter the vitamin A cycle [17]. After several enzymatic steps, the retinol ester is converted to 11-cis-retinal esters and stored in the RPE retinoid pool. After rhodopsin bleaching, 11-cis retinal is released from the RPE retinoid pool for delivery to photoreceptors and the rate of this transfer is related to the S2 gradient [18, 19]. It should be noted that recovery is dependent on the release of stored 11-cis retinal from the retinoid pool in the RPE and not on the reconversion of released all-trans retinal to 11-cis retinal.

Abnormalities in the sequence of events described above following a light flash offer plausible mechanisms for reduced S2 gradients in AMD. In some AMD patients, the presence of deposits between the RPE and receptors known as reticular pseudodrusen (RPD) is likely to impede the rapid transport of 11-cis retinal from the RPE to photoreceptors, reducing the S2 gradient [12, 15, 16]. Mutations in the members of the enzymatic and transport machinery of the vitamin A cycle are known to result in slowed S2 gradients but none have yet been reported in AMD [20]. Finally, the level of retinoids in the RPE pool is an important factor for determining the initial rate of transfer of 11-cis retinal to the photoreceptor. A reduction in the level of retinoids is expected to reduce S2 gradients.

If the vitamin A cycle was 100% efficient and all released AT-RL (from rhodopsin) was converted to 11-cis retinal, then there would be no change in the retinoid pool in the RPE. However, several factors are known that can modify the retinoid pool (**Figure 3**). First, released AT-RL can react with phosphatidylethanolamine to form

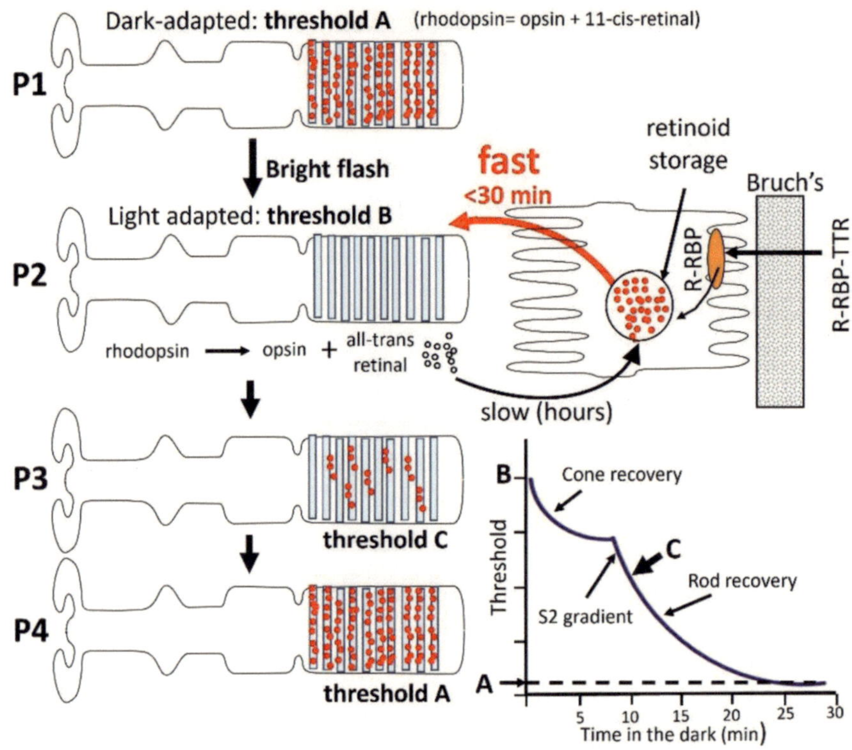

Figure 2.
Rapid deployment of 11-cis retinal from RPE stores for regeneration of rhodopsin and recovery in rod photoreceptor sensitivity following a bright flash. See text for an explanation of the rod recovery process. R-RBP, retinol-retinol binding protein; R-RBP-TTR. Retinol-retinol binding protein-transthyretin complex.

N-retinylidene-phosphatidylethanolamine (NRPE), which then reacts with a second molecule of AT-RL generating a variety of toxic bis-retinoids, compromising the retinoid pool [21, 22]. Second, the highly oxidative environment within photoreceptor outer segments leads to peroxidation of lipid such as polyunsaturated fatty acids (PUFA), resulting in lipid aggregates, lipid-protein complexes, and protein cross-link formation [23, 24]. These damaged outer segment discs are phagocytosed by the RPE and inefficient processing and extrusion onto Bruch's membrane lead to further loss of retinoids. Within the RPE, the bis-retinoids undergo further modification, resulting in the production of A2E, the fluorophore of lipofuscin. Some of the A2E is voided onto Bruch's membrane and the extent of retinoid loss can be judged by the age-related exponential increase in A2E content of the membrane [25].

Thus, to maintain the retinoid pool in the RPE, this loss must be compensated for by delivery of plasma retinol across Bruch's membrane. Retinol is transported across Bruch's membrane as a trimeric complex of retinol, retinol binding protein, and transthyretin of aggregate molecular weight (MW) of 75 kDa [26].

3. Ageing and loss of transport across Bruch's membrane

Normal ageing of Bruch's membrane is associated with gross structural alterations due to the accumulation of lipid-rich debris, damaged and trapped transitory

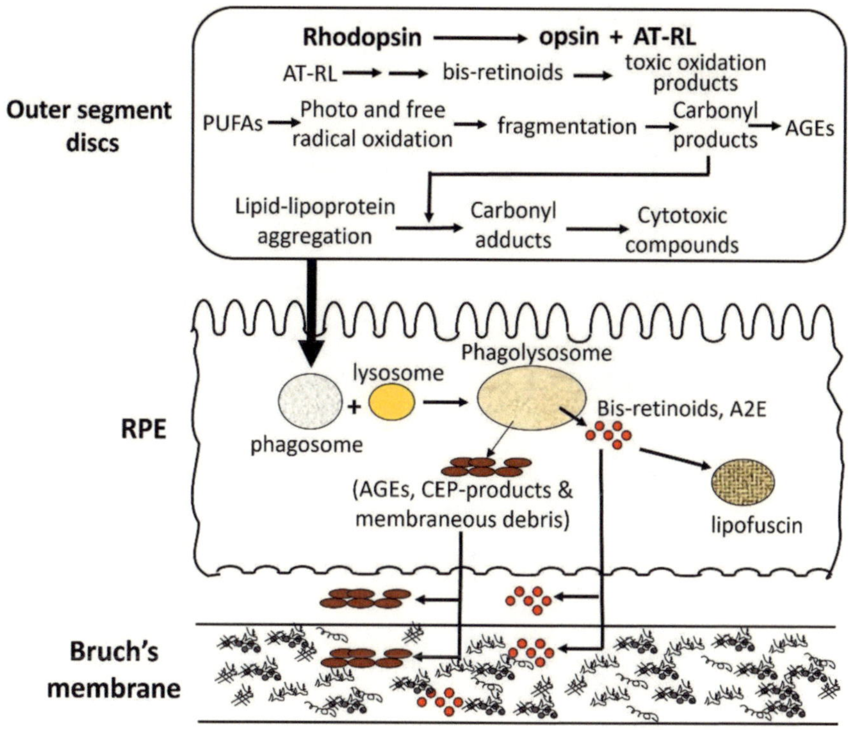

Figure 3.
Mechanisms underlying the reduction in the retinoid pool of the RPE in normal ageing and AMD. In the photoreceptor outer segment, the major loss of retinoids is due to the conversion of AT-RL to bis-retinoids. Oxidatively damaged outer segment discs cannot be digested effectively in the RPE and the degradation products are either stored as lipofuscin particles or extruded onto Bruch's membrane constituting a secondary loss of retinoids. PUFA, polyunsaturated fatty acids; A2E, the fluorophore of lipofuscin.

protein species, and extensive cross-linking of collagenous fibres, increasing its thickness and therefore reducing the driving diffusional gradients across the membrane [24, 27, 28].

The hydraulic and diffusional transport functions of human donor Bruch's membrane have been assessed as a function of age. Diffusional processes were assessed using the albumin molecule (MW 64 kDa) of similar molecular weight to the carrier for retinol (MW 75 kDa) and other carrier proteins for vitamins, anti-oxidants, and metals. In normal ageing, transport functions across Bruch's membrane showed an exponential decline with a half-life of 16–18 years, i.e., transport capacity was halved for every 16–18 years of life (**Figure 4**) [29–31]. In the elderly, transport capacities were reduced by nearly 10-fold. Such a reduction may compromise the delivery of retinol leading to a slight reduction in S2 gradients observed in the elderly [32, 33]. In the advanced ageing scenario of AMD, the diffusional transport across Bruch's membrane is further reduced (compared to age-matched controls) and may reflect the reduced transport of retinol and subsequent deficits in S2 gradients [30].

The reduction in transport across Bruch's membrane will not only affect the movement of retinol but will impact on all other carrier-mediated metabolites such as essential lipids, vitamins, anti-oxidants, and metals involved in the enzymatic protection machinery for dealing with oxidants and free radicals. The outward removal

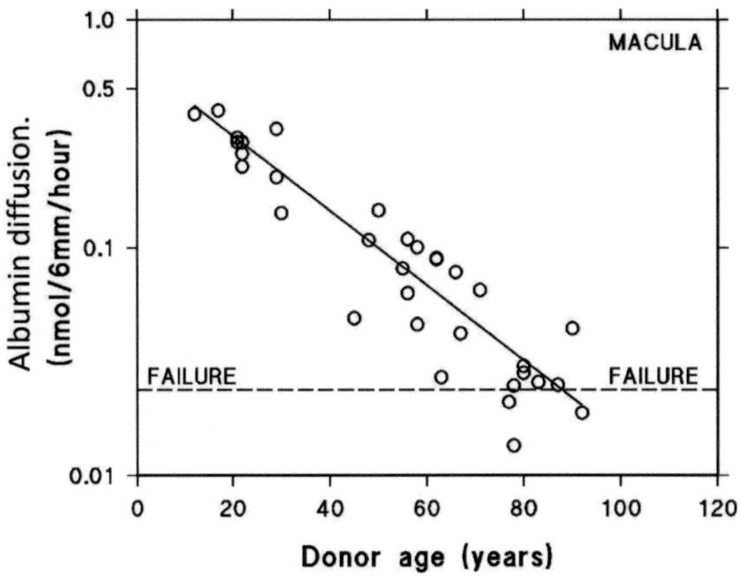

Figure 4.
Age-related reduction in the transport properties of human Bruch's membrane. Diffusional status of albumin across Bruch's membrane declines exponentially with age with transport capacities being halved for every 16–18 years of life (after Lee et al., 2015, Ref. [29]).

of toxic metabolites will also be affected, leading to their accumulation in Bruch's membrane and triggering inflammatory mediators and thereby undermining the survival of the photoreceptor-RPE complex.

4. Regeneration of Bruch's membrane

As mentioned earlier, ageing of Bruch's membrane is associated with accumulation of lipid-rich debris that essentially forms a barrier to the transport of metabolites. Reactive lipid fragments, bis-retinoid products, and free radicals lead to adducted and denatured proteins and cross-linking of the collagenous framework of the membrane. In elderly Bruch's membrane, nearly 50% of the collagen was found to be in a damaged state [24]. Normally, these ageing alterations are dealt with by continuous coupled processes of synthesis and degradation of the matrix, the latter process mediated by proteolytic enzymes called the matrix metalloproteinases (MMPs). These enzymes are released by the RPE in a latent form and following activation, can degrade most components of the matrix. Pro-matrix metalloproteinase 2 (Pro-MMP2) is the homeostatic enzyme in the system. For activation, proMMP2 and tissue inhibitor of metalloproteinase 2 (TIMP2) diffuse through Bruch's membrane to form a trimeric complex with matrix metalloproteinase 14 (MMP14) (membrane bound) on the basal surface of the RPE (proMMP2-TIMP2-MMP14). A second molecule of MMP14 then cleaves the inhibitory peptide on pro-MMP2 to release activated-matrix metalloproteinase 2 (MMP2) [34]. This system works well in the young but deteriorates with age, leading to a reduction in the level of activated MMP2 [35]. This is due most likely to slowed diffusional processes in ageing Bruch's membrane that restrict the formation of the trimeric complex for activation of proMMP2. In addition, released activated-MMP2 is most likely to be constrained and trapped within the grossly altered matrix of Bruch's membrane. In the advanced ageing of AMD, the level of activated-MMP2 in Bruch's membrane was about 50% of that in age-matched controls [36].

5. Potential target for intervention in AMD

From the above, it is obvious that any intervention must address the diminishing transport functions of Bruch's membrane. One possibility for overcoming the deficit in transport is to increase the diffusional gradient of metabolites across the membrane. Since oxidative damage in the RPE and photoreceptors is the primary driver of ageing changes, anti-oxidant and vitamin supplement regimes have been devised as a possible interventionist measure to reduce oxidative stress and hopefully slow the progression of AMD [37]. Thus, the Age-Related Eye Disease Study (AREDS) dietary supplementation cocktail was devised (vitamin C (500 mg), vitamin E (400 international units (IU)), beta-carotene (15 mg), zinc oxide (80 mg), and cupric oxide (2 mg)). Despite the wide use of AREDS supplements for over 20 years, controversy remains as to its usefulness since it does not prevent legal blindness in advanced AMD [38]. It has been pointed out that the earlier reported decrease in progression was related to the occurrence of neovascularisation rather than slowing the progression of dry AMD [39].

Given the fact that the diffusion of metabolites across Bruch's membrane is reduced by nearly 10-fold in the elderly, and more so in AMD, one must question the likely effectiveness of such dietary supplementation. The major problem with supplementation therapies is that they do not address transport in the opposite direction across Bruch's membrane, i.e., the removal of toxic metabolites that are the likely triggers of neovascular and inflammatory episodes.

The alternative to supplementation therapies is to improve the bidirectional transport pathways across Bruch's membrane. This would require the destabilisation and dispersal of the lipid-rich debris and the removal of normal and damaged proteinaceous deposits. Such a strategy would also release trapped activated MMP enzymes that could participate in hydrolysing the altered collagenous components. The expected improvement in intra-membrane mobility would favour greater activation of pro-MMP2, kick-starting the normal rejuvenation machinery in Bruch's membrane. Essentially, we would need to reverse the ageing process, i.e., elevate the decaying transport curves shown in **Figure 4** so that they no longer crossed the failure threshold within the lifetime of an individual.

6. Saponin-mediated improvement in the transport properties of Bruch's membrane

In vitro, surfactant molecules such as sodium dodecyl sulphate (SDS) can remove lipids and denatured, damaged, and aggregated proteins from Bruch's membrane and have been used to isolate proteins for SDS-PAGE (polyacrylamide gel electrophoresis). However, this class of surfactants is extremely toxic and cannot be considered for clinical intervention. Saponins, on the other hand, are naturally occurring amphipathic molecules, with the major source being the ginseng plant (*Panax ginseng*) and marine sea cucumbers (*Apostichopus japonicus*). In the Far East, saponin extracts have been used as tonics for thousands of years to promote general well-being without any

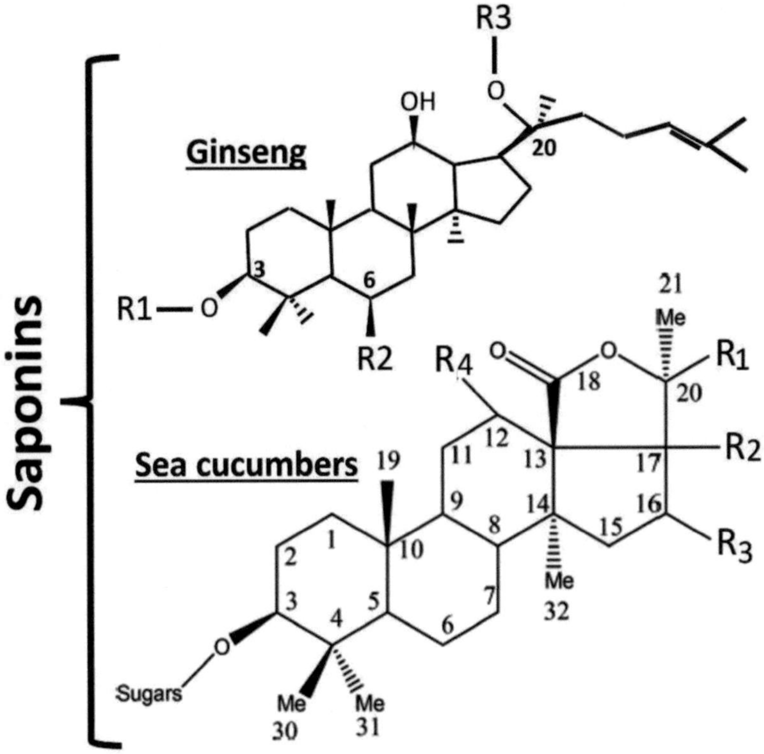

Figure 5.
Molecular structures of saponins derived from the ginseng plant and sea cucumbers. Saponins from ginseng have a 4-membered aglycone ring, whereas those from sea cucumbers have a 5-membered ring. The ring structures impart hydrophobic properties to the molecules. The several attachment sites containing primarily various glycosidic units represent the hydrophilic domain. The amphipathic nature of these molecules allows the solubilisation of lipoidal and proteinaceous deposits.

side effects. Structurally, saponins from the ginseng plant have a 4-membered ring in the hydrophobic domain, whereas sea cucumber saponins have a 5-membered ring (**Figure** 5). The incorporation of different chemical groups at the R1, R2, R3, and R4 attachment sites (sugars, hydroxyl, hydrogen, and alkane chains) gives rise to a myriad of compounds and over 400 have been characterised [40–42]. The amphipathic nature of saponins (containing hydrophilic and hydrophobic domains) allows them to readily partition into lipid structures such as liposomes, micelles, membranes, or lipoidal deposits and assist dispersal [43, 44].

Using isolated human donor Bruch's membrane preparations, we have shown that a single perfusion with saponins results in the release of various classes of lipid deposits, and attached and trapped proteinaceous material [29]. The released protein component also contained active-MMP2 enzymes. Release of this debris was associated with improvements in the transport of albumin-sized molecules across Bruch's membrane (**Figure 6A**). A dose-response curve for saponin-mediated improvement in hydraulic conductivity of Bruch's membrane showed hyperbolic saturation kinetics with the maximum improvement being 2-fold over basal levels (**Figure 6B**). With the *in vitro* work, saponins were capable of removing lipoidal and deposited proteinaceous debris from Bruch's membrane. However, they did not target the cross-linked collagenous fibres of the matrix. *In vivo*, improved diffusional

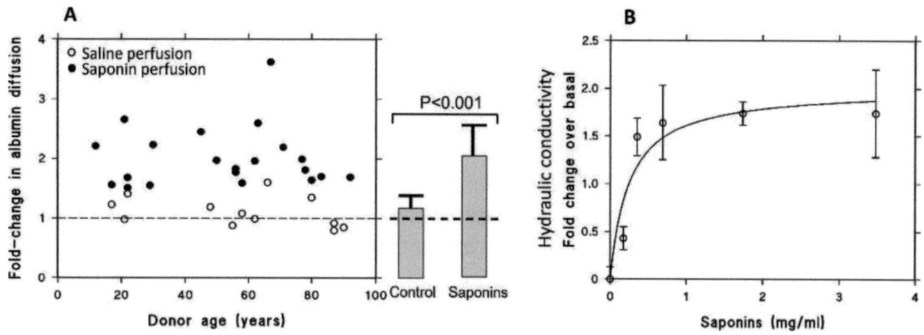

Figure 6.
Saponin-mediated improvement in the transport properties of human Bruch's membrane. (A): Incubation of Bruch's membrane with saponins improved the diffusional transport of albumin 2-fold (p < 0.001), open circles. Control; filled circles, saponin treated. (B): Dose-response curve for saponin-mediated improvement in hydraulic transport across Bruch's membrane. After Lee et al., 2015, Ref. [29].

status of Bruch's membrane would allow greater mobility of proMMP2 and TIMP2 for interaction with MMP14 on the RPE basal membrane, resulting in increased levels of activated-MMP2 to target the damaged collagenous network, leading to greater improvement in transport.

7. Saponins and dark adaptation

Saponin-mediated improvement in transport across Bruch's membrane could provide an interventionist strategy in AMD. Improved transport of retinol would augment the retinoid pool in the RPE, leading to improvement in S2 gradients. To assess this possibility, we have undertaken a pilot study with six AMD patients.

The dosage of saponins to use in this preliminary study was estimated as follows. Based on the bioavailability of saponins as 1.12 ± 1.6%, the half-life of a given saponin (Rb1) in plasma of 19.5 h, and the dose-response curve of **Figure 6B**, we calculated that a daily oral dose of 200 mg saponins should achieve a 0.5–1.0-fold improvement in transport across Bruch's membrane in our subjects over a period of 2–5 months [29, 45–48]. This dosage is similar to those of the saponin products marketed in the Far East for general health. Rather than using a single saponin species, we decided to use a wide mixture so that the varied nature of deposits in Bruch's membrane could be targeted. Thus, the final mixture of 200 mg saponins per day contained 50 mg of ginseng saponins and 150 mg of sea cucumber saponins.

Dark-adaptation curves were obtained using a Humphrey Field Analyser (HFA) (Series II, Model 750i, Zeiss). Use of the HFA to obtain dark-adaptation curves has previously been described [32, 33, 49]. In clinics, the HFA is normally used to monitor the progression of glaucoma. For this purpose, the viewing globe in the HFA has a background illumination of 10 candelas per square meter (cd m^{-2}) to suppress rod function, allowing the monitoring of cone responses. To obtain dark-adaptation curves (i.e., both rod and cone responses), we could have temporarily removed the background illumination. However, restoring background illumination takes a long time for stabilisation of light levels and this would interfere with the normal operation of the glaucoma clinic. The alternative to switching off the background illumination was to ask our AMD subjects to wear light-tight goggles incorporating

3.0 neutral density filters. The highest light intensity of the test spot offered by the HFA was 3185 cd/m^2. With the 3.0 ND goggles, this energy was reduced to 3.185 cd/m^2, providing a sufficient test range to obtain rod and cone dark-adaptation curves, as shown in **Figure 1**.

Altogether, seven test spots were utilised to measure sensitivity, three on the vertical meridian going through the fovea (yellow cross) and two on either side of the meridian (**Figure 7**). The seven spot locations were chosen to (a) allow random presentation of the test spots within the bleached area and (b) to obtain an average sensitivity change over the bleached region.

Following dilation, subjects were dark-adapted for 30 min. Dark-adapted thresholds were measured several times so as to familiarise the patient with the operational procedure of the HFA. After obtaining the dark-adapted thresholds, the goggles were removed and the patient was moved to an adjacent table and positioned in front of a box housing the bleaching apparatus. This box contained a red limit-emitting diode (LED) for fixation, a coupled-charge device (CCD) camera for monitoring fixation, and a flash unit (Speedlight SB-800, Tokyo, Japan). The patient was asked to look at the fixation light, and once confirmed, a flash of white light of integrated intensity 7.53 log scotopic Troland seconds (log sc td) was delivered inducing a calculated bleach of ~98% [50]. The bleached rectangular area subtended a width of 10.4° and a height of 6.6° and was located in the superior macula, just under the arcades (**Figure 7**). After the bleach, neutral density goggles were replaced and the patient was moved to the HFA to undergo repeated threshold assessments every 2 min for a period of 30–40 min.

At each time point, data from the seven fundal locations were averaged to produce a mean ± SD and plotted to obtain a dark-adaptation curve. Both rod and cone portions were fitted separately to an exponential function of the type $dB = a + (b^{*}\exp.(-t/k))$ where a, b, and k are constants and t is the time (in minutes) after flash using the add-in Solver module of the Microsoft EXCEL spreadsheet (EXCEL Microsoft, Redmond, WA, USA) [13]. The intersection of the rod and cone curves was taken as

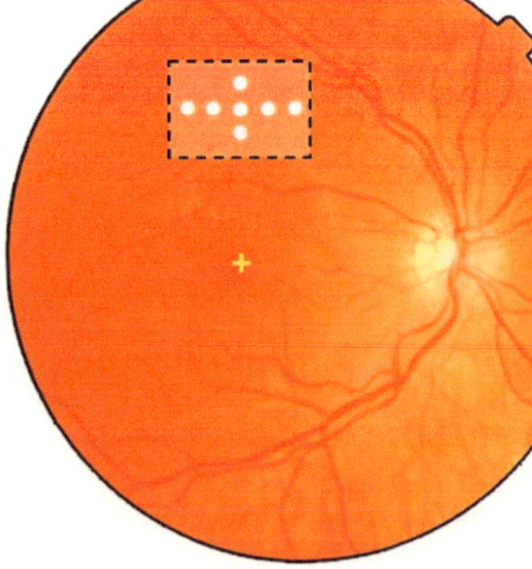

Figure 7.
Fundus bleaching region and location of test spots. The bleached area in the upper hemisphere enclosed by the dashed rectangle subtended a width of 10.4° and a height of 6.6°.

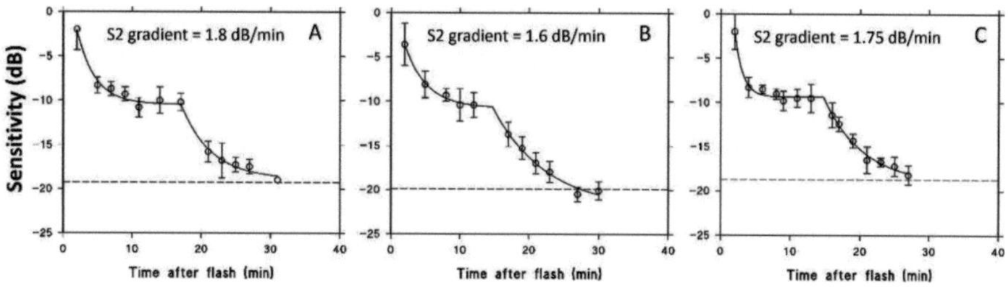

Figure 8.
Reproducibility of the dark-adaptation procedure. A control subject was tested three times over a period of 6 months and demonstrated little variability in S2 gradients.

the CRB time (min). Differentiation of the above equation with respect to time was used to calculate the gradient of the rod fit at time of the CRB and designated as the initial S2 gradient. In the absence of a rod portion within the 30–40 min of testing, the S2 gradient was designated as zero, S2 = 0.

In 10 control subjects, the S2 gradient was determined as 1.98 ± 0.16 dB/min, values equivalent to 0.2 log cd m^{-2}, similar to those reported in the literature [18, 51–53]. The reproducibility of the dark-adaptation technique was confirmed following repeated assessments in a control subject over a period of 6 months, showing little variation in S2 gradients, over the three visits (**Figure 8**).

Dark-adaptation curves for all the AMD patients are shown in **Figure 9**. On the basal visit, the six patients in the present study had S2 gradients of 0.6 ± 0.38 dB/min, considerably reduced compared to controls. One of the patients (subject F) did not show the presence of a rod component on the basal visit, i.e., S2 = 0. After basal determination of S2 gradients, all subjects were started on the saponin supplementation for a period of 2-months. Dark-adaptation curves were repeated on these patients after 2-months and the five patients who showed the presence of a rod component at the basal visit displayed improved S2 gradients following saponin supplementation.

Changes in S2 gradients following saponin supplementation are given in **Figure 10**. In this figure, basal S2 gradients are plotted against gradients after 2 months on saponins. The diagonal line in the figure is the line of no change. AMD patients on the saponin treatment showed significant improvements in their S2 gradients ($p < 0.005$, paired t-test). Patient F who lacked the rod component on the basal visit now demonstrated its presence after saponin intervention, with a S2 gradient of 0.43 dB/min.

8. Conclusions

In this preliminary study, saponin intervention (200 mg/day) for 2 months considerably improved S2 gradients in AMD patients, enhancing the rate of recovery in rod photoreceptor sensitivity following a bright flash. We and others had hypothesised that the delayed recovery in rod sensitivity following a bleach was most likely due to reduced transport of retinol across Bruch's membrane, compromising the retinoid pool in the RPE. Saponins have been shown to remove lipoidal and proteinaceous debris from Bruch's membrane improving its transport functions. This most likely underlies the improved transport of retinol leading to the observed improvement in S2 gradients in these AMD patients.

The proposed improvement in retinol transport across Bruch's membrane has implications for all other carrier-mediated metabolites and waste products. Thus, transport

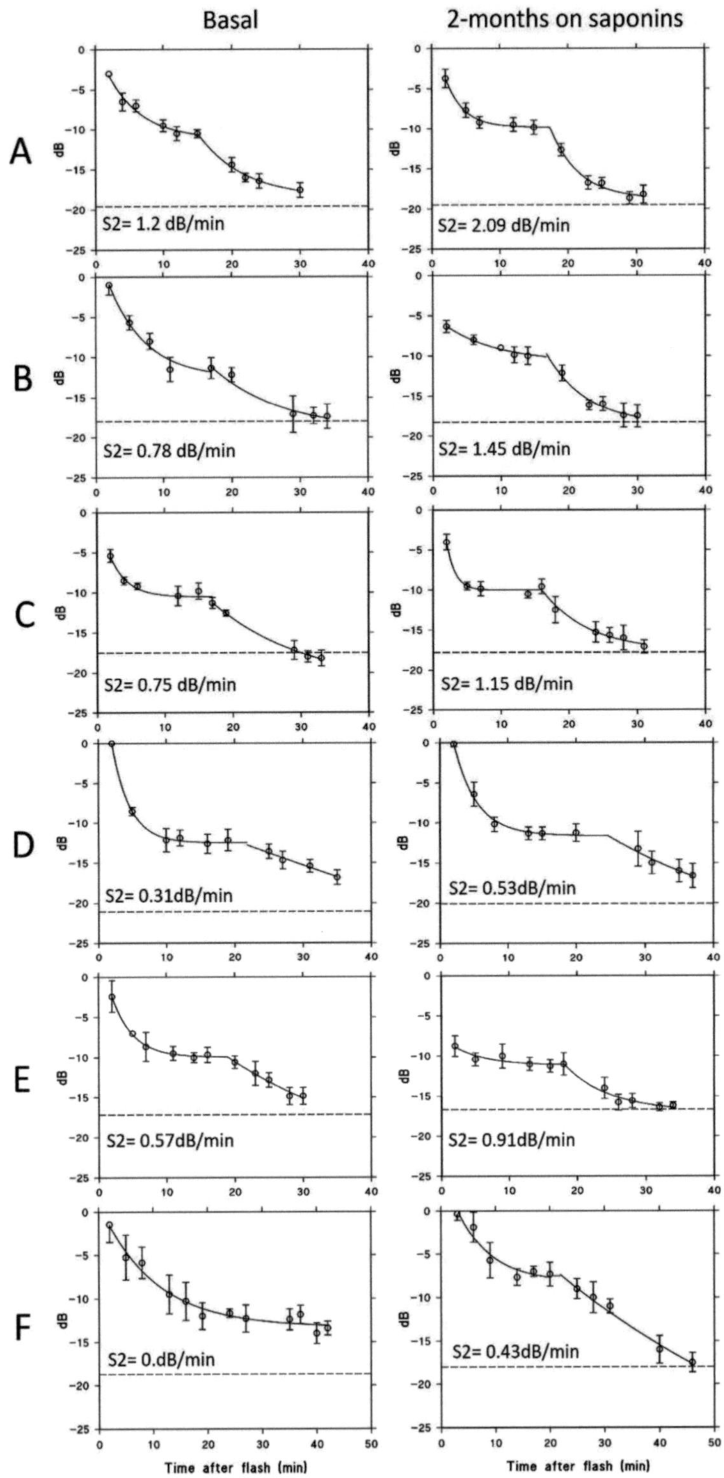

Figure 9.
Plots of dark-adaptation curves at basal visit and after 2 months on the saponin supplementation for all subjects in the study. All patients showed improved S2 gradients after saponin treatment. The horizontal dashed lines represent the pre-flash dark-adapted threshold.

DOI: http://dx.doi.org/10.5772/intechopen.1003081

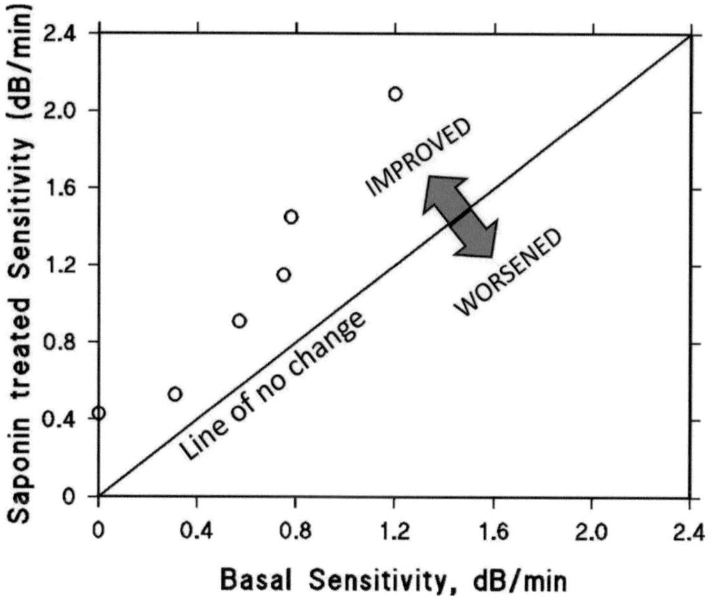

Figure 10.
Effect of oral supplementation of saponins over a period of 2 months on rod S2 gradients in AMD subjects. The oral supplementation regime showed improved S2 gradients in all patients ($p < 0.005$, paired t-test).

of vitamins, anti-oxidants, and essential metals that support the anti-oxidant defence machinery will be increased serving to maintain the health of the RPE-photoreceptor complex. Furthermore, improved transport across Bruch's membrane is expected to remove the accumulated toxic metabolites that are the triggers of neovascular and inflammatory processes. The current study has provided evidence for considering saponins as a potential new avenue for intervention in AMD. Further studies are now required to assess (a) if further improvements in S2 gradients can be elicited with prolonged saponin supplementation, (b) the stability of the improvement following withdrawal of the medication, (c) determining effects on the rate of progression of the disease, and (d) monitoring changes in clinical parameters such as drusen load. Given our current understanding of mechanisms underlying AMD, the saponin intervention is expected to slow, arrest, or reverse the progression of the disease.

Author details

Yunhee Lee[1*] and Ali A. Hussain[2]

1 AltRegen Co., Ltd., Beotkkot-ro, Geumcheon-gu, Seoul, Republic of Korea

2 Rescue, Repair and Regeneration Theme, UCL Institute of Ophthalmology, London, UK

*Address all correspondence to: eye.yunhee@gmail.com

References

[1] Klein R, Peto T, Bird A, Vannewkirk MR. The epidemiology of age-related macular degeneration. American Journal of Ophthalmology. 2004;**137**:486-495

[2] Li JQ, Welchowski T, Schmid M, Mauschitz MM, Holz FG, Finger RP. Prevalence and incidence of age-related macular degeneration in Europe: A systematic review and meta-analysis. The British Journal of Ophthalmology. 2020;**104**(8):1077-1084

[3] Ambati J, Ambati BK, Yoo SH, Ianchulev S, Adamis AP. Age-related macular degeneration: Etiology, pathogenesis, and therapeutic strategies. Survey of Ophthalmology. 2003;**48**:257-292

[4] Majewski J, Schultz DW, Weleber RG, Schain MB, Edwards AO, et al. Age-related macular degeneration – A genome scan in extended families. American Journal of Human Genetics. 2003;**73**:540-550

[5] Seddon JM, Santangelo SL, Book K, Chong S, Cote J. A genome wide scan for age-related macular degeneration provides for linkage to several chromosomal regions. American Journal of Human Genetics. 2003;**73**:780-790

[6] Edwards AO, Ritter R III, Abel KJ, Manning A, Panhuysen C, Farrer LA. Complement factor H polymorphism and age-related macular degeneration. Science. 2005;**308**:421-424

[7] Neale BM, Fagerness J, Reynolds R, et al. Genome-wide association study of advanced age-related macular degeneration identifies a role of the hepatic lipase gene (LIPC). PNAS. 2010;**107**:7395-7400

[8] Chen W, Stambolian D, Edwards AO, et al. Genetic variants near TIMP3 and high-density lipoprotein-associated loci influence susceptibility to age-related macular degeneration. PNAS. 2010;**107**:7401-7406

[9] Thakkinstian A, Bowe S, McEvoy M, et al. Association between apolipoprotein E polymorphisms and age-related macular degeneration: A HuGE review and meta-analysis. American Journal of Epidemiology. 2006;**164**:813-822

[10] Owsley C, Jackson GR, White M, et al. Delays in rod-mediated dark adaptation in early age-related maculopathy. Ophthalmology. 2002;**108**:1196-1202

[11] Dimitrov PN, Robman LD, Varsamidis M, et al. Relationship between clinical macular changes and retinal function in age-related macular degeneration. Investigative Ophthalmology & Visual Science. 2012;**53**:5213-5220

[12] Flamendorf J, Agron E, Wong WT, et al. Impairments in dark adaptation are associated with age-related macular degeneration severity and reticular pseudodrusen. Ophthalmology. 2015;**122**:2053-2062

[13] Dimitrov PN, Guymer RH, Zele AJ, Anderson AJ, Vingrys AJ. Measuring rod and cone dynamics in age-related maculopathy. Investigative Ophthalmology & Visual Science. 2008;**49**:55-65

[14] Owsley C, McGwin G, Clark ME, et al. Delayed rod-mediated dark adaptation is a functional biomarker for incident early age-related macular degeneration. Ophthalmology. 2016;**123**(2):344-351

[15] Luu CD, Tan R, Caruso E, Fletcher EL, Lamb TD, Guymer RH. Topographic rod recovery profiles after a prolonged dark adaptation in subjects with reticular pseudodrusen. Ophthalmology Retina. 2018;**2**:1206-1217

[16] Tan RS, Guymer RH, Aung KZ, Caruso E, Luu CD. Longitudinal assessment of rod function in intermediate age-related macular degeneration with and without reticular pseudodrusen. Investigative Ophthalmology & Visual Science. 2019;**60**:1511-1518

[17] Tang PH, Kono M, Koutalos Y, Ablonezy Z, Crouch RK. New insights into retinoid metabolism and cycling within the retina. Progress in Retinal and Eye Research. 2013;**32**:48-63

[18] Lamb TD, Pugh EN Jr. Dark adaptation and the retinoid cycle of vision. Progress in Retinal and Eye Research. 2004;**23**:307-380

[19] Mahroo OAR, Lamb TD. Recovery of the human photopic electroretinogram after bleaching exposures: Estimation of pigment regeneration kinetics. The Journal of Physiology. 2004;**554**:417-431

[20] Travis GH, Golczak M, Moise AR, Palczewski K. Diseases caused by defects in the visual cycle retinoids as potential therapeutic agents. Annual Review of Pharmacology and Toxicology. 2007;**47**:469-512

[21] Wu Y, Yanase E, Feng X, Siegel MM, Sparrow JR. Structural characterization of bis-retinoid A2E photocleavage products and implications for age-related macular degeneration. Proceedings of the National Academy of Sciences. 2010;**107**:7275-7280

[22] Sparrow JR, Gregory-Roberts E, Yamamoto K, et al. The bis-retinoids of retinal pigment epithelium. Progress in Retinal and Eye Research. 2012;**31**:121-135

[23] Liu A, Chang J, Lin Y, Shen Z, Bernstein PS. Long-chain and very long chain polyunsaturated fatty acids in ocular ageing and age-related macular degeneration. Journal of Lipid Research. 2010;**51**:3217-3229

[24] Karwatowski WSS, Jefferies TE, Duance VC, Albon J, Bailey AJ, Easty DL. Preparation of Bruch's membrane and analysis of the age-related changes in the structural collagens. The British Journal of Ophthalmology. 1995;**79**:944-952

[25] Murdaugh LS, Wang Z, Del Priore LV, Dillon J, Gaillard ER. Age-related accumulation of 3-nitrotyrosine and nitro-A2E in human Bruch'smembrane. Experimental Eye Research. 2010;**90**:564-571

[26] Bok D. Retinal photoreceptor-pigment epithelium interactions. Friedenwald lecture. Investigative Ophthalmology & Visual Science. 1985;**26**:1659-1694

[27] Okubo A, Rosa RH, Bunce CV, Alexander RA, Fan JT, et al. The relationships of age changes in retinal pigment epithelium and Bruch's membrane. Investigative Ophthalmology & Visual Science. 1999;**40**:443-449

[28] Holz FG, Sheraidah GS, Pauleikhoff D, Bird AC. Analysis of lipid deposits extracted from human macular and peripheral Bruch's membrane. Archives of Ophthalmology. 1994;**112**:402-406

[29] Lee Y, Hussain AA, Seok J-H, Kim S-H, Marshall J. Modulating the transport characteristics of Bruch's membrane with steroidal glycosides and its relevance to age-related macular degeneration

(AMD). Investigative Ophthalmology & Visual Science. 2015;**56**:8403-8418

[30] Hussain AA, Starita C, Hodgetts A, Marshall J. Macromolecular diffusion characteristics of ageing human Bruch's membrane: Implications for age-related macular degeneration (AMD). Experimental Eye Research. 2010;**90**:703-710

[31] Moore DJ, Clover GM. The effect of age on the macromolecular permeability of human Bruch's membrane. Investigative Ophthalmology & Visual Science. 2001;**42**:2970-2975

[32] Jackson GR, Owsley C, Cordle EP, Finley CD. Aging and scotopic sensitivity. Vision Research. 1998;**38**:3655-3662

[33] Jackson GR, Owsley C, McGwin G. Aging and dark adaptation. Vision Research. 1999;**39**:3975-3982

[34] Butler GS, Butler MJ, Atkinson SJ, Will H, Tamura T, et al. The TIMP-2 membrane type I metalloproteinase 'receptor' regulates the concentration and efficient activation of progelatinase A: A kinetic study. The Journal of Biological Chemistry. 1998;**273**:871-880

[35] Guo L, Hussain AA, Limb GA, Marshall J. Age-dependent variation in metalloproteinase activity of isolated human Bruch's membrane and choroid. Investigative Ophthalmology & Visual Science. 1999;**40**:2676-2682

[36] Hussain AA, Lee Y, Zhang JJ, Marshall J. Disturbed matrix metalloproteinase activity of Bruch's membrane in age-related macular degeneration. Investigative Ophthalmology & Visual Science. 2011;**52**:4459-4466

[37] Age-Related Eye Disease Study Research Group. A randomized, placebo controlled, clinical trial of high-dose supplementation with vitamins C and E, beta carotene, and zinc for age-related macular degeneration and vision loss: AREDS report no. 8. Archives of Ophthalmology. 2001;**119**:1417-1436

[38] Evans JR, Lawrenson JG. Antioxidant vitamin and mineral supplements for preventing age-related macular degeneration. Cochrane Database of Systematic Reviews. 2017;**7**(7):CD000253

[39] Desmettre T. Geographic atrophy and micronutritional supplements: A complex relationship. Journal Français d'Ophtalmologie. 2019;**42**(10):1111-1115

[40] Park JD, Rhee DK, Lee YH. Biological activities and chemistry of saponins from Panax ginseng Z. A. Meyer. Phytochemistry Reviews. 2005;**4**:159-175

[41] Mondol MAM, Shin HJ, Rahman MA, Islam MT. Sea cucumber glycosides: Chemical structures, producing species and important biological properties. Marine Drugs. 2017;**15**:317. DOI: 10:3390/md15100317

[42] Shi ZY, Zeng JZ, Wong AST. Chemical structures and pharmacological profiles of ginseng saponins. Molecules. 2019;**24**:2443

[43] Yu BS, Kim A, Chung HH, Yoshikawa W, Akutsu H, Kyogoku Y. Effects of purified ginseng saponins on multilamellar liposomes. Chemico-Biological Interactions. 1985;**56**:303-319

[44] Lee SJ, Lee MH, Lee K. Surface activities of ginseng saponins and their interactions with biomolecules. I. Separations and surface activities of major saponins from fresh ginseng roots. Korean Biochemical Journal. 1985;**14**:1

[45] Liu H, Yang J, Du F, et al. Absorption and disposition of ginsenosides after oral

administration of Panax notoginseng extract to rats. The American Society for Pharmacology and Experimental Therapeutics. 2009;**37**:2290-2298

[46] Han M, Sha X, Wu Y, Fang X. Oral absorption of ginsenoside Rb1, using in vitro and in vivo models. Planta Medica. 2005;**71**:398-404

[47] Xu QF, Fang XL, Chen DF. Pharmacokinetics and bioavailability of ginsenoside Rb-1 and Rg (1) from Panax notoginseng in rats. Journal of Ethnopharmacology. 2003;**84**(2-3):187-192

[48] Li L, Sheng Y, Zhang J, Wang C, Guo D. HPLC determination of four active saponins from Panax notoginseng in at serum and its application to pharmacokinetic studies. Biomedical Chromatography. 2004;**18**:849-856

[49] Owsley C, McGwin G, Jackson GR, Kallies K, Clark M. Cone- and rod-mediated dark adaptation impairment in age related maculopathy. Ophthalmology. 2007;**114**:1728-1735

[50] Rushton WAH, Powell DS. The rhodopsin content and the visual threshold of human rods. Vision Research. 1972;**12**:1073-1081

[51] Patryas L, Parry NRA, Carden D, Baker DH, Kelly JMF, et al. Assessment of age changes and repeatability for computer-based rod dark adaptation. Graefe's Archive for Clinical and Experimental Ophthalmology. 2013;**251**:1821-1827

[52] Tahir HJ, Rodrigo-Diaz E, Parry NRA, Kelly JMF, Carden D, Murray IJ. Slowed dark adaptation in older eyes: Effect of location. Experimental Eye Research. 2017;**155**:47-53

[53] Ruseckaite R, Lamb TD, Pianta MJ, Cameron AM. Human scotopic dark adaptation: Comparison of recoveries of psychophysical threshold and ERG b-wave sensitivity. Journal of Vision. 2011;**11**(8):2

Chapter 2

Central Serous Chorioretinopathy

Natalia Lobanovskaya

Abstract

Central serous chorioretinopathy (CSC) is characterized by neurosensory retinal detachment and vision deterioration at the posterior pole mostly in working-age men. The exact molecular pathogenesis of CSC remains unclear. It is proposed that leakage into subretinal space is caused by increased permeability of choroidal vessels and outer blood-retinal barrier breakdown. The majority of CSC cases are self-limited for a few months with a good visual prognosis. However, if neuroretinal detachment persists longer than 4–6 months, the condition requires treatment because chronic disease induces progressive and irreversible photoreceptor and retinal pigment epithelium (RPE) damage leading to reduced visual acuity. Treatment of CSC aims at achieving a complete resolution of subretinal fluid, and preservation of photoreceptor and RPE. There have been a number of interventions proposed for CSC management. However, treatment of this disease is still a subject of controversy. The purpose of this chapter is to overview pathophysiological hypotheses, diagnosing, and current treatment options for CSC.

Keywords: central serous chorioretinopathy, subretinal fluid, pachychoroid spectrum disorders, subthreshold micropulse laser, photodynamic therapy

1. Introduction

Central serous chorioretinopathy (CSC) is a disease characterized by idiopathic serous detachment of the neurosensory retina occurring in the macula over one or more areas of leakage from the choroid through the defects in the retinal pigment epithelium (RPE) and may be associated with retinal pigment epithelium detachments (PED). CSC is the fourth most common maculopathy associated with fluid leakage after neovascular age-related macular degeneration, diabetic macular edema, and retinal vein occlusion. CSC has been known for a long time and likely this disease was described first by Albert Von Graefe in 1866 who called it "recurrent central retinitis". CSC is usually unilateral and mainly affects young or middle-aged adults 30–60 years with the peak being in the age 35–45 years [1, 2]. It was found that men are affected 2–6 times more frequently than women [1–4].

2. Risk factors

Certain predisposing factors were found to be associated with CSC. Strong risk factors are treatment with corticosteroids or endogenous hypercortisolism (Cushing's disease) [1, 5, 6]. CSC, when related to exposure to exogenous glucocorticoids has a

 IntechOpen

less prominent male predisposition, often bilateral, and manifests more frequently with a chronic form. Psychological stress, which is associated with increased levels of catecholamines, is also recognized as a significant risk factor for CSC development [7]. Type-A personality features such as sense of urgency, competitive behavior, impulsiveness, emotional instability, and aggressive nature were observed in patients suffering from CSC [8]. Type-A personality is characterized by increased basal production of catecholamines [9]. A high incidence of primary hyperaldosteronism was detected in patients with CSC, as well as RPE changes resembling findings typical for inactive CSC are often seen in patients with primary hyperaldosteronism [10, 11]. This indicates that mineralocorticoid-dependent pathways might be involved in the pathogenesis of CSC. Genetic predisposition may play a role in the development of CSC, possibly via the complement factor H (CFH) gene [12, 13].

3. Pathogenesis

The primary molecular mechanism of CSC remains uncertain and seems to be multifactorial.

CSC is considered a pachychoroid spectrum disorder which includes features such as choroidal thickening, choroidal hyperpermeability, and RPE dysfunction [14, 15]. Choroid forms a rich vascular network plexus lying between the sclera and the retina, consisting of five layers starting from the sclera: suprachoroidea, three layers with vessels of decreasing size: Haller's layer of large blood vessels, Sattler's layer of medium and small size vasculature, and the choriocapillaris adjacent to the Bruch's membrane [16, 17]. The basement membrane of capillary endothelial cells forms the outermost fibrous layer of Bruch's membrane. The choriocapillaris is fenestrated and permeable to proteins that create a high oncotic pressure in the extravascular environment, which influences the movement of fluid from the retina to the choroid [18]. The choroidal circulation supplies oxygen and nutrients such as glucose and amino acid through the RPE to the outer retina [16, 19]. It has been proposed that abnormalities of choroidal vasculature such as dilation, congestion, and leakage lead to disruption of RPE barrier functions resulting in accumulation of subretinal fluid, PED, neurosensory retinal detachment, and RPE atrophy [20–22]. Intake of glucocorticoids is the most recognized risk factor for CSC development. It was suggested that mineralocorticoid receptor-dependent pathways are probably involved in the pathogenesis of CSC. Mineralocorticoid receptors (MRs) can bind both aldosterone and glucocorticoid hormones with similar high affinity [23]. MRs are expressed in the human RPE, in the choroidal endothelium, and also in the photoreceptors [24, 25]. It was shown that the overactivation of MRs mediates pathological effects such as oxidative stress, vascular inflammation, endothelial dysfunction, neovascularization, and fibrosis in the retina and other tissues [24, 26, 27]. Increased levels of glucocorticoid hormones induce excessive occupancy of MRs in choroidal vasculature and RPE that could mediate pathogenic effects leading to CSC. It was demonstrated in rats that intravitreal injection of aldosterone or high doses of glucocorticoids leads to choroidal vessel dilation and leakage due to upregulation of endothelial vasodilatory K channels KCa2.3 i [25]. Interestingly, low doses of glucocorticoids, widely used for intravitreal injections in ophthalmological practice, did not induce choroidal vasodilation [25]. Transgenic mice overexpressed the human MRs demonstrated dilatation of choroidal vessels, local alterations of the RPE, and outer blood barrier function disruption, resembling changes in retinal diseases of pachychoroid spectrum in humans [28]. Overactivation of MRs in RPE leads to up-regulation of *CXCR4* and *PTGER2* genes, inducing RPE migration and contraction leading to outer barrier structure malfunction and inhibition of rod outer segments phagocytosis by RPE cells [28]. On the other hand, MR-induced down-regulation of somatostatin (*SST*) and gap junction protein delta-2 (*GJD2*) genes could also cause destabilization of the RPE barrier [28]. Thereby, components of the outer retinal barrier were regulated towards disruption of its structure and function by overactivation of MRs.

Evidence suggests that patients with CSC may have functional changes in the regulation of choroidal blood flow which could be induced by emotional stress [29–32]. Neural control, provided by sympathetic or parasympathetic nerve endings, is important for choroid [33]. Increased sympathetic stimulation may reduce blood flow in the choroid [34]. Thereby sympathetic dysregulation of choroidal blood vessels, possibly stress-related, might induce focal choroidal ischemia, which may cause RPE damage. Localized ischemia can also induce increased vessel exudation leading to serous PED, breakdown of the outer blood-retinal barrier, and finally detachment of the neurosensory retina [30, 35]. The choroid can regulate its blood flow by the release of nitric oxide (NO) [36–38]. The vasodilatory impact of NO can be regulated in part by prostaglandins [39, 40]. It was suggested that the choroidal vascular hyperpermeability seen in CSC might be induced partly by abnormalities in the autoregulation of the blood flow in the choroid. Corticosteroids influence the production of NO and prostaglandins and thereby may affect the autoregulation of blood flow in the choroid leading to vessels hyperpermeability [41].

4. Classification

CSC classically is divided into acute and chronic forms based on the duration of subretinal fluid and the structural changes visible on multimodal imaging. The threshold that differentiates acute CSC (aCSC) and chronic CSC (cCSC) is set between 4 and 6 months in most published studies. This time is critical because self-resolution of the disease is no longer expected and treatment intervention can be considered.

Acute CSC has been found to be self-resolved in most cases [42]. Recurrent CSC is characterized by several spontaneously resolving episodes, whereas patients with chronic form of CSC keep subretinal fluid for at least 4–6 months [43]. Recurrence of the disease was approximately 30–50% depending on the study and happened within a year of the first episode [44–47]. Chronic CSC accounted for approximately 5% of all CSC cases [46]. General progression from aCSC to cCSC was established in around 16% of cases [48].

5. Diagnosis

5.1 Clinical presentation of CSC

Patients suffering from CSC usually complain of blurred vision or defects in the central visual field in the involved eye. Other symptoms could include metamorphopsia, micropsia, and mild dyschromatopsia. However, CSC can also be asymptomatic. The visual acuity of patients with aCSC decreases slightly or moderately and varies widely in cCSC. Amsler grid test reveals distortion of the straight lines in the majority of the cases of CSC [49]. Fundus ophthalmoscopic changes are characterized by around or oval-shaped focus of serous fluid under the neurosensory retina (**Figure 1A**) [50]. The area of the sensory retina detachment is described from less than 1 to more than 4 disc diameters [49]. The macula is affected in most cases, but the lesion can be located elsewhere, including the nasal retinal field [49]. Small pigment epithelium detachment (PED) can be seen behind the larger elevation of the sensory retina. PEDs are distinguishable by their grayish color. Subretinal precipitates are observed sometimes by biomicroscopy as multiple dot-like yellowish material under the neurosensory retina [51]. Fundoscopic examination shows focalized RPE mottling in aCSC. Persistence of serous neural retina detachment in cCSC is associated with more pronounced and diffused abnormalities in RPE including RPE hypertrophy, atrophy, and finally decompensation of RPE function and deterioration of vision [48, 52]. RPE defects can be observed as well in unaffected eyes.

5.2 Multimodal images

Spectral-domain optical coherence tomography (SD-OCT) confirms serous detachment of neurosensory retina which usually presents as dome-shaped in aCSC (**Figure 1E**) and tends to be shallower in cCSC (**Figure 2D, E**) [50].

In aCSC the outer retinal layers are usually well-observed and preserved. Sometimes protrusion of outer segments of detached photoreceptors and focal defects in the RPE at the leaking point can be noticed [53]. In contrast, in cCSC, SD-OCT demonstrates thinning of the outer retinal layers with poor visualization of the ellipsoid zone referring to photoreceptor inner segments which are tightly packed with mitochondria and therefore are very important for the photoreceptor health and function [54]. In cCSC cystoid macular degeneration can be developed. Serous retinal detachment can be associated with different types of PEDs including, dome-shaped, flat, and irregular PEDs [55, 56]. Spectral-domain enhanced depth imaging OCT (SD-OCT EDI) technique, which provides a deeper insight into the choroidal morphology, demonstrates an increased choroidal thickness in patients with CSC (**Figure 1E** on the right; **Figure 2D, E**). Interestingly, thick choroid is often seen in both eyes, even if the disease was developed in one eye [57].

Fluorescein angiography (FAG) allows to observe leakage of fluid into the subretinal space through the defects in RPE [58]. In CSC, usually, two types of patterns can be seen. Pinpoint hyperfluorescence appears in the early stage and subsequently increases in size and intensity into a large dot within the site of neuroretinal detachment called inkblot type (**Figures 1C, D** and **2C**). A smokestack pattern with dye rising superiorly within the subretinal space is thought to be related to the higher concentration of proteins in the subretinal fluid and was found in approximately 10–20% of cases. Acute CSC usually presents with one or a few focal leaks (so-called hot spots) which induce an isolated dome-shaped neuroretinal detachment. Chronic CSC is associated with multifocal leakage. If subretinal fluid persists, it tends to move toward the lower part of the macula inducing gravitational dystrophy of the RPE (**Figure 2C** on the left). Focal or geographic RPE window defects referring to past episodes of neurosensory retina detachment may also be observed.

Indocyanine green angiography (ICGA) shows hypofluorescent areas in early transit followed by late hyperfluorescence and pooling of indocyanine green

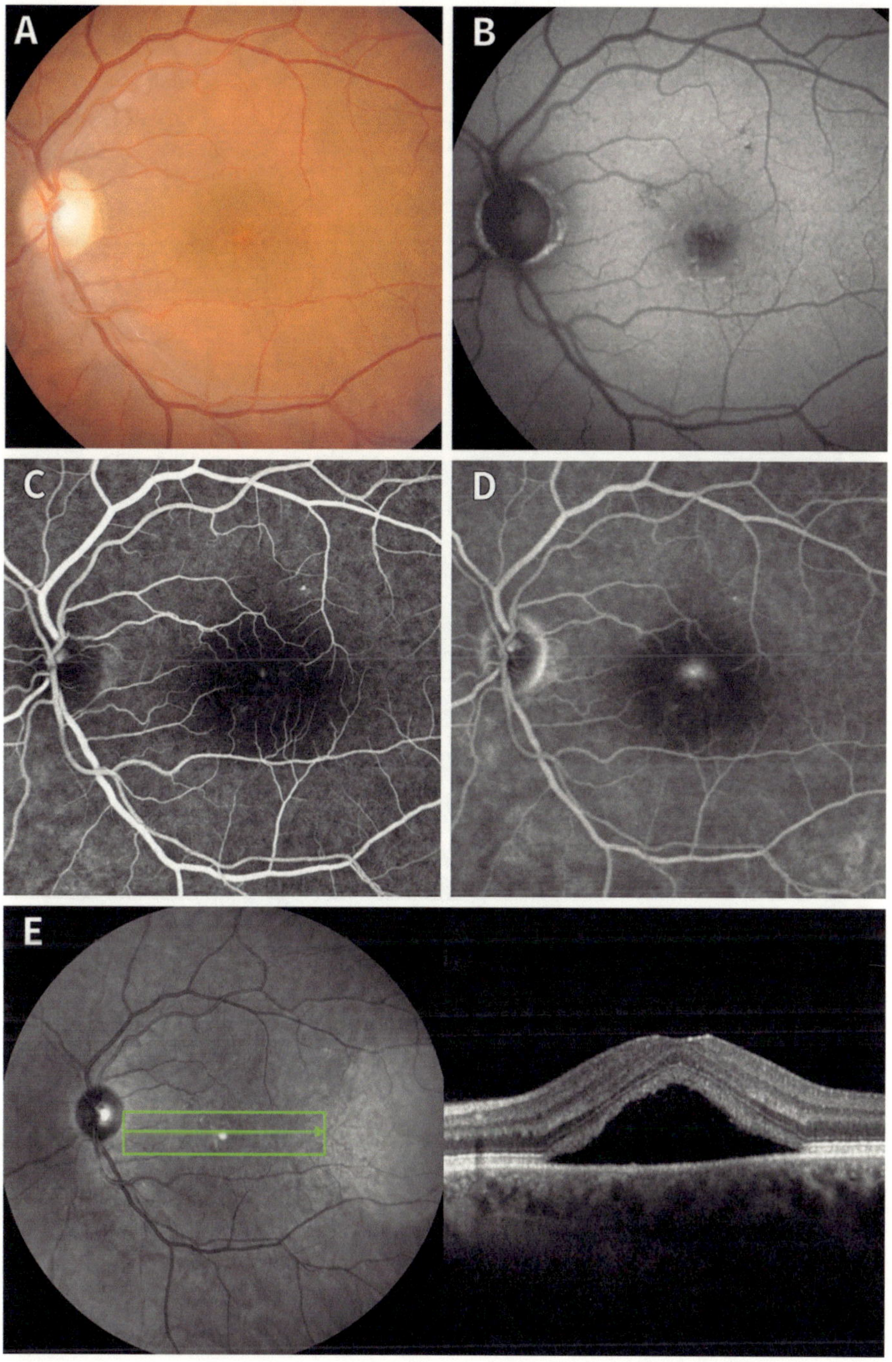

Figure 1.
Acute central serous chorioretinopathy, multimodal imaging. Color fundus photography shows serous retina detachment in the macula (A). Fundus autofluorescence shows a gentle circular area of increased autofluorescence (B). There is a focal area of hyperfluorescent dye leakage which gradually increases on fluorescein angiography (C, D). Spectral-domain optical coherence tomography enhanced depth imaging (SD-OCT EDI) detected a high dome-shaped serous neuroretina detachment at the fovea, overlying a thick choroid (E).

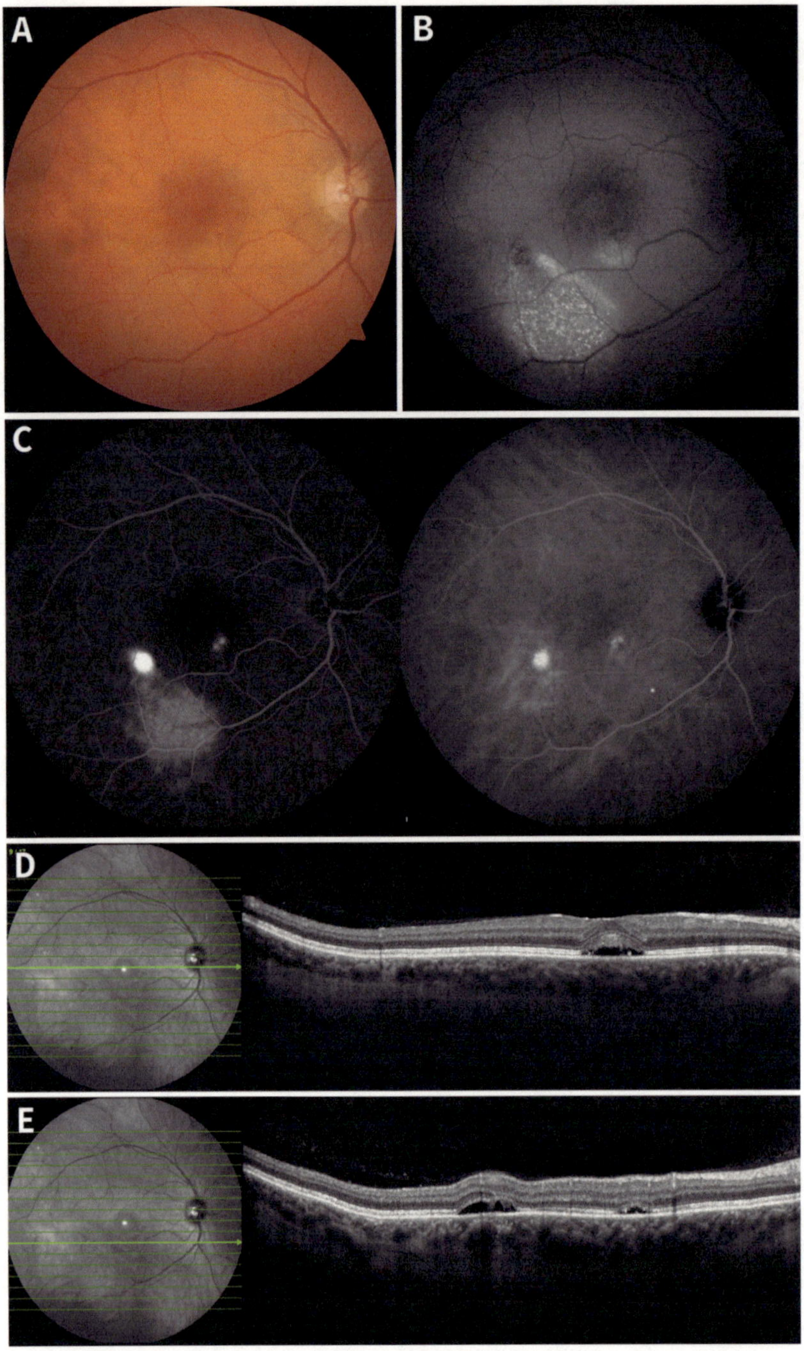

Figure 2.
Chronic central serous chorioretinopathy, multimodal imaging. Color fundus photography shows mild pigmentary abnormalities, which correspond to the areas of neuroretinal detachment and leakage (A). Fundus autofluorescence showing areas of speckled hyperautofluorescence suggesting chronic retinal pigment epithelium changes and the presence of subretinal fluid (B). Clear areas of focal leakage (inkblot pattern of leakage) can be seen on fluorescein angiography (C on the left). Indocyanine green angiography shows a similar leakage pattern with additional hyperfluorescent areas of choroidal vascular hyperpermeability (C on the right). Spectral-domain optical coherence tomography enhanced depth scan (SD-OCT EDI) showing the presence of subretinal fluid (including the fovea) and increased choroidal thickness (D, E).

which corresponds to atrophic and elevated RPE areas or leakage points on FAG (**Figure 2C** on the right) [35, 59].

Spectral-domain optical coherence tomography angiography (OCTA) and swept-source optical coherence tomography angiography (SS-OCTA) are advanced non-invasive imaging technologies that enable imaging, segmentations, and quantifications of blood flow in the retina and choroid. Some studies focused on comparisons between ICGA and OCTA imaging of CSC and found that abnormalities in the choroidal vasculature visible on OCTA correspond to ICGA changes in CSC [59, 60]. Therefore, OCTA is a promising noninvasive tool for visualization and follow-up quantifications of the choroidal vasculature in patients with CSC.

Fundus autofluorescence (FAF) helps in the diagnosis of CSC. RPE lipofuscin produces short-wavelength autofluorescence thereby FAF indicates structural and metabolic condition of the RPE cells in the macula.

Regions of granular hyper- and hypo-autofluorescence are visualized in CSC. Circumferential areas of hyperautofluorescence can be seen reflecting the presence of subretinal fluid (**Figure 1B**). Multiple gravitational tracks are seen as granular areas of hyper- and hypo-autofluorescence and are distinguishable for cCSC (**Figure 2B**).

6. Treatment

The treatment of CSC is a subject of controversy. Large prospective, randomized, controlled trials are particularly important to elicit the most effective treatment methods for CSC because of the relatively high percentage of spontaneous resolution of this disease which can be taken for treatment success in small, retrospective studies.

Acute CSC is essentially a benign disorder and in most cases, observation without treatment is generally recommended as initial management because subretinal fluid can resolve spontaneously within six months and visual acuity usually returns to normal [49]. However, small clinical sequelae can remain due to pre-existing irreversible retinal damage, including RPE alterations, complaints of darkening of the central visual field, color vision changes, metamorphopsia, and micropsia. Chronic and severe recurrent variants of CSC are associated with progressive vision loss [52]. The treatment aim for CSH is to achieve full resolution of neuroretinal detachment in order to restore normal anatomical and functional photoreceptor-RPE interactions because even a small amount of persisting subretinal fluid induces damage to photoreceptors [61, 62]. Treatment targets for CSC are the choroidal vascular network and RPE. Available treatment methods are aimed at accelerating the ability of RPE to absorb subretinal fluid, reducing leakage from the choroidal vasculature, and decreasing the flow of fluid through the RPE barrier into the subretinal space. Traditionally, continuous-wave thermal laser has been a treatment choice for CSC [63]. This method of laser treatment is directed to the site of fluorescein dye leakage and attempts to seal the focal defects in the outer blood-retinal barrier. Other benefits could be due to the migration of adjacent healthy RPE cells after injury and stimulation of the pumping function of RPE near the treated sites. Laser photocoagulation should be limited to extrafoveal leakage points because subjective scotoma can develop in the treated area. The long-term prospective randomized study compared argon laser photocoagulation with no treatment in the management of CSC revealed that direct photocoagulation reduces the duration of retinal detachment, however found no evidence that this treatment can significantly improve best corrected visual acuity (BCVA) and reduce a recurrence rate [44]. Robertson and

Ilstrup demonstrated that laser photocoagulation shortened the duration of CSC and decreased the rate of recurrences at the site of treatment as compared with sham treatment [63]. Navigated laser photocoagulation of the focal leakage point on FAG showed accuracy and effectiveness of subretinal fluid resolution [64]. Adverse events observed with laser photocoagulation include subretinal neovascularization and the development of progressive atrophy over time at the treatment site [63, 65].

Two commonly performed treatments for CSC are high-density subthreshold micropulse laser (HSML) and photodynamic therapy (PDT) with verteporfin (Visudyne (Novartis, Basel, Switzerland). HSML energy is delivered to the retina in a series of extremely short (microseconds) repetitive pulses allowing dissemination of the heart between the pulses and keeping the temperature below the threshold for denaturation of tissue proteins. Therefore, no laser-visible thermal damage to neural retina and choroid is induced. Subthreshold micropulse laser energy is absorbed mostly by melanin of RPE. It is proposed that HSML treatment increases the expression of heat shock proteins in targeted cells, which could activate endogenous protective mechanisms, decrease injury, and improve RPE functions [66]. It was demonstrated the effectiveness of HSML for CSC treatment, especially presented with point source leakage, in terms of resolution of subretinal fluid and improvement of BCVA [67, 68]. Another option available for CSC management is photodynamic therapy (PDT). The rationale for applying verteporfin PDT is a photochemical mechanism that induces occlusion of choriocapillaris leading to vascular remodeling and reduction of choroidal hyperpermeability [69–71] However, PDT can induce complications such as RPE atrophy and CNV [72, 73]. The PLACE trial is a large, prospective multicentre randomized controlled study comparing 810 nm HSML with half-dose PDT in patients with cCSC [74]. In this trial, half-dose PDT was superior to HSML in terms of complete resolution of SRF and improvement of BCVA. Measuring the value of HSML for CSC treatment is significantly complicated by the wide range of treatment regimens and laser wavelengths that have been reported [75]. Treatment with MR antagonists such as eplerenone and spironolactone has been associated with complete resolution of subretinal fluid and improved BCVA [76–78]. Eplerenone passes an increased MR selectivity compared to spironolactone and therefore has less antiandrogenic activity. Spectra trial is a prospective multicentre randomized controlled study designed to compare half-dose PDT with eplerenone in cCSC treatment regarding achieving complete resolution of SRF and improving the BCVA. In this study, PDT was found to be superior to eplerenone treatment in patients with cCSC [79]. VICI trial is a large randomized placebo-controlled double-blinded trial designed to assess the efficacy of eplerenone in cCSC [80]. VICI trial showed that eplerenone was not superior to placebo for the treatment of cCSC. Interestingly, the selective MR antagonist eplerenone has not demonstrated expected effect in the treatment of CSC in large trials. Efficiency of spironolactone was not assessed in large prospective randomized trials. Clinical and experimental evidence suggests that anti-VEGF agents could be used for CSC treatment due to their anti-hyperpermeability effect on the choroidal endothelial cells and ability to reduce choroidal blood flow [81, 82]. However, the use of anti-VEGF compounds for CSC treatment is generally off-label [75].

7. Conclusion

CSC is an enigmatic disease. Despite the fact that CSC has been known for more than 150 years, primary molecular pathogenesis and clear treatment strategy for this condition remain to be elucidated.

DOI: http://dx.doi.org/10.5772/intechopen.1004076

Author details

Natalia Lobanovskaya[1,2]

1 Ida-Viru Central Hospital, Ahtme, Ida-Viru County, Estonia

2 Tartu University Hospital, Tartu, Estonia

*Address all correspondence to: natalia.lobanovskaya@gmail.com

References

[1] Tittl MK, Spaide RF, Wong D, Pilotto E, Yannuzzi LA, Fisher YL, et al. Systemic findings associated with central serous chorioretinopathy. American Journal of Ophthalmology. 1999;**128**(1):63-68. DOI: 10.1016/s0002-9394(99)00075-6

[2] Tsai DC, Chen SJ, Huang CC, Chou P, Chung CM, Huang PH, et al. Epidemiology of Idiopathic Central Serous Chorioretinopathy in Taiwan, 2001-2006: A Population-based Study. PLoS One. 2013;**8**(6):e66858. DOI: 10.1371/ journal.pone.0066858

[3] Kitzmann AS, Pulido JS, Diehl NN, Hodge DO, Burke JP. The incidence of central serous chorioretinopathy in Olmsted County, Minnesota, 1980-2002. Ophthalmology. 2008;**115**(1):169-173. DOI: 10.1016/j.ophtha.2007.02.032

[4] Spaide RF, Campeas L, Haas A, Yannuzzi LA, Fisher YL, Guyer DR, et al. Central serous chorioretinopathy in younger and older adults. Ophthalmology. 1996;**103**(12):2070-2079; discussion 2079-2080. DOI: 10.1016/s0161-6420(96)30386-2

[5] Brinks J, van Haalen FM, van Rijssen TJ, Biermasz NR, Meijer OC, Pereira AM, et al. Central serous chorioretinopathy in active endogenous Cushing's syndrome. Scientific Reports. 2021;**11**:2748. DOI: 10.1038/s41598-021-82536-2

[6] Van Dijk EHC, Dijkman G, Biermasz NR, Van Haalen FM, Pereira AM, Boon CJF. Chronic Central Serous Chorioretinopathy as a Presenting Symptom of Cushing Syndrome. European Journal of Ophthalmology. 2016;**26**(5):442-448. DOI: 10.5301/ejo.5000790

[7] Gelber GS, Schatz H. Loss of vision due to central serous chorioretinopathy following psychological stress. The American Journal of Psychiatry. 1987;**144**(1):46-50. DOI: 10.1176/ajp.144.1.46

[8] Spahn C, Wiek J, Burger T, Hansen L. Psychosomatic aspects in patients with central serous chorioretinopathy. The British Journal of Ophthalmology. 2003;**87**(6):704-708. DOI: 10.1136/bjo.87.6.704

[9] Williams RB, Lane JD, Kuhn CM, Melosh W, White AD, Schanberg SM. Type A behavior and elevated physiological and neuroendocrine responses to cognitive tasks. Science (New York, N.Y.). 1982;**218**(4571):483-485. DOI: 10.1126/science.7123248

[10] Valverde-MegíasA,Montolío-MarzoE, Runkle I, Fernández-Vigo JI. Primary hyperaldosteronism in Acute Central Serous Chorioretinopathy: A real need for screening? Graefe's Archive for Clinical and Experimental Ophthalmology. 2023;**261**(11):3193-3200. DOI: 10.1007/s00417-023-06185-z

[11] van Dijk EHC, Nijhoff MF, de Jong EK, Meijer OC, de Vries APJ, Boon CJF. Central serous chorioretinopathy in primary hyperaldosteronism. Graefe's Archive for Clinical and Experimental Ophthalmology = Albrecht Von Graefes Archiv Fur Klinische Und Experimentelle Ophthalmologie. 2016;**254**(10):2033-2042. DOI: 10.1007/s00417-016-3417-8

[12] Miki A, Kondo N, Yanagisawa S, Bessho H, Honda S, Negi A. Common variants in the complement factor H gene confer genetic susceptibility

to central serous chorioretinopathy. Ophthalmology. 2014;**121**(5):1067-1072. DOI: 10.1016/j.ophtha.2013.11.020

[13] Mohabati D, Schellevis RL, van Dijk EHC, Fauser S, den Hollander AI, Hoyng CB, et al. Genetic risk factors in severe, nonsevere and acute phenotypes of central serous chorioretinopathy. Retina (Philadelphia, Pa.). 2020;**40**(9):1734-1741. DOI: 10.1097/IAE.0000000000002682

[14] Borooah S, Sim PY, Phatak S, Moraes G, Wu CY, Cheung CMG, et al. Pachychoroid spectrum disease. Acta Ophthalmologica. 2021;**99**(6):e806-e822. DOI: 10.1111/aos.14683

[15] Cheung CMG, Lee WK, Koizumi H, Dansingani K, Lai TYY, Freund KB. Pachychoroid disease. Eye (London, England). 2019;**33**(1):14-33. DOI: 10.1038/s41433-018-0158-4

[16] Nickla DL, Wallman J. The multifunctional choroid. Progress in Retinal and Eye Research. 2010;**29**(2):144-168. DOI: 10.1016/j.preteyeres.2009.12.002

[17] Ramrattan RS, van der Schaft TL, Mooy CM, de Bruijn WC, Mulder PG, de Jong PT. Morphometric analysis of Bruch's membrane, the choriocapillaris, and the choroid in aging. Investigative Ophthalmology & Visual Science. 1994;**35**(6):2857-2864

[18] Bill A. Aspects of the regulation of the uveal venous pressure in rabbits. Experimental Eye Research. 1962;**1**(3):193-199. DOI: 10.1016/S0014-4835(62)80001-3

[19] Bill A, Törnquist P, Alm A. Permeability of the intraocular blood vessels. Transactions of the Ophthalmological Societies of the United Kingdom. 1980;**100**(3):332-336

[20] Giovannini A, Scassellati-Sforzolini B, D'Altobrando E, Mariotti C, Rutili T, Tittarelli R. Choroidal findings in the course of idiopathic serous pigment epithelium detachment detected by indocyanine green videoangiography. Retina (Philadelphia, Pa.). 1997;**17**(4):286-293. DOI: 10.1097/00006982-199707000-00002

[21] Guyer DR, Yannuzzi LA, Slakter JS, Sorenson JA, Ho A, Orlock D. Digital indocyanine green videoangiography of central serous chorioretinopathy. Archives of Ophthalmology (Chicago, Ill.: 1960). 1994;**112**(8):1057-1062. DOI: 10.1001/archopht.1994.01090200063023

[22] Shakib M, Rutkowski P, Wise GN. Fluorescein angiography and the retinal pigment epithelium. American Journal of Ophthalmology. 1972;**74**(2):206-218. DOI: 10.1016/0002-9394(72)90536-3

[23] Arriza JL, Weinberger C, Cerelli G, Glaser TM, Handelin BL, Housman DE, et al. Cloning of human mineralocorticoid receptor complementary DNA: Structural and functional kinship with the glucocorticoid receptor. Science (New York, N.Y.). 1987;**237**(4812):268-275. DOI: 10.1126/science.3037703

[24] Behar-Cohen F, Zhao M. Mineralocorticoid pathway in retinal health and diseases. British Journal of Pharmacology. 2022;**179**(13):3190-3204. DOI: 10.1111/bph.15770

[25] Zhao M, Célérier I, Bousquet E, Jeanny J-C, Jonet L, Savoldelli M, et al. Mineralocorticoid receptor is involved in rat and human ocular chorioretinopathy. The Journal of Clinical Investigation. 2012;**122**(7):2672-2679. DOI: 10.1172/JCI61427

[26] Jaisser F, Farman N. Emerging Roles of the Mineralocorticoid Receptor in Pathology: Toward New Paradigms in Clinical Pharmacology. Pharmacological Reviews. 2016;**68**(1):49-75. DOI: 10.1124/pr.115.011106

[27] Wilkinson-Berka JL, Tan G, Jaworski K, Harbig J, Miller AG. Identification of a retinal aldosterone system and the protective effects of mineralocorticoid receptor antagonism on retinal vascular pathology. Circulation Research. 2009;**104**(1):124-133. DOI: 10.1161/CIRCRESAHA.108.176008

[28] Canonica J, Zhao M, Favez T, Gelizé E, Jonet L, Kowalczuk L, et al. Pathogenic Effects of Mineralocorticoid Pathway Activation in Retinal Pigment Epithelium. International Journal of Molecular Sciences. 2021;**22**(17):9618. DOI: 10.3390/ijms22179618

[29] Cardillo Piccolino F, Lupidi M, Cagini C, Fruttini D, Nicolò M, Eandi CM, et al. Choroidal Vascular Reactivity in Central Serous Chorioretinopathy. Investigative Ophthalmology & Visual Science. 2018;**59**(10):3897-3905. DOI: 10.1167/iovs.18-23995

[30] Hayreh SS. Submacular choroidal vascular pattern. Experimental fluorescein fundus angiographic studies. Albrecht Von Graefes Archiv Fur Klinische Und Experimentelle Ophthalmologie. Albrecht Von Graefe's Archive for Clinical and Experimental Ophthalmology. 1974;**192**(3):181-196. DOI: 10.1007/BF00416865

[31] Nathaniel Roybal C, Sledz E, Elshatory Y, Zhang L, Almeida DRP, Chin EK, et al. Dysfunctional autonomic regulation of the choroid in central serous chorioretinopathy. Retina (Philadelphia, Pa.). 2018;**38**(6): 1205-1210. DOI: 10.1097/IAE.0000000000001677

[32] Tittl M, Maar N, Polska E, Weigert G, Stur M, Schmetterer L. Choroidal hemodynamic changes during isometric exercise in patients with inactive central serous chorioretinopathy. Investigative Ophthalmology & Visual Science. 2005;**46**(12):4717-4721. DOI: 10.1167/iovs.05-0268

[33] Bill A, Nilsson SF. Control of ocular blood flow. Journal of Cardiovascular Pharmacology. 1985;7(Suppl. 3): S96-102. DOI: 10.1097/00005344-198500073-00011

[34] Bill A, Sperber GO. Control of retinal and choroidal blood flow. Eye (London, England). 1990;**4**(Pt 2): 319-325. DOI: 10.1038/eye.1990.43

[35] Prünte C, Flammer J. Digital indocyanine-green angiography in chorioretinal disorders. American Journal of Ophthalmology. 1996;**121**(1):26-34. DOI: 10.1016/s0002-9394(14)70531-8

[36] Deussen A, Sonntag M, Vogel R. L-arginine-derived nitric oxide: A major determinant of uveal blood flow. Experimental Eye Research. 1993;**57**(2):129-134. DOI: 10.1006/exer.1993.1107

[37] Luksch A, Polak K, Beier C, Polska E, Wolzt M, Dorner GT, et al. Effects of systemic NO synthase inhibition on choroidal and optic nerve head blood flow in healthy subjects. Investigative Ophthalmology & Visual Science. 2000;**41**(10):3080-3084

[38] Schmetterer L, Polak K. Role of nitric oxide in the control of ocular blood flow. Progress in Retinal and Eye Research. 2001;**20**(6):823-847. DOI: 10.1016/s1350-9462(01)00014-3

[39] Hardy P, Nuyt AM, Abran D, St-Louis J, Varma DR, Chemtob S. Nitric

oxide in retinal and choroidal blood flow autoregulation in newborn pigs: Interactions with prostaglandins. Pediatric Research. 1996;**39**(3):487-493. DOI: 10.1203/00006450-199603000-00017

[40] Salvemini D, Misko TP, Masferrer JL, Seibert K, Currie MG, Needleman P. Nitric oxide activates cyclooxygenase enzymes. Proceedings of the National Academy of Sciences of the United States of America. 1993;**90**(15):7240-7244

[41] Khanduja KL, Kaushik G, Khanduja S, Pathak CM, Laldinpuii J, Behera D. Corticosteroids affect nitric oxide generation, total free radicals production, and nitric oxide synthase activity in monocytes of asthmatic patients. Molecular and Cellular Biochemistry. 2011;**346**(1-2):31-37. DOI: 10.1007/s11010-010-0588-1

[42] Brancato R, Scialdone A, Pece A, Coscas G, Binaghi M. Eight-year follow-up of central serous chorioretinopathy with and without laser treatment. Graefe's Archive for Clinical and Experimental Ophthalmology = Albrecht Von Graefes Archiv Fur Klinische Und Experimentelle Ophthalmologie. 1987;**225**(3):166-168. DOI: 10.1007/BF02175443

[43] Hanumunthadu D, Tan ACS, Singh SR, Sahu NK, Chhablani J. Management of chronic central serous chorioretinopathy. Indian Journal of Ophthalmology. 2018;**66**(12):1704-1714. DOI: 10.4103/ijo.IJO_1077_18

[44] Ficker L, Vafidis G, While A, Leaver P. Long-term follow-up of a prospective trial of argon laser photocoagulation in the treatment of central serous retinopathy. The British Journal of Ophthalmology. 1988;**72**(11):829-834

[45] Gilbert CM, Owens SL, Smith PD, Fine SL. Long-term follow-up of central serous chorioretinopathy. The British Journal of Ophthalmology. 1984;**68**(11):815-820. DOI: 10.1136/bjo.68.11.815

[46] Liew G, Quin G, Gillies M, Fraser-Bell S. Central serous chorioretinopathy: A review of epidemiology and pathophysiology. Clinical & Experimental Ophthalmology. 2013;**41**(2):201-214. DOI: 10.1111/j.1442-9071.2012.02848.x

[47] Yap EY, Robertson DM. The long-term outcome of central serous chorioretinopathy. Archives of Ophthalmology (Chicago, Ill.: 1960). 1996;**114**(6):689-692. DOI: 10.1001/archopht.1996.01100130681007

[48] Castro-Correia J, Coutinho MF, Rosas V, Maia J. Long-term follow-up of central serous retinopathy in 150 patients. Documenta Ophthalmologica. Advances in Ophthalmology. 1992;**81**(4):379-386. DOI: 10.1007/BF00169099

[49] Klein ML, Van Buskirk EM, Friedman E, Gragoudas E, Chandra S. Experience with nontreatment of central serous choroidopathy. Archives of Ophthalmology (Chicago, Ill.: 1960). 1974;**91**(4):247-250. DOI: 10.1001/archopht.1974.03900060257001

[50] Semeraro F, Morescalchi F, Russo A, Gambicorti E, Pilotto A, Parmeggiani F, Central Serous Chorioretinopathy: Pathogenesis and Management. Clinical Ophthalmology (Auckland, N.Z.). 2019;**13**:2341-2352. DOI: 10.2147/ OPTH.S220845

[51] Kon Y, Iida T, Maruko I, Saito M. The optical coherence tomography-ophthalmoscope for examination of central serous chorioretinopathy with

precipitates. Retina (Philadelphia, Pa.). 2008;**28**(6):864-869. DOI: 10.1097/IAE.0b013e3181669795

[52] Gawęcki M, Jaszczuk-Maciejewska A, Jurska-Jaśko A, Kneba M, Grzybowski A. Impairment of visual acuity and retinal morphology following resolved chronic central serous chorioretinopathy. BMC Ophthalmology. 2019;**19**:160. DOI: 10.1186/s12886-019-1171-5

[53] Yu H, Xia G, Gao M, Yu J, Zhang Y. Morphologic changes in acute central serous chorioretinopathy evaluated by spectral domain optical coherence tomography. [Zhonghua Yan Ke Za Zhi] Chinese Journal of Ophthalmology. 2011;**47**(6):508-515

[54] Tao LW, Wu Z, Guymer RH, Luu CD. Ellipsoid zone on optical coherence tomography: A review. Clinical & Experimental Ophthalmology. 2016;**44**(5):422-430. DOI: 10.1111/ceo.12685

[55] Hirami Y, Tsujikawa A, Sasahara M, Gotoh N, Tamura H, Otani A, et al. Alterations of retinal pigment epithelium in central serous chorioretinopathy. Clinical & Experimental Ophthalmology. 2007;**35**(3):225-230. DOI: 10.1111/j.1442-9071.2006.01447.x

[56] Kaye R, Chandra S, Sheth J, Boon CJF, Sivaprasad S, Lotery A. Central serous chorioretinopathy: An update on risk factors, pathophysiology and imaging modalities. Progress in Retinal and Eye Research. 2020;**79**:100865. DOI: 10.1016/j.preteyeres.2020.100865

[57] Imamura Y, Fujiwara T, Margolis R, Spaide RF. Enhanced depth imaging optical coherence tomography of the choroid in central serous chorioretinopathy. Retina (Philadelphia, Pa.). 2009;**29**(10):1469-1473. DOI: 10.1097/IAE.0b013e3181be0a83

[58] Mohanty A, Mahapatra SK. Funduscopy-guided fluorescein angiography-free focal laser photocoagulation for central serous chorioretinopathy. Indian Journal of Ophthalmology. 2022;**70**(3):890. DOI: 10.4103/ijo.IJO_2006_21

[59] Zeng Q, Yao Y, Li S, Yang Z, Qu J, Zhao M. Comparison of swept-source OCTA and indocyanine green angiography in central serous chorioretinopathy. BMC Ophthalmology. 2022;**22**:380. DOI: 10.1186/s12886-022-02607-4

[60] Kim HC, Cho WB, Chung H. Morphologic Changes in Acute Central Serous Chorioretinopathy Using Spectral Domain Optical Coherence Tomography. Korean Journal of Ophthalmology: KJO. 2012;**26**(5):347-354. DOI: 10.3341/kjo.2012.26.5.347

[61] Chowers G, Cohen M, Marks-Ohana D, Stika S, Eijzenberg A, Banin E, et al. Course of Sodium Iodate-Induced Retinal Degeneration in Albino and Pigmented Mice. Investigative Ophthalmology & Visual Science. 2017;**58**(4):2239-2249. DOI: 10.1167/iovs.16-21255

[62] Winkler BS. Glycolytic and oxidative metabolism in relation to retinal function. The Journal of General Physiology. 1981;**77**(6):667-692. DOI: 10.1085/ jgp.77.6.667

[63] Robertson DM, Ilstrup D. Direct, indirect, and sham laser photocoagulation in the management of central serous chorioretinopathy. American Journal of Ophthalmology. 1983;**95**(4):457-466. DOI: 10.1016/0002-9394(83)90265-9

[64] Chhablani J, Rani PK, Mathai A, Jalali S, Kozak I. Navigated focal laser photocoagulation for central serous chorioretinopathy. Clinical Ophthalmology. 2014;**8**:1543-1547. DOI: 10.2147/OPTH.S67025

[65] Chhablani J, Pichi F, Silva R, Casella AM, Murthy H, Banker A, et al. King Khaled Eye Specialist Hospital International Collaborative Retina Study Group. Antiangiogenics in choroidal neovascularization associated with laser in central serous chorioretinopathy. Retina (Philadelphia, Pa.). 2016;**36**(5):901- 908. DOI: 10.1097/IAE.0000000000000804

[66] Morimura Y, Okada AA, Hayashi A, Fujioka S, Hashida N, Kawahara S, et al. Histological effect and protein expression in subthreshold transpupillary thermotherapy in rabbit eyes. Archives of Ophthalmology (Chicago, Ill.: 1960). 2004;**122**(10):1510-1515 10.1001/archopht.122.10.1510

[67] Chen S-N, Hwang J-F, Tseng L-F, Lin C-J. Subthreshold diode micropulse photocoagulation for the treatment of chronic central serous chorioretinopathy with juxtafoveal leakage. Ophthalmology. 2008;**115**(12):2229-2234. DOI: 10.1016/j.ophtha.2008.08.026

[68] Lanzetta P, Furlan F, Morgante L, Veritti D, Bandello F. Nonvisible subthreshold micropulse diode laser (810 nm) treatment of central serous chorioretinopathy. A pilot study. European Journal of Ophthalmology. 2008;**18**(6):934-940. DOI: 10.1177/112067210801800613

[69] Cardillo Piccolino F, Eandi CM, Ventre L, Rigault de la Longrais RC, Grignolo FM. Photodynamic therapy for chronic central serous chorioretinopathy. Retina (Philadelphia, Pa.). 2003;**23**(6):752-763. DOI: 10.1097/00006982-200312000-00002

[70] Schmidt-Erfurth U, Michels S, Barbazetto I, Laqua H. Photodynamic effects on choroidal neovascularization and physiological choroid. Investigative Ophthalmology & Visual Science. 2002;**43**(3):830-841

[71] Yannuzzi LA, Slakter JS, Gross NE, Spaide RF, Costa DLL, Huang SJ, et al. Indocyanine green angiography-guided photodynamic therapy for treatment of chronic central serous chorioretinopathy: A pilot study. Retina (Philadelphia, Pa.). 2003;**23**(3):288-298. DOI: 10.1097/00006982-200306000-00002

[72] Chan W-M, Lam DSC, Lai TYY, Tam BSM, Liu DTL, Chan CKM. Choroidal vascular remodelling in central serous chorioretinopathy after indocyanine green guided photodynamic therapy with verteporfin: A novel treatment at the primary disease level. The British Journal of Ophthalmology. 2003;**87**(12):1453-1458. DOI: 10.1136/bjo.87.12.1453

[73] Ober MD, Yannuzzi LA, Do DV, Spaide RF, Bressler NM, Jampol LM, et al. Photodynamic therapy for focal retinal pigment epithelial leaks secondary to central serous chorioretinopathy. Ophthalmology. 2005;**112**(12):2088-2094. DOI: 10.1016/j.ophtha.2005.06.026

[74] van Dijk EHC, Fauser S, Breukink MB, Blanco-Garavito R, Groenewoud JMM, Keunen JEE, et al. Half-Dose Photodynamic Therapy versus High-Density Subthreshold Micropulse Laser Treatment in Patients with Chronic Central Serous Chorioretinopathy: The PLACE Trial. Ophthalmology. 2018;**125**(10):1547-1555. DOI: 10.1016/j.ophtha.2018.04.021

[75] Van Rijssen TJ, Van Dijk EHC, Yzer Y, Ohno-Matsui K, Keunen JEE, Schlingemann RO, et al. Central serous

chorioretinopathy: Towards an evidence-based treatment guideline. Progress in Retinal and Eye Research. 2019;**73**:100770. DOI: 10.1016/j.preteyeres.2019.07.003

[76] Cakir B, Fischer F, Ehlken C, Bühler A, Stahl A, Schlunck G, et al. Clinical experience with eplerenone to treat chronic central serous chorioretinopathy. Graefe's Archive for Clinical and Experimental Ophthalmology = Albrecht Von Graefes Archiv Fur Klinische Und Experimentelle Ophthalmologie. 2016;**254**(11):2151-2157. DOI: 10.1007/s00417-016-3373-3

[77] Pichi F, Carrai P, Ciardella A, Behar-Cohen F, Nucci P, Central Serous Chorioretinopathy Study Group. Comparison of two mineralcorticosteroids receptor antagonists for the treatment of central serous chorioretinopathy. International Ophthalmology. 2017;**37**(5):1115-1125. DOI: 10.1007/s10792-016-0377-2

[78] Rahimy E, Pitcher JD, Hsu J, Adam MK, Shahlaee A, Samara WA, et al. A randomized double-blind placebo-control pilot study of eplerenone for the treatment of central serous chorioretinopathy (ecselsior). Retina (Philadelphia, Pa.). 2018;**38**(5):962-969. DOI: 10.1097/IAE.0000000000001649

[79] van Rijssen TJ, van Dijk EHC, Tsonaka R, Feenstra HMA, Dijkman G, Peters PJH, et al. Half-Dose Photodynamic Therapy Versus Eplerenone in Chronic Central Serous Chorioretinopathy (SPECTRA): A Randomized Controlled Trial. American Journal of Ophthalmology. 2022;**233**:101-110. DOI: 10.1016/j.ajo.2021.06.020

[80] Lotery A, Sivaprasad S, O'Connell A, Harris RA, Culliford L, Ellis L, et al. Eplerenone for chronic central serous chorioretinopathy in patients with active, previously untreated disease for more than 4 months (VICI): A randomised, double-blind, placebo-controlled trial. Lancet (London, England). 2020;**395**(10220):294-303. DOI: 10.1016/S0140-6736(19)32981-2

[81] Peters S, Julien S, Heiduschka P, Grisanti S, Ziemssen F, Adler M, et al. Antipermeability and antiproliferative effects of standard and frozen bevacizumab on choroidal endothelial cells. The British Journal of Ophthalmology. 2007;**91**(6):827-831. DOI: 10.1136/bjo.2006.109702

[82] Torres-Soriano ME, García-Aguirre G, Kon-Jara V, Ustariz-Gonzáles O, Abraham-Marín M, Ober MD, et al. A pilot study of intravitreal bevacizumab for the treatment of central serous chorioretinopathy (case reports). Graefe's Archive for Clinical and Experimental Ophthalmology = Albrecht Von Graefes Archiv Fur Klinische Und Experimentelle Ophthalmologie. 2008;**246**(9):1235-1239. DOI: 10.1007/s00417-008-0856-x

Chapter 3

Age-Related Macular Degeneration and Its Current Treatment Strategies: An Updated Review

Brijesh Gelat, Krupali Trivedi, Pooja Malaviya, Pooja Rathaur, Binita Patel, Rahul Gelat and Kaid Johar

Abstract

The retinal pigment epithelium (RPE), which is crucial for good vision, supports the health and function of photoreceptors or Bruch's membrane (BM). The two most prevalent retinal vascular disorders that account for the majority of blindness in people in their working years and older are diabetic macular edema (DME) and neovascular age-related macular degeneration (nAMD). The blood-retinal barrier (BRB), cell differentiation, autophagy, growth factors (GFs), and other complex signaling pathways all play a role in maintaining morphology, and their disruption by harmful substances affects RPE function. It is urgent to gain a better understanding of the molecular mechanisms underlying the pathogenesis of AMD and identify potential targets as leads for creating potent therapies because there are currently no effective treatments for the early-AMD and late-AMD forms of the disease. For this reason, it is vital to identify molecular targets and therapies that can stop RPE deterioration in AMD and restore RPE function. Currently, the first-line treatment for nAMD and DME involves anti-vascular endothelial growth factor (VEGF) medications that inhibit VEGF family ligands, such as ranibizumab, bevacizumab (off-label usage), brolucizumab, and aflibercept. However, because nAMD and DME have complicated pathophysiological backgrounds, further research is still needed to determine the causes of non-response, resistance to anti-VEGF treatment, and disease relapses.

Keywords: age-related macular degeneration, oxidative stress, epithelial-mesenchymal transition, ranibizumab, aflibercept, brolucizumab, faricimab

1. Introduction

The main factor in blindness among the elderly in industrialized nations is age-related macular degeneration (AMD), which causes central vision loss. Choroidoidal neovascularization (CNV) is a hallmark of neovascular age-related macular degeneration (nAMD). In people with nAMD, a complicated mechanism involving the signal protein vascular endothelial growth factor A (VEGF-A) promotes the formation of new blood vessels. Ranibizumab, bevacizumab, and aflibercept are examples of anti-VEGF medications that inhibit this protein [1–3]. Retinal vascular disease has been treated with anti-VEGF medication; however, because VEGF plays a role in pathophysiology, its efficacy is restricted. The anti-VEGF-A impact has several effects, including suppression of neovascularization, reduction of vascular permeability, and inhibition of endothelial proliferation. The identification of alternative targets has led to the discovery of the function of angiopoietin (Ang), which binds to tyrosine kinase (Tie-2) endothelium receptors in two different isoforms, Ang-1 and Ang-2, to control vasculogenesis (**Figure 1**) [4, 5]. AMD, the main cause of vision loss in the elderly, is frequently a precursor and driver of ocular degenerative illnesses, such as retinal pigment epithelium (RPE) phenotypic alteration [1–3].

A lack of effective treatments and a poor knowledge of its pathophysiology make AMD, the primary cause of visual impairment in the aging population [6]. AMD first manifests as atrophic changes in the RPE, followed by the development of lysosomal lipofuscin and extracellular drusen deposits. Geographic atrophy (GA), choroidal neovascularization (CNV), and fibrosis may result from injury brought on by long-term oxidative stress, protein aggregation, inflammation, and epithelial-mesenchymal transition of RPE [3, 6, 7]. More importantly, the epithelial-mesenchymal transition and oxidative stress are highly involved in the occurrence of AMD [8]. Numerous *in vitro*, *in vivo*, and clinical investigations have shown that several regulators are implicated in AMD. It is yet unknown how exactly these transcription factors or regulators affect RPE and cause AMD at the molecular level [7]. To better comprehend molecular processes, establish intercellular signal network profiles, and identify cellular function-specific biomarkers and therapeutic targets are required [9]. This

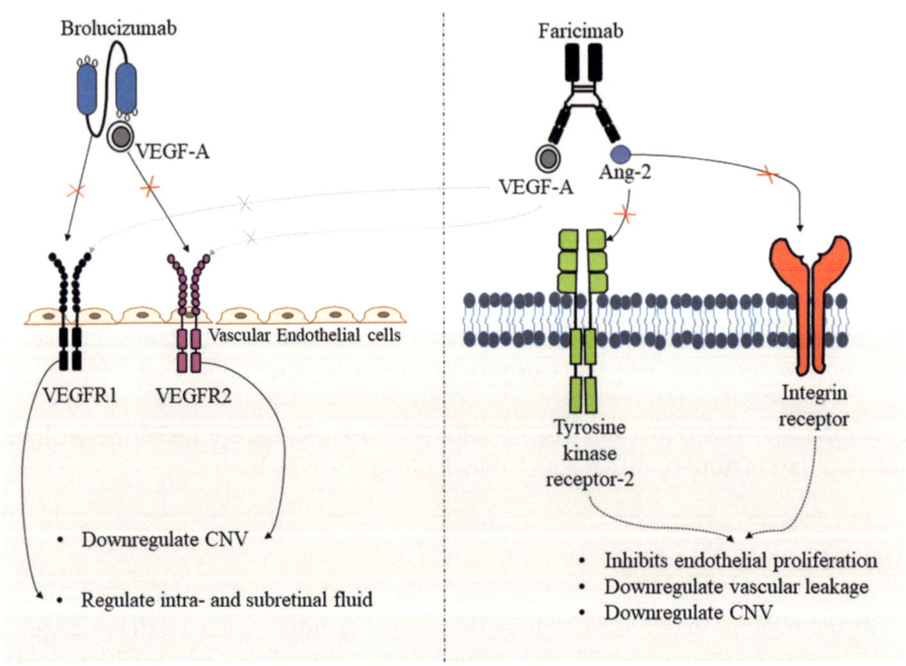

Figure 1.
The relative mechanisms of action of drugs agents for maculopathy, including faricimab and brolucizumab. Faricimab is a bispecific antibody that functions by simultaneously inhibiting vascular endothelial growth factor a and angiopoietin-2. In the world of ophthalmology, brolucizumab represents an important development. When tested in the same laboratory under the same circumstances, brolucizumab bound to all VEGF-A isoforms with strong affinity, with a comparable but numerically greater affinity than aflibercept or ranibizumab.

chapter briefly addresses the mechanisms of epithelial-mesenchymal transition and oxidative stress in the altered functioning of ocular RPE cells, as well as the current prospective pharmaceutical therapies for AMD.

2. Retinal pigment epithelium and age-related macular degeneration

The choroid and photoreceptors are separated by a monolayer of highly polarized, terminally differentiated RPE (**Figure 2**) [3, 10]. The presence of tight connections, melanosomes, a basal nucleus, and basal proteins in morphologically polarized RPE can be explained by their arrangement apically. RPE and choroidal vasculature are distinguished by the extracellular matrix (ECM) membrane known as Bruch's membrane (BM), which is basally situated and made up of several ECM proteins such collagen-IV, laminin, and fibronectin [3, 8, 11]. The maintenance of healthy retinal physiology and a variety of signaling cascades required for good vision are greatly influenced by RPE [12]. Additionally, they are crucial for the movement of nutrients from the choroid to the inner retinal membranes as well as for absorbing extra dispersed light to prevent photooxidation [8, 11]. Furthermore, it produces growth factors (GFs), which are crucial for the survival and development of the neuronal retina [13]. An outer blood-retinal barrier (BRB) is the RPE in the structural arrangements of the eyes [11]. For effective retinal homeostasis, the BRB is very crucial [10, 14]. Due to the necessity of

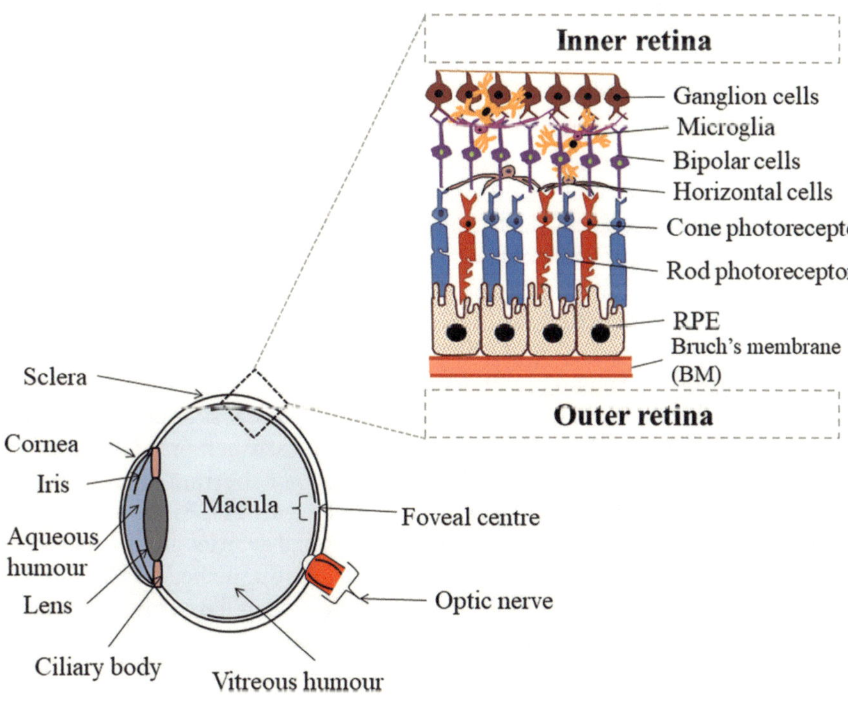

Figure 2.
The structure of the eye with the position of RPE and the layers of the retina has been shown schematically. The outer plexiform layer, outer nuclear membrane, outer limiting membrane, bipolar cells layer, rods-cones cells, and finally retinal pigment epithelial cells (RPE) make up the outer retinal layers. The RPE has tight connections and rests on the choroid's Bruch's membrane, serving as a barriers between the blood and the retina as well as performing a variety of other essential functions.

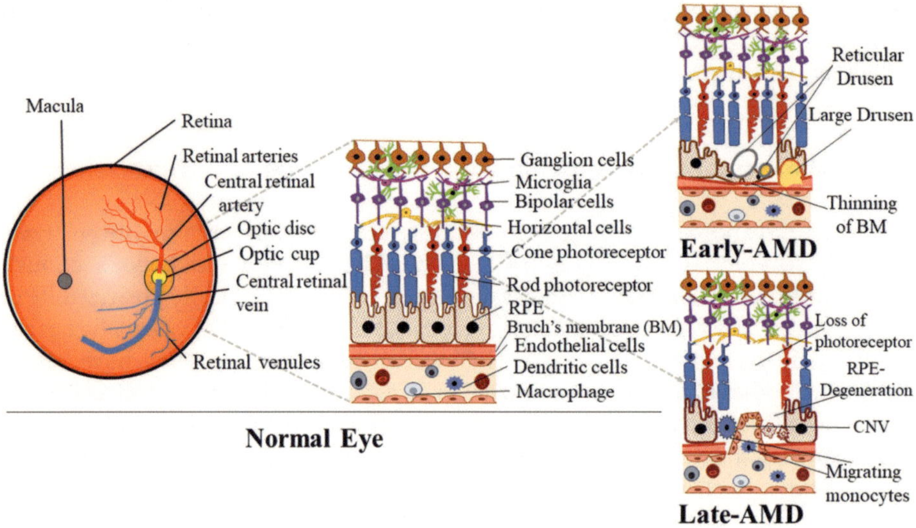

Figure 3.
Schematic representation of the normal retina, dry age-related macular degeneration, and wet age-related macular degeneration. Drusen, a debris-like substance that accumulates under the RPE on Bruch's membrane over time. During a funduscopic eye examination, drusen can be seen. These deposits are known as either soft drusen or hard drusen, which are clinical terms that define their relative size, abundance, and morphology. Drusen may be prevalent in the peripheral retina of normal eyes even if the macula is usually devoid of them. It is thought to be a significant risk factor for AMD to have multiple or confluent soft drusen in the macula.

cell connections like tight junctions and adherens junctions, the BRB is essential for maintaining proper visual acuity [15, 16]. Other oxidative changes, such as tyrosine nitration, which appears to be controlled by light in rat retina, are expected to be observed in drusen due to the high photooxidative stress in the retina (**Figure 3**) [17].

The primary cause of normal vision loss in older people is AMD. In general, it is described as the loss of RPE cells in the macular area [18, 19]. The macular area of the retina contains the greatest concentration of photoreceptors [20]. Due to its multifactorial nature, AMD is referred to as a multifactorial retinopathy. The factors that cause it include genetic predisposition, aberrant physiological inflammation, and oxidative stress (**Figure 4**) [19]. AMD is classified into two types: dry and wet. Progressive atrophy of the retinal pigment epithelium, choriocapillaris, and photoreceptors occurs in dry AMD, leading to slow but progressive loss of central vision. Drusen, or yellow lipid deposits under the macula, is an early symptom of AMD [8]. Wet AMD is distinguished by the formation of new yet aberrant blood vessels underneath the macula. Vascular endothelial growth factor (VEGF) is one of the growth factors involved in the formation of new choroidal arteries and the expansion of vascular permeability. Wet-AMD and dry-AMD are distinguished by CNV and GA, respectively [19, 21]. The term GA implies aberrant choriocapillaris, photoreceptor disruption, and RPE [19, 22]. CNV is defined as the creation of new blood vessels with scarring tissue around the RPE [23, 24]. This can cause early vision loss due to macular edema, hemorrhage, and scarring. Visual distortion (straight lines seem wavy), a central scotoma, or a blurry patch are frequent symptoms [8, 25, 26]. Furthermore, oxidative stress has been identified as the primary disease-causing factor in AMD [23]. Aside from oxidative stress, additional environmental variables including smoking, sunlight exposure, and inadequate dietary antioxidants also contribute to AMD development (**Figure 4**) [27–29].

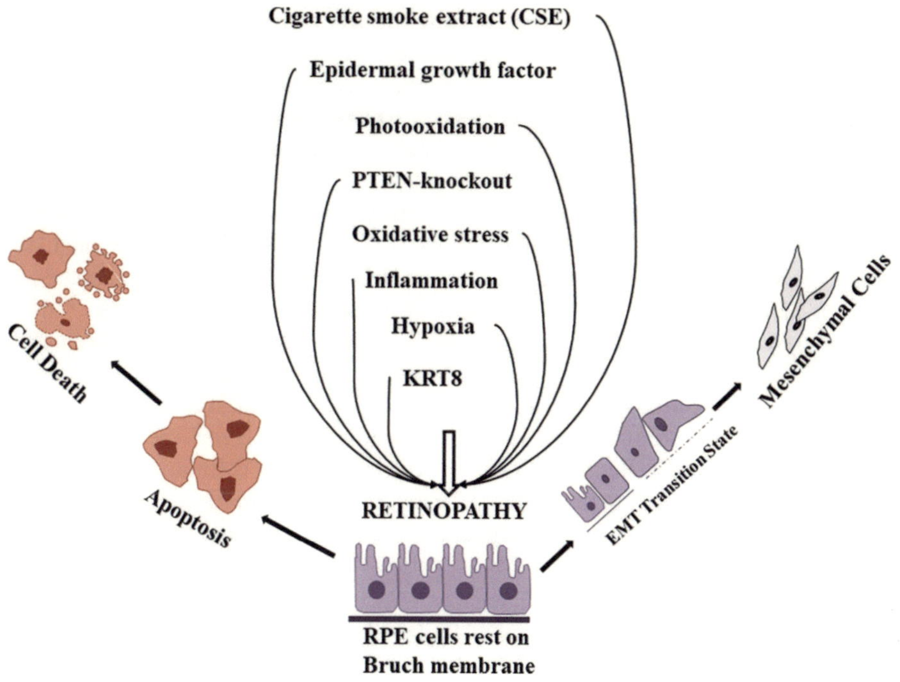

Figure 4.
Diagrammatic representation of factors involved to alter fate of normal retinal pigment epithelium. The normal retinal pigment epithelium is prone to epithelial-mesenchymal transition or stress-mediated cell death, both of which are responsible for retinopathies such as age-related macular degeneration, under the impact of different stimuli such as photooxidation, oxidative stress, and altered growth hormones microenvironment.

3. Oxidative stress (OS) and age-related macular degeneration

The oxidative stress (OS) concept is built on an oxidation-reduction process [23]. OS is caused by an imbalance in the ratio of reactive oxygen species (ROS) generation to antioxidants [20, 30, 31]. The fact that ROS displayed critical biological processes such as cell proliferation, inflammation, apoptosis, certain gene expressions, survival, and migration explains the favorable influence of ROS in the simplest words [20, 32]. To sustain signal transduction and cell cycle control for healthy cellular homeostasis, ROS functions as a secondary messenger [20, 33, 34]. The intracellular concentration of ROS is essential for both the induction and inhibition of apoptosis [20, 35]. Recent research suggests that a decreased ROS concentration, particularly in the eye, aided in maintaining normal defenses against conditions that could threaten vision [36]. The ROS-mediated defense against pathogenic infection in the eye is provided by macrophages, neutrophils, and microglia [36]. A contributing element in age-related illnesses is the cumulative OS damage to essential macromolecules [37, 38]. Because of its increased oxygen tension, constant exposure to light, and presence of rich polyunsaturated fatty acids (PUFAs), the retina in particular is exceptionally susceptible to OS-induced harm [39]. According to observations, numerous ocular health conditions, including AMD and DR, have a significant association with OS [38, 40, 41]. Therefore, RPE is more likely to develop OS and cause a variety of degenerative disorders such as AMD, DR, and proliferative vitreoretinopathy (PVR) [42–45]. One of the most significant pathogenic factors in AMD is oxidative stress, as previously mentioned. Due to physiological sources of oxidative stress, including the high metabolic activity of RPE cells and the phagocytosis of photoreceptor outer segments, as well as specific sources of photooxidative stress brought on by high UV exposure, RPE cells are exposed to an especially high oxidative cellular environment [46, 47]. Aging-related declines in the ability to neutralize ROS and lower autophagy ability expose degenerative RPE cells to particularly large accumulations of ROS [47].

Oxidized lipoproteins that affect RPE are one possible common target. It is well known that oxidized low-density lipoproteins preferentially collect in the macular area and are key participants in the etiology of AMD [48, 49]. By increasing the buildup of ROS, oxidized low-density lipoproteins play a significant role in oxidative stress and inflammation in AMD [50, 51]. ROS must be eliminated from the body for organisms to survive [34]. Antioxidants are essential for preventing the accumulation of ROS [20, 52]. To combat the harm caused by ROS, antioxidants are available naturally and are also found in the body [52]. By neutralizing the free radicals from blood, it shields the macromolecules by preventing the oxidation of cellular macromolecules [49, 52–54]. The antioxidants neutralize ROS by a variety of methods, including chelation, electron transfer, and hydrogen atom transfer from molecules [52, 55, 56].

4. Epithelial-mesenchymal transition (EMT) and age-related macular degeneration

Epithelial-mesenchymal transition (EMT), the trans-differentiation of epithelial cells into mesenchymal-like cells, plays a role in a number of biological processes, such as cell migration, wound healing, and development. Different substances, such as TGFβ, CTGF, epidermal growth factor, and fibroblast growth factor-2, cause EMT, which enhances cell motility and results in an invasive phenotype [8, 57, 58].

There are three different categories of EMT: type I, type II, and type III. In particular, type II-EMT is involved in retinopathy [8, 59]. Tissue fibrosis is caused by an unfavorable microenvironment and inappropriate stimulation of the pathological state [60]. Given that EMT is present in retinopathies and is particularly present in the RPE, it is believed to represent the fundamental underlying mechanism for severe retinal diseases. In particular, type II-EMT is involved in retinopathy [8, 61]. Epithelial cells must undergo a complex cellular reorganization and reprogramming the process that communicates new biochemical directives in order to become mesenchymal cells [62]. During EMT, desmosomes, adherent or tight junctions, and apical-basal polarity are all eliminated [63].

According to the *in vivo* investigation, the formation of mesenchymal cells in the vitreous cavity, which contributes to EMT, is mostly caused by the loss of cell-cell connections in RPE [64]. The RPE encounters altered apoptosis, dedifferentiation, and loss of epithelial polarity in pathological situations, which allows it to persist even in an abnormal microenvironment [12]. A few retinal disease symptoms, such as scarring and the development of the proliferative membrane, which compromise visual acuity, were evident during the clinical examination [65, 66]. Additionally, the *in vitro* research revealed that during the epithelial-mesenchymal transition of retinal pigment epithelium (RPE-EMT), the RPE demonstrates aberrant migratory ability, which is not desired for normal vision [64, 67, 68]. AMD, DR, rhegmatogenous retinal detachment (RRD), PVR, diabetic macular edema (DME), and GA are some of the oculopathies where EMT is implicated in RPE [66, 67, 69–73]. Clinical data also suggest that RPE fibrosis in PVR and DR [65, 66, 71].

During a full clinical evaluation of AMD patients, non-apoptotic degraded RPE was discovered, which was hypothesized to be the outcome of epithelial-mesenchymal transition of retinal pigment epithelium [51, 74, 75]. According to a clinical examination, a lesion brought on by abnormal pathological fluid buildup resulted in hyperreflective foci (HRF) [76, 77]. As a result, the HRF and RPE-EMT are interconnected [78]. The other research also revealed that HRF is a byproduct of RPE, further illuminating the HRF-RPE-EMT connection [78, 79]. In addition, another study found a connection between HRF severity and AMD, including GA and CNV [80]. Intriguingly, HRF content is protectively suppressed by anti-VEGF in AMD patients [78, 81]. The prevalence of drusen-burden and aberrant pigment is taken into consideration by the Age-Related Eye Disease Study (AREDS) when assessing the severity of the disease condition. A higher risk of illness is indicated by more drusen as well as more depigmented RPE [82]. However, it is not yet known how their molecular mechanism contributes to the development of diseases.

5. Current treatment strategy of age-related macular degeneration

The major objective of nAMD therapy is to improve visual acuity. To accomplish this purpose, the damaged retina must prevent new blood vessel formation and minimize fluid leakage [83]. CNV is exacerbated by VEGF [84]. Antagonism of vascular endothelial growth factor has been found to decrease CNV in mouse and nonhuman primate models of neovascularization [85]. CNV can be delayed by inhibiting VEGF from attaching to its receptor, VEGF receptor-2, in blood vessels, which is the main proangiogenic pathway [85]. Antibodies that neutralize VEGF binding to its receptor (anti-VEGF drugs) diminish fluid leakage from the CNV, restrict growth, and result in CNV regression (**Figure 5**). The development of the anti-VEGF agent therapeutic class has substantially improved visual results and prognosis for people with nAMD [86, 87]. A variety of treatments have been utilized to treat neovascular AMD. Before the development of anti-VEGF antibody therapy, laser treatment, including laser coagulation and photodynamic therapy (PDT), was employed. Anti-VEGF medicines that block VEGF family ligands, including ranibizumab, bevacizumab (off-label usage), brolucizumab, and aflibercept, are being used as first-line therapy for nAMD and DME [88].

5.1 Ranibizumab

The first anti-VEGF medication, ranibizumab (Lucentis), a humanized recombinant monoclonal antibody fragment, was demonstrated to improve visual acuity (VA) in individuals with wet-AMD and DME. Based on MARINA and ANCHOR studies, it obtained regulatory permission for the use of ranibizumab [89, 90]. Furthermore, the release of ranibizumab (Lucentis; Genentech, South San Francisco, CA, USA) in 2006 was one of the most significant advancements in the treatment of CNV in AMD [1]. Ranibizumab inhibits cell proliferation, prevents the development of new blood vessels, and reduces vascular leakage [91]. Intravitreal ranibizumab treatment for 2 years prevented vision loss and improved mean visual acuity in patients with minimally classic or occult (no classic lesions) choroidal neovascularization secondary to age-related macular degeneration [92].

Ranibizumab was found to be more effective than verteporfin as an intravitreal therapy for primarily classic nAMD, with fewer significant ocular side effects

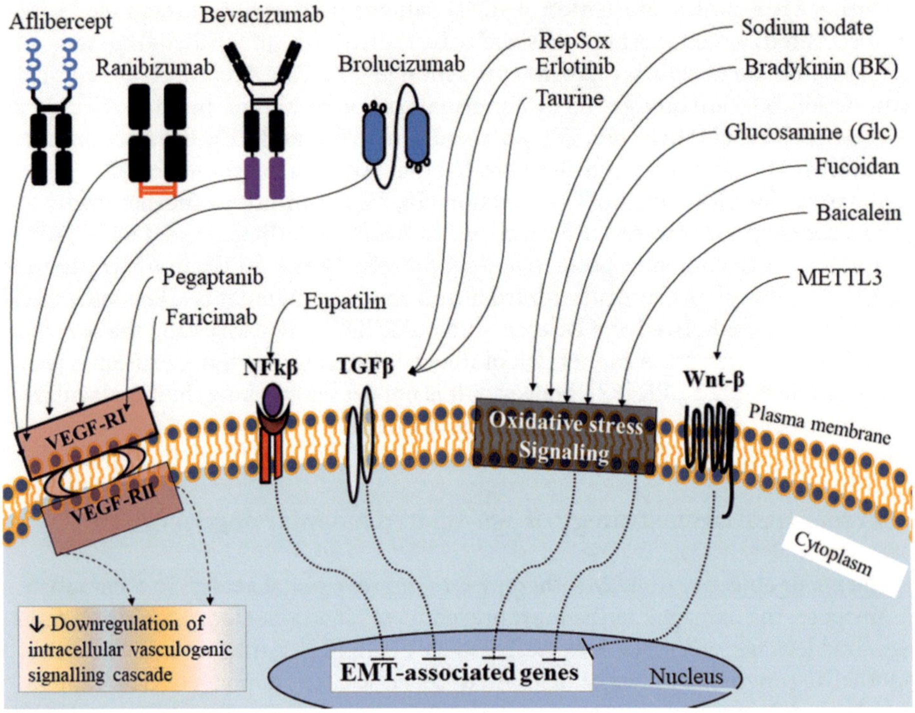

Figure 5.
Diagrammatic representation of mechanism of various drugs or compounds utilized for the treatment of retinopathies such as age-related macular degeneration. For the treatment of age-related macular degeneration, different compounds are utilized. the VEGF-inhibitors include substances such as aflibercept, ranibizumab (Lucentis), and pegaptanib. additional compounds, including non-lethal sodium iodate (NaI), bradykinin (BK), and glucosamine (Glc), downregulate the epithelial-mesenchymal transition of the retinal pigment epithelium by acting through different signaling pathways.

based on one study of 1 year, the treatment increased visual acuity on average [92]. Ranibizumab has improved the treatment of nAMD and gives millions of people hope. Outcomes of clinical trials indicate that ranibizumab was efficacious and well tolerated in patients [91]. Razumab™ (the world's first biosimilar ranibizumab) was well-tolerated and dramatically improved visual acuity in individuals with wet-AMD [93, 94]. Razumab™ (biosimilar ranibizumab), has been approved by the highest Indian regulatory authority "Drugs Controller General of India (DCGI)" for the treatment of neovascular wet-AMD, DME, macular edema following retinal vein occlusion (RVO), and visual impairment due to CNV secondary to pathologic myopia [94]. According to the findings of this study, lowered blood VEGF and TGFβ-1 concentrations were seen following combination therapy, suggesting that the condition is well managed and visual acuity is improved. Photodynamic therapy can block existing CNV, and ranibizumab is capable of resisting VEGF and suppressing CNV, therefore combining the two treatments appears to improve clinical effectiveness [94].

Based on clinical data, most guidelines prescribe three consecutive monthly intravitreal injections of ranibizumab [95, 96]. In other words, the pivotal trials MARINA, ANCHOR, and subsequently Pronto, SUSTAIN, and IVAN planned three loading doses of ranibizumab as the first therapy [89, 90, 97–99]. Their findings demonstrate that after the first three injections, visual acuity improves. The current ranibizumab product features summary recommendations to begin therapy with a loading phase consisting of three consecutive months of monthly injections of 0.5 mg ranibizumab. However, the comparisons of age-related macular degeneration treatment trials (CATT)-protocol recently discovered that after the first year, ranibizumab administered as needed without the use of three necessary loading doses was similar to ranibizumab given monthly [98, 100]. Ranibizumab is being studied further as a potential treatment for various conditions such as DME, retinal vein occlusion, and probable ocular histoplasmosis syndrome [89, 90].

In brief, the development of VEGF inhibitors has dramatically improved the prognosis of this life-threatening oculopathy, and ranibizumab, which targets VEGF-A, has become the gold standard in its therapy. Large randomized controlled studies, however, have revealed that ranibizumab therapy necessitates long-term treatment regimens and repeated intravitreal injections. This rigorous therapy is expensive for both the patient and the healthcare system. This burden, as well as the potential side effects of intraocular administration, is driving research toward individualized dosing strategies and multimodal treatment combinations aimed at combating the complex pathogenesis responsible for CNV and potentially reducing the frequency of retreatment required for optimal results [101].

5.2 Brolucizumab

Brolucizumab is a humanized, single-chain variable fragment (scFv) that inhibits VEGF-A [102, 103]. It is also known as "RTH258" (and was formerly known as "ESBA1008"). In other words, Brolucizumab is a newly created, humanized single-chain fragment of a monoclonal antibody that binds all VEGF-A isoforms and was recently authorized for the treatment of neovascular AMD [102, 103]. By producing equivalent therapeutic results with fewer clinic visits, intravitreal brolucizumab holds the potential to lessen the burden of therapy for individuals with nAMD. Its application to the management of more difficult maculopathies, such as DME, also seems promising [104]. These brolucizumab molecules are composed of a small protein fragment, about 26 kDa, that is formed by joining the heavy and light chain domains of a monoclonal antibody together with a flexible linker [102]. Single-chain variable fragments are a desirable form for pharmacologic treatment due to their small size and lack of a fragment crystallizable area [102]. Small molecules have shown better penetration into target tissues than full-sized immunoglobulin-G. This can lead to increased local efficacy, extended duration of action, and decreased systemic exposure, all of which can minimize side effects [87, 102].

Following an intravitreal injection of 1 or 6 mg of the medication into each of the two eyes of cynomolgus monkeys, the pharmacokinetics of Brolucizumab were examined *in vivo*. According to estimates made by the researchers, the concentration of brolucizumab in the central retina and choroid after delivery was 42 and 18%, respectively, of the vitreous concentration. The maximum concentration of brolucizumab in serum was found to be almost 3500 times lower than the concentration in the vitreous, and its serum clearance was 51.0 hours. According to these study findings, brolucizumab has a low systemic penetration rate and can enter the choroid through the retina. Intravitreal administration of brolucizumab in monkeys showed no ocular or systemic harm and only mild ocular inflammation [87]. Brolucizumab systemic exposure was shown to be limited, as in earlier studies. The quick systemic clearance by brolucizumab is thought to be due to its short molecular size and lack of an Fc-region [87, 104, 105].

These preclinical trials in nonhuman monkey species demonstrate brolucizumab as an anti-VEGF drug that has a minimal systemic concentration and little to no side effects, which might ease the treatment of nAMD patients burden because it would be given more rarely [87].

The MERLIN research, which began in 2018, compares the effectiveness of 6 mg brolucizumab with 2 mg-aflibercept delivered in a 4-week dose schedule following the loading phase in nAMD patients with persisting retinal fluid despite anti-VEGF therapy. MERLIN one-year data showed that brolucizumab was non-inferior to aflibercept in mean best corrected visual acuity change and had superior anatomic outcomes. In the brolucizumab group, however, 4-week treatment intervals were linked with a greater reported frequency of significant ocular adverse events such as ocular inflammation, retina vasculitis, and retina occlusion. As a result, Novartis stated that the MERLIN research will be terminated in May 2021 owing to patient safety concerns [106]. Ogura and colleagues presented the 96-week visual and anatomic results of brolucizumab treatment compared to aflibercept in Japanese eyes diagnosed with polypoidal choroidal vasculopathy in a HAWK research subanalysis [104, 106]. HAWK and HARRIER were two-year, randomized, double-masked, multicenter phase 3 studies that evaluated the safety and effectiveness of brolucizumab intravitreal injections for the treatment of nAMD to aflibercept [107–109]. The KESTREL and KITE trials were the first to compare the effectiveness of brolucizumab vs. aflibercept in DME patients. In 52-week findings from KITE and KESTREL, 6 mg-brolucizumab was shown to be non-inferior to 2 mg-aflibercept in mean Best Corrected Visual Acuity change from baseline (**Table 1**) [106, 125]. Similar phase III trials, TENAYA and LUCERNE, are randomized, double-masked, active comparator-controlled, and lasted 112 weeks when it came to faricimab treatment for nAMD. Throughout the trial, patients were randomized to either aflibercept or faricimab. Throughout weeks 40, 44, and 48, the mean change in best-corrected visual acuity (BCVA) from baseline was the main effectiveness objective. According to some investigations safety outcomes comprised the frequency and severity of retinal and other ocular adverse events [110, 112].

Experimental research on non-human primates has demonstrated that brolucizumab binds to all VEGF-A isoforms. According to Gaudreault and coworkers, it has been demonstrated to prevent VEGF from binding to its receptor, VEGFR2 [134]. The suggested dosage of brolucizuab is 6 mg (0.05 mL of solution, or 120 mg/mL) for the treatment of both DME and non-alcoholic AMD. Intravitreal injections into the vitreous cavity are used to deliver brolucizumab. It is advised to have injections into the afflicted eye or eyes once a month for the first three loading doses. Based on the clinician's assessment of the patient"s condition, a dosage interval of 8–12 weeks is advised subsequently [108]. According to the European Society of Retina Specialists (EURETINA) guidelines, fluid on an OCT scan indicates an active illness that has to be treated with an anti-VEGF medication. Brolucizumab has been shown in other trials to be beneficial in patients whose subretinal fluid did not resolve after prior anti-VEGF therapy. Studies using brolucizumab have demonstrated higher rates of fluid resolution and more persistent decreases in central subfield thickness, suggesting morphological and structural benefits [4, 109, 118].

As previously noted, injection frequency may be decreased without sacrificing therapeutic efficacy when using brolucizumab, an intravitreal anti-VEGF medication approved for the treatment of nAMD and DME [135]. The FDA, USA authorized brolucizumab in October 2019 for the treatment of neovascular AMD. Two phase 3

Name of the study (Name of the drug/treatment agent/year of study)	Type of the study (Type of oculopathy/ retinopathy)	Outcome of the study/ investigation	References
The BREW study (Brolucizumab, year-2020)	Real-world study (nAMD)	• No inflammation or vasculitis • No other adverse ocular outcome	[4]
The STAIRWAY study (Faricumab, year-2020)	Phase-II, Real-world study (nAMD)	• No other adverse ocular	[110, 111]
The TENAYA and LUCERNE study (Faricumab, year-2020)	Phase-III, Real-world clinical trials (nAMD)	• No retinal vasculitis • No retinal occlusion	[112]
The BOURLEVARD study (Faricumab, year-2020)	Phase-III, Real-world randomized study (DME)	• No adverse effects observed	[113]
Kushuhara et al., study (Faricumab, year-2023)	Real-world retrospective study (DME)	• No adverse effects reported	[114]
The YOSHEMITE and RHINE study (Faricumab, year-2022)	Phase-III, Real-world clinical trials (DME)	• Very few retinal adverse effects reported	[115]
The TRUCKEE study (Faricumab, year-2023)	Real-world study (Multicentre) (nAMD)	• Intraocular inflammation reported	[110, 111]
Mukai et al., (Faricumab, year-2023)	Real-world study (nAMD-	RPE-detachment observed	[116]
Enrique study (Brolucizumab, year-2023)	Real-world study (Case study) (nAMD)	• Intraocular inflammation reported • Adverse ocular outcome observed	[117]
Bulirsch et al., (Brolucizumab, year-2021)	Real-world study (observational study) (nAMD)	• Intraocular inflammation observed • Retinal vasculitis observed	[118]
The REBA study	Real-world study (observational, multicentric study) (nAMD)	• Vascular occlusions reported • Macular hole observed	[119, 120]
The BRAILLE study (Brolucizumab, year-2021)	Real world study (non-randomized, uncontrolled study) (nAMD)	• Subretinal hemorrhage • RPE-tear observed • No intraocular inflammation reported	[121]
Matsumoto et al., (Brolucizumab, year-2021)	Real-world study (Retrospective study) (nAMD)	• Intraocular inflammation reported • Adverse ocular outcome observed	[122]
Bilgic et al., The PROBE Study (Brolucizumab, year-2021)	Real-world study (observational) (nAMD)	• No ocular adverse events reported	[119, 123]
Montesel et al. (Brolucizumab, year-2021)	Real-world study (observational, monocentric) (nAMD)	• Few patients developed intraocular inflammation	[124]

Name of the study (Name of the drug/treatment agent/year of study)	Type of the study (Type of oculopathy/retinopathy)	Outcome of the study/investigation	References
Michalska-Małecka et al. (Brolucizumab, year-2021)	Real-world study (observational, monocentric) (nAMD)	No ocular adverse events reported	[125]
Tamashiro et al. (Brolucizumab, year-2022)	Real-world study (multicentre) (nAMD)	• Inflammation of iris observed	[126]
Avaylon et al. (Brolucizumab, year-2022)	Real-world study(nAMD)	• No ocular adverse events reported	[127]
Haensli et al. (Brolucizumab, year-2021)	Real-world study(nAMD)	• Intraocular inflammation with ocular occlusion but no vision loss reported	[128]
Hussain et al. (Brolucizumab, year-2021)	Real-world study(nAMD)	• No vascular inflammation reported	[129]
Awh et al. Brolucizumab, year-2022)	Real-world study (nAMD)	• Intraocular inflammation observed additionally other retinal inflammation observed	[130]
Matsumoto et al. (Brolucizumab, year-2021)	Real-world study (Polypoidal choroidal vasculopathy)	• Suppression of lesions	[122]
Fukuda et al. (Brolucizumab, year-2021)	Real-world study (Polypoidal choroidal vasculopathy)	• Intraocular inflammation observed	[131]
Chakraborty et al. (Brolucizumab, year-2021)	Real-world study (DME)	• No Intraocular inflamma-tion reported	[121, 132]
The SEE study (Brolucizumab)	Clinical trials (nAMD)	• Occasional adverse ocular events observed	[102]
The OWL study (Brolucizumab)	Clinical trials (nAMD)	• Positive treatment response observed	[133]
The OSPREY study (aflibercept, Brolucizumab, year-2017)	Clinical trials (nAMD)	• Adverse ocular events observed	[108, 109]
HAWK and HARRIER (aflibercept, Brolucizumab, year-2020)	Clinical trials, Phase-III (nAMD)	• Well tolerated range of Brolucizumab observed	[108]
KESTREL and KITE (aflibercept, Brolucizumab, year-2022)	Clinical trials, Phase-III (DME)	• Very low severe ocular adverse events reported	[125]

Table 1.
List of treatment agents/drugs utilized for retinopathy condition.

randomized clinical studies, HAWK and HARRIER, were conducted concurrently to examine brolucizumab [136]. The BCVA change from baseline at week 48 served as the main outcome [107–109]. As of week 96, in the HAWK and HARRIER investigations, conjunctival bleeding, impaired visual acuity, cataracts, vitreous floaters, dry eye, and eye discomfort were the most common ocular adverse events (>5% of patients for the whole research group). While 47% of brolucizumab patients in the HARRIER trial reported experiencing at least one ocular adverse event, 61% of patients in the HAWK trial reported experiencing at least one ocular adverse event. The eye inflammation, uveitis, chorioretinitis, iridocyclitis, keratitis precipitates, anterior chamber cell, vitreous haze, retinal vasculitis, anterior chamber flare, and vitritis were adverse outcomes associated with intraocular inflammation. In the HAWK trial, the most frequent conditions were uveitis (2.2%) and iritis (2.5%) (**Table 1**) [105].

In brief, both individuals with newer to treatment and switch therapy patients respond well to intravitreal brolucizumab therapy. The drug, however, does entail an insignificant but evident risk [119]. Patients with nAMD may have less treatment burden as a result of the preclinical and clinical results on brolucizumab, which show maintained disease management with longer injection intervals [87]. With concentrated molar dose, brolucizumab has proven to be a highly effective therapeutic molecule that outperforms other anti-VEGFs licensed for the treatment of patients with nAMD in terms of clarity of vision, fluid adjustment, and duration of impact. Additionally, there is evidence that brolucizumab can lessen treatment burden by permitting longer injection intervals with sustained disease control, as demonstrated by the OSPREY study and the key studies HAWK and HARRIER. By lessening the burden of medication, improving patient adherence, and assisting in the management of patients who are under control with the anti-VEGFs that are already on the market, this is anticipated to enhance long-term results. In the upcoming years, more data on the clinical effectiveness of brolucizumab and its influence on clinical practice in other anti-VEGF-responsive diseases are anticipated, underscoring the potential of compound significance in applications other than nAMD [87, 102, 108].

5.3 Faricimab

The FDA approved faricimab, also known as RG7716 in preclinical testing, in January 2021 for the treatment of nAMD and DME. Faricimab is the first bispecific monoclonal antibody created for intravitreal administration [137]. Unlike conventional monospecific antibodies, bispecific heterodimeric antibodies may attach to two distinct targets because they contain independent light chains in each of the fragment antigen-binding (Fab) domains. During the drug design phase, a knob and hole mechanism between the heavy chains was used to achieve these properties utilizing the CrossMAb CH1-CL technology, which was first described in 2011 [138]. Due to its distinct structural characteristics, faricimab has one VEGF-binding domain and one Ang-2-binding domain, enabling simultaneous and independent neutralization [88, 137, 139, 140]. Similar to this, the FDA, USA approved faricimab-svoa (Vabysmo™, Genentech, San Francisco, CA) in January 2022 for the treatment of DME and nAMD. This medication has simultaneous and independent binding on both VEGF-A and angiopoietin-2 (Ang-2) [111]. It is hypothesized that the anti-Ang 2 impact will increase vascular stability and desensitize the vessels to the effects of VEGF-A. One chance to target two mediators of retinal vascular disease with a single molecule was provided by the use of monoclonal antibodies in anti-VEGF treatment. With CrossMAb (Roche, Basel, Switzerland), a patented method that enables the antibody to have two distinct antigen-binding domains (Fab), these bispecific antibodies may be created. Facitimab, formerly known as RG7716, was developed with the aid of CrossMAb [4, 5, 141, 142]. As was previously noted, faricimab has been shown to be able to inhibit VEGF-A and the detrimental effects of Ang-2 on human vascular endothelial cells *in vitro*. Additionally, compared to VEGF and Ang-2 inhibitors used separately, the combined reduction of VEGF and Ang-2 activity significantly decreased vascular permeability and retinal edema, neuronal death, and macrophage infiltration of neovascular lesions in JR5558 mice with spontaneous CNV [88]. Intravitreal faricimab was able to significantly reduce the levels of pro-inflammatory IL-6 in the aqueous humor and was more effective than ranibizumab in decreasing leaky lesions in monkeys with laser-induced CNV [143]. In replication research, Foxton and associates confirmed similar results [88, 143].

Faricimab is administered intravitreally at a dosage of 6 mg from 0.05 mL of a 120 mg/mL solution. One regimen for nAMD is 6 mg intravitreal every 4 weeks for the first four doses, then the same dose 8 or 12 weeks later depending on the results of optical coherence tomography (OCT) and visual acuity assessments [110]. Faricimab has been tested in a number of clinical studies to determine its safety and effectiveness. YOSEMITE and RHINE are phase III clinical studies of faricimab in individuals with DME who have never received anti-VEGF therapy. The primary effectiveness outcome is the mean change from baseline in best-corrected visual acuity averaged across weeks 48, 52, and 56 [144]. BOULEVARD and STAIRWAY are faricimab phase II clinical studies for DME and nAMD, respectively. Faricimab phase III studies RHINE and YOSEMITE are underway in DME. Similarly, faricimab phase III trials in nAMD are TENAYA and LUCERNE [4, 110, 111]. BOULEVARD is a phase II, 36-week, randomized, and double-blinded, multicenter study of 229 DME patients who have not previously received therapy. The 6.0 mg faricimab cohort showed better letter improvement in visual perception, a decrease in central subfield thickness, and an improvement in the diabetic retinopathy severity score. The findings showed that combined suppression of Ang-2 and VEGF-A might improve visual gain and have a longer duration in individuals with DME [112, 113, 145].

In brief, targeting the angiopoietin/Tie (Ang/Tie) signaling cascade beyond the VEGF pathway may be a promising therapeutic technique that has the ability to address some of the previously described complications. Faricimab is a novel bispecific antibody that targets both VEGF-A and the Ang-Tie/pathway. Faricimab can sustain clinical effectiveness with more prolonged treatment regimens compared to aflibercept (12 or 16 weeks) with a favorable safety profile, according to results from phase III studies TENAYA and LUCERNE (nAMD) and RHINE and YOSEMITE (DME) profile [112, 146]. In comparison to earlier anti-VEGF medications, faricimab is believed to have a more enduring impact and inhibits both VEGF-A and Ang-2. Faricimab injection, like all intravitreal anti-VEGF injections, can cause thromboembolic events, endophthalmitis, hypersensitivity, retinal detachment, vitreous hemorrhage, subconjunctival hemorrhage, and elevated intraocular pressure, among other possible side effects. In about 8–10% of instances, the potential immunogenicity of the drug may result in an occurrence of an anti-faricimab immunoglobulin. The usage of this medication in pregnant women has not been thoroughly studied. Effective contraception is suggested for women of reproductive potential who use this medication, as the impact of the drug on human fertility is uncertain. After the final faricimab dose, the contraception should be used for at least three more months [146, 147].

5.4 Aflibercept

Aflibercept is a new recombinant fusion protein composed of VEGF receptor (R1) and VEGFR2 extracellular domains fused to the Fc-region of human immunoglobulin G1. It binds all VEGF isoforms and has a greater affinity for VEGF-A/B. Aflibercept's effectiveness was evaluated in two randomized, double-blind, multicenter, active-controlled studies in patients with choroidal neovascularization owing to exudative age-related macular degeneration (AMD) [1, 103]. The findings of phase 1 and 2 studies demonstrated effective short-term suppression of choroidal neovascularization in individuals with exudative age-related macular degeneration and revealed that aflibercept had longer durability when compared to other anti-VEGF medications [1].

Aflibercept was studied in multiple preclinical trials before entering clinical trials. In these investigations, VEGF-Trap inhibited the growth of bovine vascular endothelial cells in a manner analogous to ranibizumab [148]. The effectiveness of aflibercept in preventing CNV formation was subsequently evaluated in rodent and non-human primate models [149, 150]. In adult rats with CNV caused by subretinal Matrigel injection, two systemic treatments of aflibercept, 2 days before and 6 days after Matrigel administration, inhibited the formation of CNV. Aflibercept, on the other hand, inhibited collagen production and thus prevented the creation of new neovascular lesions and the regression of existing lesions, leukocyte infiltration, and the development of fibrosis in CNV that developed over 10 days [149]. Another study found that subcutaneous and intravitreal aflibercept inhibited CNV growth in mice with laser photocoagulation-induced BM-damage. Aflibercept's inhibitory impact on CNV development after subcutaneous injection in transgenic mice with enhanced VEGF expression inside the photoreceptor layer was also verified. This experiment also demonstrated the protective properties of aflibercept against BRB by limiting its damage in the presence of increased VEGF concentrations in the vitreous, both after administration of recombinant VEGF and in transgenic mice with VEGF overexpression [150].

VEGF-Trap has also been studied for its capacity to prevent and cure laser-induced CNV in cynomolgus monkeys [151]. The results demonstrated that aflibercept, delivered weekly intravenously at doses of 3 and 10 mg/kg, as well as intravitreal at doses of 50, 250, and 500 g at two-week intervals, effectively protected the investigated eyes from developing CNV. Furthermore, it was demonstrated during the trial that a single intravitreal injection of aflibercept at a dosage of 500 g reversed neovascular alterations generated by laser 2 weeks earlier and strongly reduced the establishment of advanced vascular leakage sites [88, 151]. In the real world, aflibercept has equivalent effects to ranibizumab for treatment-naive nAMD and may be more beneficial for individuals with poorer initial visual acuity [152]. In a cohort of neovascular AMD patients resistant to chronic bevacizumab and/or ranibizumab injections, switching to intravitreal aflibercept treatment can result in considerable visual improvement in the near term and persistent decrease of central macular thickness over a year of follow-up [103].

5.5 Pegaptanib

Pegaptanib (Macugen; OSI/Eyetech Pharmaceuticals, New York, NY, USA) was the first VEGF inhibitor to get FDA clearance for CNV in AMD in 2004. Pegaptanib is an RNA aptamer with excellent affinity and specificity for human VEGF [153]. However, the medication did not bind to other active VEGF isoforms like VEGF121. However, the results of the investigation were encouraging, with 70% of patients losing fewer than three lines of vision compared to 55% of controls (p 0.001) [1, 153]. In 2004, the FDA authorized Macugen™ (Pegaptanib sodium) as the first anti-VEGF therapy for AMD. Pegaptanib, an aptamer that binds to the heparin-binding site of VEGF-165, prevents it from connecting with its endothelial cell receptor. The Fab portion of an anti-VEGF isoform-A antibody was used to create Lucentis™ [154]. It was authorized for use in AMD patients because it retained 95% of vision while improving visual gain [155]. Avastin™ (bevacizumab), derived from the same antibody as Lucentis™, is being used to treat AMD [92]. Anecortave acetate (Retaane™), a steroid, squalene, triamcinolone, Visudyne™, and other VEGF inhibitors are now being researched *in vivo* and *in vitro* [155–157].

5.6 Other regulators of epithelial-mesenchymal transition and age-related macular degeneration

Lampalizumab, a drug in clinical trials, has been demonstrated to be ineffective against AMD and GA [158]. Laser photocoagulation, intravenous anti-VEGF, and other steroid medicines are used to treat ocular diseases. Pan-retinal photocoagulation (PRP) is used to treat PDR. PRP has been demonstrated to have various beneficial benefits, including lessening the chance of blindness later in life, and is thus commonly used as a therapy [159]. Several phase-III trials in the developed world have indicated that anti-VEGF is better than other therapies in lowering the risk of later-life vision loss and, more interestingly, improvement of vision gain in DME [158, 160, 161]. Many intravenous steroids are useful in DME, although their adverse effects are unknown [162, 163]. However, anti-VEGF is not advised for those who are unable to maintain frequent checkups. As an adverse effect of steroid medication, cataracts and glaucoma may develop. Anti-VEGF medication still fails to work in 40–50% of eyes with DME, necessitating the adoption of a non-invasive, non-surgical, and more durable remedy [164]. The production of new nucleotides was hindered by the anticancer medication methotrexate [165]. According to patient-based research, methotrexate can help persons with PVR and AMD with vision improvement [51, 166, 167]. Interestingly, phase 3 clinical studies for the treatment of PVR are being conducted using the methotrexate analog (ADX-2191) [168]. When utilized to treat AMD under *in vivo* testing, the anti-diabetic drug metformin was discovered to have a favorable association with sustaining mitochondrial health [158, 169]. The use of a light spectrum to regulate the physiological activity of tissues or cells is known as photobiomodulation (PBM) [170]. PBM is another kind of PRP. Retinopathies and PBM treatment have recently been linked clinically [171]. Despite the fact that laser therapy has many clear advantages, it cannot be considered the best option for treating sub-foveal lesions since there are significant dangers associated with vision loss in old age, particularly in the sub-foveal region, as well as a high chance of recurrence [172]. However, it can still be considered useful for treating tiny lesions in wet-AMD [173]. Because AMD is defined as either "dry" or "wet," PRP, photodynamic therapy, and anti-neovascular therapy can be used to prevent vision loss, but there is presently no therapy for dry-AMD [155].

According to research on antioxidants in peripheral blood, AMD patients had higher levels of superoxide dismutase (SOD), catalase (CAT), glutathione peroxidase (GSH-Px), and reduced GSH in their platelets as well as GSH-Px, (R-GSH), and glutathione transferase (GST) in their RBCs [174]. There is no long-term treatment for AMD at present [175, 176]. Antioxidants may be used to modify ROS-mediated apoptosis, according to several studies [38]. Antioxidants and zinc supplements have been found to slow down the course of retinopathy [38, 177]. Additionally, the National Health and Nutrition Examination Survey (NHANES) reported a favorable correlation between antioxidant-rich dietary consumption and the suppression of AMD [178].

The decline in antioxidants causes aberrant neovascularization, as shown in AMD [20, 43]. It is interesting to note that phytochemical treatment aided in maintaining cellular SOD status [179]. More intriguingly, evidence from recent studies shows that the antioxidant homologs were effective in restoring the antioxidant state [175, 180]. Antioxidants may help prevent vision loss in roughly 20–25% of injured eyes. It may be possible to develop more effective treatment plans by researching significant biological processes, hereditary factors, and metabolic procedures that are thought to be implicated in AMD. As already mentioned, epidemiological research conducted over the past 40 years has found a number of risk factors linked to AMD, including heredity, age, smoking, and obesity [181]. In 1992, the AREDS examined several AMD patients who were given antioxidant treatment or a placebo. These individuals were then categorized as having wet-AMD in one eye or mild, moderate, or severe dry-AMD in both eyes. The findings of this study, which took around 6–7 years to complete, were released in 2001 [182, 183]. According to these results, patients who got antioxidant treatment instead of a placebo had a decreased probability of developing advanced AMD. Unexpectedly, it was also demonstrated that patients still had early AMD [155].

It has been proven via numerous *in vivo* and *in vitro* experimental research that nicotinamide (NAM) suppresses TGFβ-induced EMT in human adult-retinal pigment epithelial stem cells (RPESC) [184–188]. Bone morphogenetic proteins (BMPs) demonstrated an anti-fibrotic impact in both *in vivo* and *in vitro* investigations, with BMP7 in particular contributing to the maintenance of RPE differentiation and the inhibition of TGFβ-2-induced EMT [189]. The diabetic drug pioglitazone is frequently administered. The main RPE of monkeys did not exhibit EMT-like features due to the PPAR-gamma, an agonist of pioglitazone, necessitating more investigation [66].

Rapamycin, a mTOR suppressor, demonstrated anti-RPE-EMT effects both *in vivo* and *in vitro* [67]. According to the *in vivo* mouse model research, combined treatment with bevacizumab (anti-VEGF) and shRNA (anti-CTGF) led to better vascularizations than either drug alone [190]. Dichloroacetate (DCA), an analog of pyruvate, was shown by Shukal and colleagues to have anti-RPE-EMT effects (TGFβ-2-induced EMT) that are mediated by suppressing the MAPK/Erk and PI3K/Akt signaling pathways [191]. The COX-2 antagonist (NS-398) was shown to be an anti-CNV drug in both *in vivo* and *in vitro* studies by maintaining VEGF and TGFβ expression in the RPE-ECM [192]. Clinical investigations have revealed that anti-VEGFs, anti-inflammatory factors, TGF-receptor inhibitors, PPAR-gamma agonists, and retinoic acid receptor-gamma (RAR-gamma) inhibitors all have therapeutic promise in preventing EMT in RPE [10, 78].

6. Future prospects

Although drusen are a well-established risk factor for AMD, nothing is known regarding their molecular makeup or method of production [17]. The disintegration of the BRB, the breakdown of tight junctions, and the noteworthy feature of AMD are only a few of the ways that OS has an impact on RPE cells [193]. The delayed and increasing function of OS makes it difficult to pinpoint the specific etiology of AMD [19]. Numerous *in vitro* investigations demonstrated that OS-induced damage in retinal tissue resembled AMD [175, 194–196]. Recent understandings from *in vivo* and *in vitro* experiments show that inducers, suppressors, and even miRNA may modify the RPE-EMT [78]. Even after more than 40 years of research, there are still gaps in the concrete diagnostic candidate for the management of retinopathies [78]. Although the precise mechanism affecting EMT cascades is yet unknown, research conducted *in vitro* generally indicates that altering cell density, passages, and serum deprivation induces "anti-EMT" effects in epithelial cells, especially if, and if so, to what extent, anti-fibrosis methods may affect RPE [51]. Therefore, there is a critical need for the development and improvement of therapeutic methods that could enable more satisfactory disease management and lower treatment burden, leading to a better quality of life for patients. This is because there is an increasing incidence of both nAMD and DME, both of which are associated with a marked impact on the health status of the global population.

With concentrated molar dosing and robust gains in visual acuity, superior fluid resolution, and longer effect durability than other anti-VEGFs approved for the treatment of patients with nAMD, brolucizumab has been developed into a highly effective therapeutic molecule [102, 108]. In addition, the OSPREY study and the critical HAWK and HARRIER studies show that brolucizumab can lessen the burden of therapy by enabling longer injection intervals with long-lasting disease control [102, 108]. By lessening the burden of therapy, boosting patient compliance, and assisting in the management of uncontrolled patients with the currently available anti-VEGFs, this is anticipated to enhance long-term results. In the upcoming years, more data on brolucizumab's clinical effectiveness and its effects on clinical practice in other anti-VEGF-responsive diseases are anticipated, demonstrating the drug's potential benefits beyond nAMD [105]. A minority of patients with neovascular age-related macular degeneration who display recurrent or resistant intraretinal or subretinal fluid after numerous injections with either bevacizumab or ranibizumab may benefit from aflibercept treatment [197].

After receiving a ranibizumab injection, minor and transient side effects may last for a few days. These include floaters, conjunctival hemorrhage, a feeling of a foreign body, and discomfort. Each injection has a negligible risk of endophthalmitis, a severe eye infection, of around 1 in 2000 individuals. Increased blurriness, eye discomfort, increased redness, and periocular edema are some of the signs and symptoms of endophthalmitis. An ophthalmologist must address this dangerous problem urgently. Other issues include vitreous hemorrhage, retinal detachment, and lens damage that can need surgical correction [197]. Due to the fact that the only available treatment for subretinal fibrosis is invasive surgery, it is crucial to understand the molecular pathways behind abnormal retinal wound healing in order to create non-invasive drug-based treatments [51, 198].

7. Conclusion

Inhibit epithelial-mesenchymal transition of retinal pigment epithelium is the exclusive focus of current *in vivo* and *in vitro* research, but it is crucial to comprehend how stress and RPE-EMT interact molecularly. There is an urgent need for treatments for retinopathies, which are the main factor in the loss of eyesight for millions of individuals. In conclusion, because they have a broader spectrum of activity than VEGF-A, therapy drugs including pegaptanib, ranibizumab, aflibercept, brolucizumab, and faricimab are beneficial therapeutic choices for individuals with retinal vascular disorders. The treatment load on patients and treatment facilities is decreased by intravitreal anti-angiogenic medicines, which have a sustained clinical action following intravitreal administration and enable appropriate disease management with concurrently lower injection frequency. The development of novel therapeutic strategies for nAMD and DME using cutting-edge pharmacotherapy that targets alternative pathways is crucial in the fight against the worldwide epidemic of blindness and visual impairment brought on by DME and nAMD due to the alarming prognosis of both conditions' rising incidence.

Conflict of interest

There are no conflicts of interest to report among the authors. The final draft was approved by all the authors.

Abbreviations

AMD	age-related macular degeneration
AREDS	age-related eye disease study
BCVA	best-corrected visual acuity
BK	bradykinin
BMP7	bone morphogenic protein 7
BRB	blood-retinal barrier
CAT	catalase
CNV	choroidal neovascularization
DME	diabetic macula edema
DR	diabetic retinopathy
ECM	extracellular matrix
EGF	epidermal growth factor
EGFR	epidermal growth factor (EGF) and its receptor
EMT	epithelial-mesenchymal transition
Glc-N	glucosamine
GR	glutathione reductase
GSH-Px	glutathione peroxidase
KRT8	keratin 8
LPO	lipid peroxidation
MAPKs	mitogen-activated protein kinases
MCT1	monocarboxylate transporters 1
MIF	macrophage migration inhibitory factors
mTOR	mammalian target of rapamycin
n-AMD	neovascular-age-related macular degeneration
NHANES	National Health and Nutrition Examination Survey
OCT	optical coherence tomography
OS	oxidative stress
PBM	photo biomodulation
PPAR	peroxisome proliferator-activated receptor
PPAR-γ	peroxisome proliferator-activated receptor
PVR	proliferative vitreoretinopathy
RAR-γ	retinoic acid receptor gamma
ROCK	rho-associated protein kinase
RPE	retinal pigment epithelium
RPESC	retinal pigment epithelial stem cell
Shh	sonic hedgehog
SOD	superoxide dismutase
TGFβ	transforming growth factor β
VEGF	vascular endothelial growth factor

Author details

Brijesh Gelat[1]*, Krupali Trivedi[2], Pooja Malaviya[3], Pooja Rathaur[3], Binita Patel[4], Rahul Gelat[5] and Kaid Johar[2]

1 Government Arts, Commerce, and Science College, Kachhal, Gujarat, India

2 Department of Zoology, BMTC and Human Genetics, School of Sciences, Gujarat University, Ahmedabad, India

3 Iladevi Cataract and IOL Research Centre, Ahmedabad, India

4 Department of Life Science, School of Sciences, Gujarat University, Ahmedabad, India

5 Institute of Teaching and Research in Ayurveda (ITRA), Gujarat Ayurved University, Jamnagar, India

*Address all correspondence to: gelatbrijesh004@gmail.com

References

[1] Ohr M, Kaiser PK. Aflibercept in wet age-related macular degeneration: A perspective review. Therapeutic Advances in Chronic Disease. 2012;**3**:153-161. DOI: 10.1177/2040622312446007

[2] Kaiser PK, Blodi BA, Shapiro H, Acharya NR. Angiographic and optical coherence tomographic results of the MARINA study of ranibizumab in neovascular age-related macular degeneration. Ophthalmology. 2007;**114**:1868-1875. DOI: 10.1016/j.ophtha.2007.04.030

[3] Gelat B, Malaviya P, Rathaur P, Trivedi K, Chaudhary P, Patel B, et al. Regulation of epithelial-mesenchymal transition in retinal pigment epithelium and its associated cellular signaling cascades: An updated review. Beni-Suef University Journal of Basic and Applied Sciences. 2023;**12**:1-10. DOI: 10.1186/S43088-023-00435-Z

[4] Sharma A, Kumar N, Parachuri N, Sadda SR, Corradetti G, Heier J, et al. Brolucizumab—Early real-world experience:BREWstudy.Eye.2021;**35**:1045-1047. DOI: 10.1038/s41433-020-1111-x

[5] Benest AV, Kruse K, Savant S, Thomas M, Laib AM, Loos EK, et al. Angiopoietin-2 is critical for cytokine-induced vascular leakage. PLoS One. 2013;**8**:e70459. DOI: 10.1371/journal.pone.0070459

[6] Kaarniranta K, Blasiak J, Liton P, Boulton M, Klionsky DJ, Sinha D. Autophagy in age-related macular degeneration. Autophagy. 2023;**19**:388-400. DOI:10.1080/15548627.2022.2069437

[7] Zou H, Shan C, Ma L, Liu J, Yang N, Zhao J. Polarity and epithelial-mesenchymal transition of retinal pigment epithelial cells in proliferative vitreoretinopathy. PeerJ. 2020;**8**:e10136. DOI: 10.7717/peerj.10136

[8] Gelat B, Rathaur P, Malaviya P, Patel B, Trivedi K, Johar K, et al. The intervention of epithelial-mesenchymal transition in homeostasis of human retinal pigment epithelial cells: A review. Journal of Histotechnology. 2022;**45**:148-160. DOI: 10.1080/01478885.2022.2137665

[9] Song D, Yang D, Powell CA, Wang X, Song D, Yang D, et al. Cell–cell communication: Old mystery and new opportunity. Cell Biology and Toxicology. 2019;**35**:89-93. DOI: 10.1007/S10565-019-09470-Y

[10] Naylor A, Hopkins A, Hudson N, Campbell M. Tight junctions of the outer blood retina barrier. International Journal of Molecular Sciences. 2020;**21**:211. DOI: 10.3390/ijms21010211

[11] Strauss O. The retinal pigment epithelium in visual function. In: Physiological Reviews. 2005;**85**(3):845-881. DOI: 10.1152/physrev.00021.2004

[12] Yang X, Chung JY, Rai U, Esumi N. Cadherins in the retinal pigment epithelium (RPE) revisited: P-cadherin is the highly dominant cadherin expressed in human and mouse RPE *in vivo*. PLoS One. 2018;**13**:1-20. DOI: 10.1371/journal.pone.0191279

[13] Sheedlo HJ, Li L, Turner JE. Effects of RPE-cell factors secreted from permselective fibers on retinal cells *in vitro*. Brain Research. 1992;**587**:327-337. DOI: 10.1016/0006-8993(92)91015-7

[14] Cunha-Vaz J, Bernardes R, Lobo C. Blood-retinal barrier. European Journal

of Ophthalmology. 2011;**21**:3-9. DOI: 10.5301/EJO.2010.6049

[15] Rizzolo LJ. Development and role of tight junctions in the retinal pigment epithelium. International Review of Cytology. 2007;**258**:195-234. DOI: 10.1016/S0074-7696(07)58004-6

[16] Sakakibara A, Furuse M, Saitou M, Ando-Akatsuka Y, Tsukita S. Possible involvement of phosphorylation of occludin in tight junction formation. The Journal of Cell Biology. 1997;**137**:1393-1401. DOI: 10.1083/jcb.137.6.1393

[17] Crabb JW, Miyagi M, Gu X, Shadrach K, West KA, Sakaguchi H, et al. Drusen proteome analysis: An approach to the etiology of age-related macular degeneration. Proceedings of the National Academy of Sciences of the United States of America. 2002;**99**:14682-14687. DOI: 10.1073/pnas.222551899

[18] Pascolini D, Mariotti SP, Pokharel GP, Pararajasegaram R, Etyaale D, Négrel AD, et al. Global update of available data on visual impairment: A compilation of population-based prevalence studies. Ophthalmic Epidemiology. 2002;**11**(2004):67-115. DOI: 10.1076/opep.11.2.67.28158

[19] Zhang XY, Ng TK, Brelén ME, Wu D, Wang JX, Chan KP, et al. Continuous exposure to non-lethal doses of sodium iodate induces retinal pigment epithelial cell dysfunction. Scientific Reports. 2016;**6**:1-13. DOI: 10.1038/srep37279

[20] Ung L et al. Oxidative stress and reactive oxygen species: A review of their role in ocular disease. Clinical Science. 2017;**131**:2865-2883. DOI: 10.1042/CS20171246

[21] Jager RD, Mieler WF, Miller JW. Age-related macular degeneration. The New England Journal of Medicine. 2008;**358**:2606. DOI: 10.1056/NEJMra0801537

[22] Kamoshita M, Toda E, Osada H, Narimatsu T, Kobayashi S, Tsubota K, et al. Lutein acts via multiple antioxidant pathways in the photo-stressed retina. Scientific Reports. 2016;**6**:1-10. DOI: 10.1038/srep30226

[23] Beatty S, Koh H-H, Phil M, Henson D, Boulton M. The role of oxidative stress in the pathogenesis of age-related macular degeneration. Survey of Ophthalmology. 2000;**45**:115-134. DOI: 10.1016/S0039-6257(00)00140-5

[24] Bird AC, Bressler NM, Bressler SB, Chisholm IH, Coscas G, Davis MD, et al. An international classification and grading system for age-related maculopathy and age-related macular degeneration. Survey of Ophthalmology. 1995;**39**:367-374. DOI: 10.1016/S0039-6257(05)80092-X

[25] Biasella F, Plössl K, Karl C, Weber BHF, Friedrich U. Altered protein function caused by AMD-associated variant rs704 links vitronectin to disease pathology. Investigative Ophthalmology and Visual Science. 2020;**61**:2. DOI: 10.1167/IOVS.61.14.2

[26] Patel P, Sheth V. New and innovative treatments for neovascular age-related macular degeneration (nAMD). Journal of Clinical Medicine. 2021;**10**:2436. DOI: 10.3390/jcm10112436

[27] Seddon JM, Ajani UA, Sperduto RD, Hiller R, Blair N, Burton TC, et al. Dietary carotenoids, vitamins A, C, and E, and advanced age-related macular degeneration. Journal of the American Medical Association. 1994;**272**:1413-1420. DOI: 10.1001/jama.1994.03520180037032

[28] Samiec PS, Drews-Botsch C, Flagg EW, Kurtz JC, Sternberg P, Reed RL, et al. Glutathione in human plasma: Decline in association with aging, age- related macular degeneration, and diabetes. Free Radical Biology & Medicine. 1998;**24**:699-704. DOI: 10.1016/S0891-5849(97)00286-4

[29] Smith W, Assink J, Klein R, Mitchell P, Klaver CCW, Klein BEK, et al. Risk factors for age-related macular degeneration: Pooled findings from three continents. Ophthalmology. 2001;**108**:697-704. DOI: 10.1016/S0161-6420(00)00580-7

[30] Bayir H. Reactive oxygen species. Critical Care Medicine. 2005;**33**:S498-S501. DOI: 10.1097/01.CCM.0000186787.64500.12

[31] Subrizi A, Toropainen E, Ramsay E, Airaksinen AJ, Kaarniranta K, Urtti A. Oxidative stress protection by exogenous delivery of rhhsp70 chaperone to the retinal pigment epithelium (RPE), a possible therapeutic strategy against RPE degeneration. Pharmaceutical Research. 2015;**32**:211-221. DOI: 10.1007/s11095-014-1456-6

[32] Li W, Cao L, Han L, Xu Q, Ma Q. Superoxide dismutase promotes the epithelial-mesenchymal transition of pancreatic cancer cells via activation of the H2O2/ERK/NF-κB axis. International Journal of Oncology. 2015;**46**:2613-2620. DOI: 10.3892/ijo.2015.2938

[33] Hancock JT, Desikan R, Neill SJ. Role of reactive oxygen species in cell signalling pathways. Biochemical Society Transactions. 2001;**29**:345-349. DOI: 10.1042/bst0290345

[34] Sies H, Belousov VV, Chandel NS, Davies MJ, Jones DP, Mann GE, etal. Defining roles of specific reactive oxygen species (ROS) in cell biology and physiology. Nature Reviews Molecular Cell Biology. 2022;**23**(7):499-515. DOI: 10.1038/s41580-022-00456-z

[35] Simon HU, Haj-Yehia A, Levi-Schaffer F. Role of reactive oxygen species (ROS) in apoptosis induction. Apoptosis. 2000;**5**:415-418. DOI: 10.1023/A:1009616228304

[36] Kumar A, Pandey RK, Miller LJ, Singh PK, Kanwar M. Müller glia in retinal innate immunity: A perspective on their roles in endophthalmitis. Critical Reviews in Immunology. 2013;**33**:119-135. DOI: 10.1615/CritRevImmunol.2013006618

[37] Inumaru J, Nagano O, Takahashi E, Ishimoto T, Nakamura S, Suzuki Y, et al. Molecular mechanisms regulating dissociation of cell-cell junction of epithelial cells by oxidative stress. Genes to Cells. 2009;**14**:703-716. DOI: 10.1111/j.1365-2443.2009.01303.x

[38] Yu AL, Fuchshofer R, Kook D, Kampik A, Bloemendal H, Welge-Lüssen U. Subtoxic oxidative stress induces senescence in retinal pigment epithelial cells via TGF-β release. Investigative Ophthalmology and Visual Science. 2009;**50**:926-935. DOI: 10.1167/iovs.07-1003

[39] Jain M, Rivera S, Monclus EA, Synenki L, Zirk A, Eisenbart J, et al. Mitochondrial reactive oxygen species regulate transforming growth factor-β signaling. The Journal of Biological Chemistry. 2013;**288**:770-777. DOI: 10.1074/jbc.M112.431973

[40] Plafker SM, O'Mealey GB, Szweda LI. Mechanisms for countering oxidative stress and damage in retinal pigment epithelium. International Review of Cell and Molecular Biology. 2012;**298**:135-177. DOI: 10.1016/B978-0-12-394309-5.00004-3

[41] Khandhadia S, Cree A, Lotery A. Oxidative damage and macular degeneration. In: Systems Biology of Free Radicals and Antioxidants. Heidelberg: Springer, Berlin; 2014. pp. 3625-3653. DOI: 10.1007/978-3-642-30018-9_171

[42] Huang CK, Lin Y, Su H, Ye D. Forsythiaside protects against hydrogen peroxide-induced oxidative stress and apoptosis in PC12 cell. Neurochemical Research. 2014;**40**:27-35. DOI: 10.1007/s11064-014-1461-5

[43] Zhao H, Wang R, Ye M, Zhang L. Genipin protects against H_2O_2-induced oxidative damage in retinal pigment epithelial cells by promoting Nrf_2 signaling. International Journal of Molecular Medicine. 2019;**43**:936-944. DOI: 10.3892/ijmm.2018.4027

[44] Taylor HR, West S, Muñoz B, Rosenthal FS, Bressler SB, Bressler NM. The long-term effects of visible light on the eye. Archives of Ophthalmology. 1992;**110**:99-104. DOI: 10.1001/archopht.1992.01080130101035

[45] Rosen RB, Hu DN, Chen M, McCormick SA, Walsh J, Roberts JE. Effects of melatonin and its receptor antagonist on retinal pigment epithelial cells against hydrogen peroxide damage. Molecular Vision. 2012;**18**:1640-1648

[46] Datta S, Cano M, Ebrahimi K, Wang L, Handa JT. The impact of oxidative stress and inflammation on RPE degeneration in non-neovascular AMD. Progress in Retinal and Eye Research. 2017;**60**:201-218. DOI: 10.1016/J.PRETEYERES.2017.03.002

[47] Miceli MV, Liles MR, Newsome DA. Evaluation of oxidative processes in human pigment epithelial cells associated with retinal outer segment phagocytosis. Experimental Cell Research. 1994;**214**:242-249. DOI: 10.1006/excr.1994.1254

[48] Suzuki M, Kamei M, Itabe H, Yoneda K, Bando H, Kume N, et al. Oxidized phospholipids in the macula increase with age and in eyes with age-related macular degeneration. Molecular Vision. 2007;**3**:772-778. Available from: /pmc/articles/PMC2768762/ [Accessed: September 21, 2023]

[49] Gelat B, Malaviya P, Rathaur P, Patel B, Sr KJ. Lipid peroxidation and retinal pigment epithelium: A review article. Towards Excellence. 2022;**14**: 1155-1163. DOI: 10.37867/te1403103

[50] Yamada Y, Tian J, Yang Y, Cutler RG, Wu T, Telljohann RS, et al. Oxidized low density lipoproteins induce a pathologic response by retinal pigmented epithelial cells. Journal of Neurochemistry. 2008;**105**:1187-1197. DOI: 10.1111/J.1471-4159.2008.05211.X

[51] Shu DY, Butcher E, Saint-Geniez M. EMT and ENDMT: Emerging roles in age-related macular degeneration. International Journal of Molecular Sciences. 2020;**21**(12):1-26. DOI: 10.3390/ijms21124271. Multidisciplinary Digital Publishing Institute

[52] Mitra AK. Antioxidants: A masterpiece of mother nature to prevent illness. Journal of Chemical Reviews. 2020;**2**:243-256. DOI: 10.33945/SAMI/JCR.2020.4.3

[53] Young IS, Woodside JV. Antioxidants in health and disease. Journal of Clinical Pathology. 2001;**54**:176-186. DOI: 10.1136/jcp.54.3.176

[54] Kim YW, Byzova TV. Oxidative stress in angiogenesis and vascular disease. Blood. 2014;**123**:625-631. DOI: 10.1182/blood-2013-09-512749

[55] Foyer CH, Noctor G. Redox homeostasis and antioxidant signaling: A metabolic interface between stress

perception and physiological responses. The Plant Cell. 2005;**17**:1866-1875. DOI: 10.1105/tpc.105.033589

[56] Møller IM, Jensen PE, Hansson A. Oxidative modifications to cellular components in plants. Annual Review of Plant Biology. 2007;**58**:459-481. DOI: 10.1146/annurev.arplant.58. 032806.103946

[57] Kalluri R, Weinberg RA. The basics of epithelial-mesenchymal transition. The Journal of Clinical Investigation. 2009;**119**:1420-1428. DOI: 10.1172/JCI39104

[58] Kobayashi M, Tokuda K, Kobayashi Y, Yamashiro C, Uchi SH, Hatano M, et al. Suppression of epithelial-mesenchymal transition in retinal pigment epithelial cells by an MRTF-A inhibitor. Investigative Ophthalmology and Visual Science. 2019;**60**:528-537. DOI: 10.1167/ iovs.18-25678

[59] Kalluri R, Neilson EG. Epithelial-mesenchymal transition and its implications for fibrosis. The Journal of Clinical Investigation. 2003;**112**:1776-1784. DOI: 10.1172/JCI200320530

[60] Nisticò P, Bissell MJ, Radisky DC. Epithelial-mesenchymal transition: General principles and pathological relevance with special emphasis on the role of matrix metalloproteinases. Cold Spring Harbor Perspectives in Biology. 2012;**4**:a011908. DOI: 10.1101/ cshperspect.a011908

[61] Zhang Y, Zhao D, Yang S, Yao H, Li M, Zhao C, et al. Protective effects of fucoidan on epithelial-mesenchymal transition of retinal pigment epithelial cells and progression of proliferative vitreoretinopathy. Cellular Physiology and Biochemistry. 2018;**46**:1704-1715. DOI: 10.1159/000489246

[62] Thiery JP, Acloque H, Huang RYJ, Nieto MA. Epithelial-mesenchymal transitions in development and disease. Cell. 2009;**139**:871-890. DOI: 10.1016/j. cell.2009.11.007

[63] Shook D, Keller R. Mechanisms, mechanics and function of epithelial-mesenchymal transitions in early development. Mechanisms of Development. 2003;**120**:1351-1383. DOI: 10.1016/j.mod.2003.06.005

[64] Tamiya S, Kaplan HJ. Role of epithelial - mesenchymal transition in proliferative vitreoretinopathy. Experimental Eye Research. 2016;**142**: 26-31. DOI: 10.1016/j.exer.2015.02.008

[65] Ünver YB, Yavuz GA, Bekiroğlu N, Presti P, Li W, Sinclair SH. Relationships between clinical measures of visual function and anatomic changes associated with bevacizumab treatment for choroidal neovascularization in age-related macular degeneration. Eye. 2009;**23**:453-460. DOI: 10.1038/eye.2008.349

[66] Hatanaka H, Koizumi N, Okumura N, Kay EDP, Mizuhara E, Hamuro J, et al. Epithelial-mesenchymal transition-like phenotypic changes of retinal pigment epithelium induced by TGF-γ are prevented by PPAR-γ agonists. Investigative Ophthalmology and Visual Science. 2012;**53**:6955-6963. DOI: 10.1167/iovs.12-10488

[67] Feng H, Zhao X, Guo Q, Feng Y, Ma M, Guo W, et al. Autophagy resists EMT process to maintain retinal pigment epithelium homeostasis. International Journal of Biological Sciences. 2019;**15**:507-521. DOI: 10.7150/ijbs.30575

[68] D'Amico DJ. Primary retinal detachment. The New England Journal of Medicine. 2008;**359**:2346-2354. DOI: 10.1056/nejmcp0804591

[69] Baek A, Yoon S, Kim J, Baek YM, Park H, Lim D, et al. Autophagy and

KRT8/keratin 8 protect degeneration of retinal pigment epithelium under oxidative stress. Autophagy. 2017;**13**:248-263. DOI: 10.1080/15548627.2016.1256932

[70] Tan X, Chen C, Zhu Y, Deng J, Qiu X, Huang S, et al. Proteotoxic stress desensitizes TGF-beta signaling through receptor downregulation in retinal pigment epithelial cells. Current Molecular Medicine. 2017;**17**:189-199. DOI: 10.2174/1566524017666170619113435

[71] Sivagurunathan S, Raman R, Chidambaram S. PIWI-like protein, HIWI2: A novel player in proliferative diabetic retinopathy. Experimental Eye Research. 2018;**177**:191-196. DOI: 10.1016/j.exer.2018.08.018

[72] Chen Z, Shao Y, Li X. The roles of signaling pathways in epithelial-to-mesenchymal transition of PVR. Molecular Vision. 2015;**21**:706-710

[73] Pastor JC, De La Rúa ER, Martín F. Proliferative vitreoretinopathy: Risk factors and pathobiology. Progress in Retinal and Eye Research. 2002;**21**:127-144. DOI: 10.1016/S1350-9462(01)00023-4

[74] Sarks JP, Sarks SH, Killingsworth MC. Evolution of geographic atrophy of the retinal pigment epithelium. Eye. 1988;**2**:552-577. DOI: 10.1038/eye.1988.106

[75] Zanzottera EC, Messinger JD, Ach T, Theodore Smith R, Curcio CA. Subducted and melanotic cells in advanced age-related macular degeneration are derived from retinal pigment epithelium. Investigative Ophthalmology and Visual Science. 2015;**56**:3269-3278. DOI: 10.1167/iovs.15-16432

[76] Liu Z, Li C, Kang N, Malhi H, Shah VH, Maiers JL. Transforming growth factor (TGF) cross-talk with the unfolded protein response is critical for hepatic stellate cell activation. The Journal of Biological Chemistry. 2019;**294**:3137-3151. DOI: 10.1074/jbc.RA118.005761

[77] Roy R, Saurabh K, Shah D, Chowdhury M, Goel S. Choroidal hyperreflective foci: A novel spectral domain optical coherence tomography biomarker in eyes with diabetic macular edema. The Asia-Pacific Journal of Ophthalmology. 2019;**8**:314-318. DOI: 10.1097/APO.0000000000000249

[78] Zhou M, Geathers JS, Grillo SL, Weber SR, Wang W, Zhao Y, et al. Role of epithelial-mesenchymal transition in retinal pigment epithelium dysfunction. Frontiers in Cell and Development Biology. 2020;**8**:501. DOI: 10.3389/fcell.2020.00501

[79] Chen KC, Jung JJ, Curcio CA, Balaratnasingam C, Gallego-Pinazo R, Dolz-Marco R, et al. Intraretinal hyperreflective foci in acquired vitelliform lesions of the macula: Clinical and histologic study. American Journal of Ophthalmology. 2016;**164**:89-98. DOI: 10.1016/j.ajo.2016.02.002

[80] Christenbury JG, Folgar FA, O'Connell RV, Chiu SJ, Farsiu S, Toth CA. Progression of intermediate age-related macular degeneration with proliferation and inner retinal migration of hyperreflective foci. Ophthalmology. 2013;**120**:1038-1045. DOI: 10.1016/j.ophtha.2012.10.018

[81] Aghdam KA, Pielen A, Framme C, Junker B. Correlation between hyperreflective foci and clinical outcomes in neovascular age-related macular degeneration after switching to aflibercept. Investigative Ophthalmology and Visual Science. 2015;**56**:6448-6455. DOI: 10.1167/iovs.15-17338

[82] Merry GF, Munk MR, Dotson RS, Walker MG, Devenyi RG. Photobiomodulation reduces drusen volume and improves visual acuity and contrast sensitivity in dry age-related macular degeneration. Acta Ophthalmologica. 2017;**95**:e270-e277. DOI: 10.1111/aos.13354

[83] Wykoff CC, Clark WL, Nielsen JS, Brill JV, Greene LS, Heggen CL. Optimizing anti-VEGF treatment outcomes for patients with neovascular age-related macular degeneration. Journal of Managed Care & Specialty Pharmacy. 2018;**24**:S3-S15. DOI: 10.18553/JMCP.2018.24.2-A.S3/ASSET/IMAGES/SMALL/FIG 1.GIF

[84] Bakri SJ, Thorne JE, Ho AC, Ehlers JP, Schoenberger SD, Yeh S, et al. Safety and efficacy of anti-vascular endothelial growth factor therapies for neovascular age-related macular degeneration: A report by the American Academy of Ophthalmology. Ophthalmology. 2019;**126**:55-63. DOI: 10.1016/J.OPHTHA.2018.07.028

[85] Campochiaro PA, Aiello LP, Rosenfeld PJ. Anti–vascular endothelial growth factor agents in the treatment of retinal disease: From bench to bedside. Ophthalmology. 2016;**123**:S78-S88. DOI: 10.1016/j.ophtha.2016.04.056

[86] Shibuya M. Vascular endothelial growth factor (VEGF) and its receptor (VEGFR) signaling in angiogenesis: A crucial target for anti- and pro-angiogenic therapies. Genes and Cancer. 2011;**2**:1097-1105. DOI: 10.1177/1947601911423031

[87] Nguyen QD, Das A, Do DV, Dugel PU, Gomes A, Holz FG, et al. Brolucizumab: Evolution through preclinical and clinical studies and the implications for the management of neovascular age-related macular degeneration. Ophthalmology. 2020;**127**:963-976. DOI: 10.1016/j.ophtha.2019.12.031

[88] Liberski S, Wichrowska M, Kocięcki J. Aflibercept versus Faricimab in the treatment of neovascular age-related macular degeneration and diabetic macular edema: A review. International Journal of Molecular Sciences. 2022;**23**:9424. DOI: 10.3390/ijms23169424

[89] Dhoot DS, Kaiser PK. Ranibizumab for age-related macular degeneration. Expert Opinion on Biological Therapy. 2012;**12**:371-381. DOI: 10.1517/14712598.2012.660523

[90] Ciulla TA. Therapeutic effects of ranibizumab in neovascular age-related macular degeneration. Expert Review of Ophthalmology. 2007;**2**:679-693. DOI: 10.1586/17469899.2.5.679

[91] Kourlas H, Abrams P. Ranibizumab for the treatment of neovascular age-related macular degeneration: A review. Clinical Therapeutics. 2007;**29**:1850-1861. DOI: 10.1016/j.clinthera.2007.09.008

[92] Rosenfeld PJ, Moshfeghi AA, Puliafito CA. Optical coherence tomography findings after an intravitreal injection of bevacizumab (Avastin®) for neovascular age-related macular degeneration. Ophthalmic Surgery, Lasers and Imaging Retina. 2005;**36**:331-335. DOI: 10.3928/1542-8877-20050701-14

[93] Sharma S, Gupta V, Maiti A, Natesh S, Saxena S, Dave V, et al. Safety and efficacy of Razumab™ (world's first biosimilar ranibizumab) in wet age-related macular degeneration: A post-marketing, prospective ASSET study. International Journal of Retina and Vitreous. 2021;7:24. DOI: 10.1186/s40942-021-00293-w

[94] Jiang S, Park C, Barner JC. Ranibizumab for age-related macular degeneration: A meta-analysis of dose effects and comparison with no anti-VEGF treatment and bevacizumab. Journal of Clinical Pharmacy and Therapeutics. 2014;**39**:234-239. DOI: 10.1111/jcpt.12146

[95] Thoongsuwan S, Hanutsaha P, Chantarasorn Y, Ruamviboonsuk P, Vongkulsiri S, Kungwanpongpun P. Treatment outcome of wet age-related macular degeneration management in Thailand: A retrospective real-world study (TOWER study). Ophthalmology and Therapy. 2022;**11**:739-757. DOI: 10.1007/s40123-022-00471-5

[96] Ruiz-Moreno JM, Arias-Barquet L, Armadá-Maresca F, Boixadera-Espax A, García-Layana A, Gómez-Ulla-de-Irazazábal F, et al. Guías de práctica clínica de la SERV: Tratamiento de la degeneración macular asociada a la edad (DMAE) exudativa. Archivos de la Sociedad Española de Oftalmología. 2009;**84**:333-344. Available from: https://scielo.isciii.es/scielo.php?script=sci_arttext&pid=S0365-66912009000700004&lng=es&nrm=iso&tlng=es [Accessed: September 21, 2023]

[97] Rosenfeld PJ, Brown DM, Heier JS, Boyer DS, Kaiser PK, Chung CY, et al. Ranibizumab for neovascular age-related macular degeneration. The New England Journal of Medicine. 2006;**355**:1419-1431. DOI: 10.1056/nejmoa054481

[98] García-Layana A, Figueroa MS, Arias L, Araiz J, Ruiz-Moreno JM, García-Arumí J, et al. Individualized therapy with ranibizumab in wet age-related macular degeneration. Journal of Ophthalmology. 2015;**2015**:412903. DOI: 10.1155/2015/412903

[99] Holz FG, Amoaku W, Donate J, Guymer RH, Kellner U, Schlingemann RO, et al. Safety and efficacy of a flexible dosing regimen of ranibizumab in neovascular age-related macular degeneration: The SUSTAIN study. Ophthalmology. 2011;**118**:663-671. DOI: 10.1016/j.ophtha.2010.12.019

[100] Moja L, Lucenteforte E, Kwag KH, Bertele V, Campomori A, Chakravarthy U, et al. Systemic safety of bevacizumab versus ranibizumab for neovascular age-related macular degeneration. Cochrane Database of Systematic Reviews. 2014;**2014**:CD011230. DOI: 10.1002/14651858.CD011230.pub2

[101] Spielberg L, Leys A. Treatment of neovascular age-related macular degeneration with a variable ranibizumab dosing regimen and one-time reduced-fluence photodynamic therapy: The TORPEDO trial at 2 years. Graefe's Archive for Clinical and Experimental Ophthalmology. 2010;**248**:943-956. DOI: 10.1007/s00417-009-1256-6

[102] Holz FG, Dugel PU, Weissgerber G, Hamilton R, Silva R, Bandello F, et al. Single-chain antibody fragment VEGF inhibitor RTH258 for neovascular age-related macular degeneration: A randomized controlled study. Ophthalmology. 2016;**123**:1080-1089. DOI: 10.1016/j.ophtha.2015.12.030

[103] Hamid MA, Abdelfattah NS, Salamzadeh J, Abdelaziz STA, Sabry AM, Mourad KM, et al. Aflibercept therapy for exudative age-related macular degeneration resistant to bevacizumab and ranibizumab. International Journal of Retina and Vitreous. 2021;**7**:1-13. DOI: 10.1186/s40942-021-00299-4

[104] Karasavvidou EM, Tranos P, Panos GD. Brolucizumab for the treatment of degenerative macular conditions: A review of clinical studies.

Drug Design, Development and Therapy. 2022;**16**:2659-2680. DOI: 10.2147/DDDT.S378450

[105] Tadayoni R, Sararols L, Weissgerber G, Verma R, Clemens A, Holz FG. Brolucizumab: A newly developed anti-VEGF molecule for the treatment of neovascular age-related macular degeneration. Ophthalmologica. 2021;**244**:93-101. DOI: 10.1159/000513048

[106] Michalska-Małecka K, Śpiewak D, Luksa D. Three-month results of brolucizumab intravitreal therapy in patients with wet age-related macular degeneration. International Journal of Environmental Research and Public Health. 2021;**18**:8450. DOI: 10.3390/ijerph18168450

[107] Dugel PU, Singh RP, Koh A, Ogura Y, Weissgerber G, Gedif K, et al. HAWK and HARRIER: Ninety-Six-week outcomes from the phase 3 trials of brolucizumab for neovascular age-related macular degeneration. Ophthalmology. 2021;**128**:89-99. DOI: 10.1016/J.OPHTHA.2020.06.028

[108] Dugel PU, Koh A, Ogura Y, Jaffe GJ, Schmidt-Erfurth U, Brown DM, et al. HAWK and HARRIER: phase 3, multicenter, randomized, double-masked trials of brolucizumab for neovascular age-related macular degeneration. Ophthalmology. 2020;**127**:72-84. DOI: 10.1016/j.ophtha.2019.04.017

[109] Dugel PU, Jaffe GJ, Sallstig P, Warburton J, Weichselberger A, Wieland M, et al. Brolucizumab versus aflibercept in participants with neovascular age-related macular degeneration: A randomized trial. Ophthalmology. 2017;**124**:1296-1304. DOI: 10.1016/j.ophtha.2017.03.057

[110] Khanani AM, Aziz AA, Khan H, Gupta A, Mojumder O, Saulebayeva A, et al. The real-world efficacy and safety of faricimab in neovascular age-related macular degeneration: The TRUCKEE study – 6 month results. Eye. 2023;**37**:3574-3581. DOI: 10.1038/s41433-023-02553-5

[111] Khanani AM, Patel SS, Ferrone PJ, Osborne A, Sahni J, Grzeschik S, et al. Efficacy of every four monthly and quarterly dosing of faricimab vs ranibizumab in neovascular age-related macular degeneration: The STAIRWAY phase 2 randomized clinical trial. JAMA Ophthalmology. 2020;**138**:964-972. DOI: 10.1001/jamaophthalmol.2020.2699

[112] Heier JS, Khanani AM, Ruiz CQ, Basu K, Ferrone PJ, Brittain C, et al. Efficacy, durability, and safety of intravitreal faricimab up to every 16 weeks for neovascular age-related macular degeneration (TENAYA and LUCERNE): Two randomised, double-masked, phase 3, non-inferiority trials. Lancet. 2022;**399**:729-740. DOI: 10.1016/S0140-6736(22)00010-1

[113] Sahni J, Patel SS, Dugel PU, Khanani AM, Jhaveri CD, Wykoff CC, et al. Simultaneous inhibition of angiopoietin-2 and vascular endothelial growth factor-a with faricimab in diabetic macular edema: BOULEVARD phase 2 randomized trial. Ophthalmology. 2019;**126**:1155-1170. DOI: 10.1016/j.ophtha.2019.03.023

[114] Kusuhara S, Kishimoto-Kishi M, Matsumiya W, Miki A, Imai H, Nakamura M. Short-term outcomes of intravitreal faricimab injection for diabetic macular edema. Medicina. 2023;**59**:665. DOI: 10.3390/medicina59040665

[115] Wykoff CC, Abreu F, Adamis AP, Basu K, Eichenbaum DA, Haskova Z, et al. Efficacy, durability, and safety of intravitreal faricimab with extended

dosing up to every 16 weeks in patients with diabetic macular oedema (YOSEMITE and RHINE): Two randomised, double-masked, phase 3 trials. Lancet. 2022;**399**:741-755. DOI: 10.1016/S0140-6736(22)00018-6

[116] Mukai R, Kataoka K, Tanaka K, Miyara Y, Maruko I, Nakayama M, et al. Three-month outcomes of faricimab loading therapy for wet age-related macular degeneration in Japan. Scientific Reports. 2023;**13**:8747. DOI: 10.1038/s41598-023-35759-4

[117] Enríquez AB, Baumal CR, Crane AM, Witkin AJ, Lally DR, Liang MC, et al. Early experience with Brolucizumab treatment of neovascular age-related macular degeneration. JAMA Ophthalmology. 2021;**139**:441-448. DOI: 10.1001/jamaophthalmol.2020.7085

[118] Bulirsch LM, Saßmannshausen M, Nadal J, Liegl R, Thiele S, Holz FG. Short-term real-world outcomes following intravitreal brolucizumab for neovascular AMD: SHIFT study. The British Journal of Ophthalmology. 2022;**106**:1288-1294. DOI: 10.1136/bjophthalmol-2020-318672

[119] Bilgic A, Kodjikian L, de Ribot FM, Vasavada V, Gonzalez-Cortes JH, Abukashabah A, et al. Real-world experience with brolucizumab in wet age-related macular degeneration: The reba study. Journal of Clinical Medicine. 2021;**10**:2758. DOI: 10.3390/jcm10132758

[120] Bilgic A, Kodjikian L, Srivastava S, Dwivedi S, Banker AS, Abukashabah A, et al. Initial pro re nata brolucizumab for exudative AMD: The PROBE study. Journal of Clinical Medicine. 2021;**10**:4153. DOI: 10.3390/jcm10184153

[121] Chakraborty D, Maiti A, Sheth JU, Boral S, Mondal S, Nandi K, et al. Brolucizumab in neovascular age-related macular degeneration – Indian real-world experience: The BRAILLE study. Clinical Ophthalmology. 2021;**15**:3787-3795. DOI: 10.2147/OPTH.S328160

[122] Matsumoto H, Hoshino J, Mukai R, Nakamura K, Akiyama H. Short-term outcomes of intravitreal brolucizumab for treatment-naïve neovascular age-related macular degeneration with type 1 choroidal neovascularization including polypoidal choroidal vasculopathy. Scientific Reports. 2021;**11**:6759. DOI: 10.1038/s41598-021-86014-7

[123] Bilgic A, Kodjikian L, Vasavada S, Jha S, Srivastava S, Sudhalkar A, et al. Brolucizumab for choroidal neovascular membrane with pigment epithelial tear and subretinal fluid. Journal of Clinical Medicine. 2021;**10**:2425. DOI: 10.3390/jcm10112425

[124] Montesel A, Bucolo C, Sallo FB, Eandi CM. Short-term efficacy and safety outcomes of brolucizumab in the real-life clinical practice. Frontiers in Pharmacology. 2021;**12**:720345. DOI: 10.3389/fphar.2021.720345

[125] Brown DM, Emanuelli A, Bandello F, Barranco JJE, Figueira J, Souied E, et al. KESTREL and KITE: 52-week results from two phase III pivotal trials of brolucizumab for diabetic macular edema. American Journal of Ophthalmology. 2022;**238**:157-172. DOI: 10.1016/j.ajo.2022.01.004

[126] Tamashiro T, Tanaka K, Itagaki K, Nakayama M, Maruko I, Wakugawa S, et al. Subfoveal choroidal thickness after brolucizumab therapy for neovascular age-related macular degeneration: A short-term multicenter study. Graefe's Archive for Clinical and Experimental Ophthalmology. 2022;**260**:1857-1865. DOI: 10.1007/s00417-021-05517-1

[127] Avaylon J, Lee S, Gallemore RP. Case series on initial responses to intravitreal brolucizumab in patients with recalcitrant chronic wet age-related macular degeneration. International Medical Case Reports Journal. 2020;**13**:145-152. DOI: 10.2147/IMCRJ.S252260

[128] Haensli C, Pfister IB, Garweg JG. Switching to brolucizumab in neovascular age-related macular degeneration incompletely responsive to ranibizumab or aflibercept: Real-life 6 month outcomes. Journal of Clinical Medicine. 2021;**10**:2666. DOI: 10.3390/jcm10122666

[129] Sharma A, Kumar N, Parachuri N, Sadda SR, Corradetti G, Heier J, et al. Brolucizumab—early real-world experience: BREW study. In Eye (Basingstoke). 2021;**35**(4):1045-1047. DOI: 10.1038/s41433-020-1111-x. Springer Nature

[130] Awh CC, Davis EC, Thomas MK, Thomas AS. Short-term outcomes after interim treatment with brolucizumab: A retrospective case series of a single center experience. Retina. 2022;**42**:899-905. DOI: 10.1097/IAE.0000000000003418

[131] Fukuda Y, Sakurada Y, Kashiwagi K, Matsubara M, Hasebe Y, Sugiyama A, et al. Comparison of outcomes between 3 monthly brolucizumab and aflibercept injections for polypoidal choroidal vasculopathy. Biomedicine. 2021;**9**:1164. DOI: 10.3390/biomedicines9091164

[132] Chakraborty D, Mondal S, Parachuri N, Kumar N, Sharma A. Brolucizumab—Early experience with early extended interval regime in chronic centre involved diabetic macular oedema. Eye. 2022;**36**:358-360. DOI: 10.1038/s41433-021-01816-3

[133] Berger BB, Yanni SE, Wenzel A, Weichselberger A, Hubschman JP. Efficacy of RTH258 (ESBA1008), an anti-VEGF agent, applied by microvolume injection or infusion in subjects with neovascular AMD. Investigative Ophthalmology & Visual Science. 2015;**56**:821. Available from: https://iovs.arvojournals.org/article.aspx?articleID=2336548 [Accessed: October 23, 2023]

[134] Gaudreault J, Gunde T, Floyd HS, Ellis J, Tietz J, Binggeli D, et al. Preclinical pharmacology and safety of ESBA1008, a single-chain antibody fragment, investigated as potential treatment for age related macular degeneration. Investigative Ophthalmology & Visual Science. 2012;**53**:3025. Available from: https://iovs.arvojournals.org/article.aspx?articleid=2354604&mod=article_inline [Accessed: October 26, 2023]

[135] Garweg JG, Blum CA, Copt RP, Eandi CM, Hatz K, Prünte CF, et al. Brolucizumab in neovascular age-related macular degeneration and diabetic macular edema: Ophthalmology and diabetology treatment aspects. Ophthalmology and Therapy. 2023;**12**:639-655. DOI: 10.1007/S40123-023-00647-7

[136] Khanani AM, Zarbin MA, Barakat MR, Albini TA, Kaiser PK, Guruprasad B, et al. Safety outcomes of brolucizumab in neovascular age-related macular degeneration: Results from the IRIS registry and komodo healthcare map. JAMA Ophthalmology. 2022;**140**:20-28. DOI: 10.1001/jamaophthalmol.2021.4585

[137] Khan M, Aziz AA, Shafi NA, Abbas T, Khanani AM. Targeting angiopoietin in retinal vascular diseases: A literature review and summary of clinical trials involving faricimab. Cell. 2020;**9**:1869. DOI: 10.3390/cells9081869

[138] Surowka M, Schaefer W, Klein C. Ten years in the making: Application

of CrossMab technology for the development of therapeutic bispecific antibodies and antibody fusion proteins. MAbs. 2021;**13**:1967714. DOI: 10.1080/19420862.2021.1967714

[139] Jakubiak P, Alvarez-Sánchez R, Fueth M, Broders O, Kettenberger H, Stubenrauch K, et al. Ocular pharmacokinetics of intravitreally injected protein therapeutics: Comparison among standard-of-care formats. Molecular Pharmaceutics. 2021;**18**:2208-2217. DOI: 10.1021/acs.molpharmaceut.0c01218

[140] Sharma A, Kumar N, Kuppermann BD, Bandello F, Loewenstein A. Faricimab: Expanding horizon beyond VEGF. Eye. 2020;**34**:802-804. DOI: 10.1038/s41433-019-0670-1

[141] Dillon M, Yin Y, Zhou J, McCarty L, Ellerman D, Slaga D, et al. Efficient production of bispecific IgG of different isotypes and species of origin in single mammalian cells. MAbs. 2017;**9**:213-230. DOI: 10.1080/19420862.2016.1267089

[142] Regula JT, Lundh von Leithner P, Foxton R, Barathi VA, Cheung CMG, Bo Tun SB, et al. Targeting key angiogenic pathways with a bispecific cross MA b optimized for neovascular eye diseases. EMBO Molecular Medicine. 2016;**8**:1265-1288. DOI: 10.15252/emmm.201505889

[143] Foxton RH, Uhles S, Grüner S, Revelant F, Ullmer C. Efficacy of simultaneous VEGF-A/ANG-2 neutralization in suppressing spontaneous choroidal neovascularization. EMBO Molecular Medicine. 2019;**11**:e10204. DOI: 10.15252/emmm.201810204

[144] Wells JA, Wykoff CC, Willis JR, Haskova Z, Lin H, Silverman D, et al. Efficacy, durability, and safety of faricimab in diabetic macular edema (DME): One-year results from the phase 3 YOSEMITE and RHINE trials. Investigative Ophthalmology & Visual Science. 2021;**62**:1037-1037

[145] Danzig CJ, Wells JA, Eichenbaum D, Lim JI, Asik K, Haskova Z, et al. 47-OR: Efficacy, durability, and safety of faricimab in diabetic macular edema: Two-year results from the phase 3 YOSEMITE and RHINE trials. Diabetes. 2022;**71**:1037-1037. DOI: 10.2337/db22-47-or

[146] Ferro Desideri L, Traverso CE, Nicolò M, Munk MR. Faricimab for the treatment of diabetic macular edema and neovascular age-related macular degeneration. Pharmaceutics. 2023;**15**:1413. DOI: 10.3390/pharmaceutics15051413

[147] Panos GD, Lakshmanan A, Dadoukis P, Ripa M, Motta L, Amoaku WM. Faricimab: Transforming the future of macular diseases treatment - a comprehensive review of clinical studies. Drug Design, Development and Therapy. 2023;**17**:2861-2873. DOI: 10.2147/DDDT.S427416

[148] Yu L, Liang XH, Ferrara N. Comparing protein VEGF inhibitors: *In vitro* biological studies. Biochemical and Biophysical Research Communications. 2011;**408**:276-281. DOI: 10.1016/j.bbrc.2011.04.014

[149] Cao J, Zhao L, Li Y, Liu Y, Xiao W, Song Y, et al. A subretinal matrigel rat choroidal neovascularization (CNV) model and inhibition of CNV and associated inflammation and fibrosis by VEGF trap. Investigative Ophthalmology and Visual Science. 2010;**51**:6009-6017. DOI: 10.1167/iovs.09-4956

[150] Saishin Y, Saishin Y, Takahashi K, Silva RLE, Hylton D, Rudge JS, et al. VEGF-TRAPR1R2 suppresses choroidal neovascularization and VEGF-induced breakdown of the blood-retinal barrier. Journal of Cellular Physiology.

2003;**195**:241-248. DOI: 10.1002/jcp.10246

[151] Nork TM, Dubielzig RR, Christian BJ, Miller PE, Miller JM, Cao J, et al. Prevention of experimental choroidal neovascularization and resolution of active lesions by VEGF trap in nonhuman primates. Archives of Ophthalmology. 2011;**129**:1042-1052. DOI: 10.1001/archophthalmol.2011.210

[152] Zhang Y, Chioreso C, Schweizer ML, Abràmoff MD. Effects of aflibercept for neovascular age-related macular degeneration: A systematic review and meta-analysis of observational comparative studies. Investigative Ophthalmology and Visual Science. 2017;**58**:5616-5627. DOI: 10.1167/iovs.17-22471

[153] Gragoudas ES, Adamis AP, Cunningham ET, Feinsod M, Guyer DR. Pegaptanib for neovascular age-related macular degeneration. The New England Journal of Medicine. 2004;**351**:2805-2816. DOI: 10.1056/NEJMOA042760

[154] Singh SAA. Randomized, controlled phase III study of ranibizumab (LucentisTM) for minimally classic or occult neovascular age–related macular degeneration: Two–year efficacy results of the MARINA study. Investigative Ophthalmology & Visual Science. 2006;**47**:2959. Available from: https://iovs.arvojournals.org/article.aspx?articleid=2392796-2959 [Accessed: January 9, 2020]

[155] Gehrs KM, Anderson DH, Johnson LV, Hageman GS. Age-related macular degeneration - emerging pathogenetic and therapeutic concepts. Annals of Medicine. 2006;**38**:450-471. DOI: 10.1080/07853890600946724

[156] Slaker JS, Miller JW, Lane AM. Anecortave acetate as monotherapy for treatment of subfoveal neovascularization in age-related macular degeneration: Twelve-month clinical outcomes. Ophthalmology. 2003;**110**:2372-2383. DOI: 10.1016/j.ophtha.2003.08.020

[157] Quiram PA, Gonzales CR, Schwartz SD. Severe steroid-induced glaucoma following intravitreal injection of triamcinolone acetonide. American Journal of Ophthalmology. 2006;**141**:580-582. DOI: 10.1016/j.ajo.2005.10.004

[158] Ferrington DA, Fisher CR, Kowluru RA. Mitochondrial defects drive degenerative retinal diseases. Trends in Molecular Medicine. 2020;**26**:105-118. DOI: 10.1016/j.molmed.2019.10.008

[159] Bochaton-Piallat ML, Kapetanios AD, Donati G, Redard M, Gabbiani G, Pournaras CJ. TGF-β1, TGF-β receptor II and ED-A fibronectin expression in myofibroblast of vitreoretinopathy. Investigative Ophthalmology and Visual Science. 2000;**41**:2336-2342. Available from: http://iovs.arvojournals.org/article.aspx?articleid=2122911

[160] Brown DM, Nguyen QD, Marcus DM, Boyer DS, Patel S, Feiner L, et al. Long-term outcomes of ranibizumab therapy for diabetic macular edema: The 36-month results from two phase III trials: RISE and RIDE. Ophthalmology. 2013;**120**:2013-2022. DOI: 10.1016/j.ophtha.2013.02.034

[161] Heier JS, Korobelnik JF, Brown DM, Schmidt-Erfurth U, Do DV, Midena E, et al. Intravitreal aflibercept for diabetic macular edema: 148-week results from the VISTA and VIVID studies. Ophthalmology. 2016;**123**:2376-2385. DOI: 10.1016/j.ophtha.2016.07.032

[162] Campochiaro PA, Brown DM, Pearson A, Chen S, Boyer D, Ruiz-Moreno J, et al. Sustained delivery

fluocinolone acetonide vitreous inserts provide benefit for at least 3 years in patients with diabetic macular edema. Ophthalmology. 2012;**119**:2125-2132. DOI: 10.1016/j.ophtha.2012.04.030

[163] Boyer DS, Yoon YH, Belfort R, Bandello F, Maturi RK, Augustin AJ, et al. Three-year, randomized, sham-controlled trial of dexamethasone intravitreal implant in patients with diabetic macular edema. Ophthalmology. 2014;**121**:1904-1914. DOI: 10.1016/j.ophtha.2014.04.024

[164] Duh EJ, Sun JK, Stitt AW. Diabetic retinopathy: Current understanding, mechanisms, and treatment strategies. JCI Insight. 2017;**2**:1-13. DOI: 10.1172/jci.insight.93751

[165] Chan ESL, Cronstein BN. Methotrexate how does it really work? Nature Reviews Rheumatology. 2010;**6**:175-178. DOI: 10.1038/nrrheum.2010.5

[166] Kurup SK, Gee C, Greven CM. Intravitrealmethotrexateintherapeutically resistant exudative age-related macular degeneration. Acta Ophthalmologica. 2010;**88**:e145-e146. DOI: 10.1111/j.1755-3768.2009.01560.x

[167] Frenkel S, Hendler K, Siegal T, Shalom E, Pe'er J. Intravitreal methotrexate for treating vitreoretinal lymphoma: 10 years of experience. The British Journal of Ophthalmology. 2008;**92**:383-388. DOI: 10.1136/bjo.2007.127928

[168] Shu DY, Butcher E, Saint-Geniez M. EMT and ENDMT: Emerging roles in age-related macular degeneration. In International Journal of Molecular Sciences. Multidisciplinary Digital Publishing Institute. 2020;**21**(12):1-26. doi: 10.3390/ijms21124271

[169] Brown EE, Ball JD, Chen Z, Khurshid GS, Prosperi M, Ash JD. The common antidiabetic drug metformin reduces odds of developing age-related macular degeneration. Investigative Ophthalmology and Visual Science. 2019;**60**:1470-1477. DOI: 10.1167/iovs.18-26422

[170] Hamblin MR. Shining light on the head: Photobiomodulation for brain disorders. BBA Clinical. 2016;**6**:113-124. DOI: 10.1016/j.bbacli.2016.09.002

[171] Tang J, Herda AA, Kern TS. Photobiomodulation in the treatment of patients with non-center-involving diabetic macular oedema. The British Journal of Ophthalmology. 2014;**98**:1013-1015. DOI: 10.1136/bjophthalmol-2013-304477

[172] Maguire MG, Klein ML, Olk RJ, Phillips DA, Alexander J, Javornik NB, et al. Persistent and recurrent neovascularization after laser photocoagulation for subfoveal choroidal neovascularization of age-related macular degeneration. Archives of Ophthalmology. 1994;**112**:489-499. DOI: 10.1001/archopht.1994.01090160065024

[173] Al-Zamil WM, Yassin SA. Recent developments in age-related macular degeneration: A review. Clinical Interventions in Aging. 2017;**12**:1313-1330. DOI: 10.2147/CIA.S143508

[174] Ulańczyk Z, Grabowicz A, Cecerska-Heryć E, Śleboda-Taront D, Krytkowska E, Mozolewska-Piotrowska K, et al. Dietary and lifestyle factors modulate the activity of the endogenous antioxidant system in patients with age-related macular degeneration: Correlations with disease severity. Antioxidants. 2020;**9**:1-19. DOI: 10.3390/antiox9100954

[175] Ni T, Yang W, Xing Y. Protective effects of delphinidin against

H_2O_2-induced oxidative injuries in human retinal pigment epithelial cells. Bioscience Reports. 2019;**39**:BSR20190689. DOI: 10.1042/BSR20190689

[176] Wolf S. Current status of anti-vascular endothelial growth factor therapy in Europe. Japanese Journal of Ophthalmology. 2008;**52**:433-439. DOI: 10.1007/s10384-008-0580-4

[177] Voloboueva LA, Liu J, Suh JH, Ames BN, Miller SS. (R)-α-lipoic acid protects retinal pigment epithelial cells from oxidative damage. Investigative Ophthalmology and Visual Science. 2005;**46**:4302-4310. DOI: 10.1167/iovs.04-1098

[178] Goldberg J, Flowerdew G, Smith E, Brody JA, Tso MOM. Factors associated with age-related macular degeneration: An analysis of data from the fi1r8t National health and nutrition examination survey. American Journal of Epidemiology. 1988;**128**:700-710. DOI: 10.1093/oxfordjournals.aje.a115023

[179] Sajeeth CI, Manna PK, Manavalan R. Antioxidant activity of polyherbal formulation on streptozotocin induced diabetes in experimental animals. Der Pharmacia Sinica. 2011;**2**:220-226

[180] Liu Y, Liu M, Zhang X, Chen Q, Chen H, Sun L, et al. Protective effect of fucoxanthin isolated from laminaria japonica against visible light-induced retinal damage both *in vitro* and *in vivo*. Journal of Agricultural and Food Chemistry. 2016;**64**:416-424. DOI: 10.1021/acs.jafc.5b05436

[181] Klein BEK, Howard KP, Lee KE, Iyengar SK, Sivakumaran TA, Klein R. The relationship of cataract and cataract extraction to age-related macular degeneration: The beaver dam eye study. Ophthalmology. 2012;**119**:1628-1633. DOI: 10.1016/j.ophtha.2012.01.050

[182] Ferris FL, Davis MD, Clemons TE, Lee LY, Chew EY, Lindblad AS, et al. A simplified severity scale for age-related macular degeneration: AREDS report no. 18. Archives of Ophthalmology. 2005;**123**:1570-1574. DOI: 10.1001/archopht.123.11.1570

[183] Sparrow JR, Hicks D, Hamel CP. The retinal pigment epithelium in health and disease. Current Molecular Medicine. 2010;**10**:802-823. DOI: 10.2174/156652410793937813

[184] Hazim RA, Volland S, Yen A, Burgess BL, Williams DS. Rapid differentiation of the human RPE cell line, ARPE-19, induced by nicotinamide. Experimental Eye Research. 2019;**179**:18-24. DOI: 10.1016/j.exer.2018.10.009

[185] Boles NC, Fernandes M, Swigut T, Srinivasan R, Schiff L, Rada-Iglesias A, et al. Epigenomic and transcriptomic changes during human RPE EMT in a stem cell model of epiretinal membrane pathogenesis and prevention by nicotinamide. Stem Cell Reports. 2020;**14**:631-647. DOI: 10.1016/j.stemcr.2020.03.009

[186] Saini JS, Corneo B, Miller JD, Kiehl TR, Wang Q, Boles NC, et al. Nicotinamide ameliorates disease phenotypes in a human iPSC model of age-related macular degeneration. Cell Stem Cell. 2017;**20**:635-647.e7. DOI: 10.1016/j.stem.2016.12.015

[187] Meng Y, Ren Z, Xu F, Zhou X, Song C, Wang VYF, et al. Nicotinamide promotes cell survival and differentiation as kinase inhibitor in human pluripotent stem cells. Stem Cell Reports. 2018;**11**:1347-1356. DOI: 10.1016/j.stemcr.2018.10.023

[188] Zhou L, Shi DP, Chu WJ, Song S, Hao XH, Yang LL, et al. Nicotinamide suppresses bevacizumab-induced epithelial-mesenchymal transition

of ARPE-19 cells by attenuating oxidative stress. International Journal of Ophthalmology. 2021;**14**:481-488. DOI: 10.18240/ijo.2021.04.01

[189] Yao H, Ge T, Zhang Y, Li M, Yang S, Li H, et al. BMP7 antagonizes proliferative vitreoretinopathy through retinal pigment epithelial fibrosis *in vivo* and *in vitro*. The FASEB Journal. 2019;**33**:3212-3224. DOI: 10.1096/fj.201800858RR

[190] Hu B, Zhang Y, Zeng Q, Han Q, Zhang L, Liu M, et al. Intravitreal injection of ranibizumab and CTGF shRNA improves retinal gene expression and microvessel ultrastructure in a rodent model of diabetes. International Journal of Molecular Sciences. 2014;**15**:1606-1624. DOI: 10.3390/ijms15011606

[191] Shukal D, Bhadresha K, Shastri B, Mehta D, Vasavada A, Johar K. Dichloroacetate prevents TGFβ-induced epithelial-mesenchymal transition of retinal pigment epithelial cells. Experimental Eye Research. 2020;**197**:108072. DOI: 10.1016/j.exer.2020.108072

[192] Zhang R, Liu Z, Zhang H, Zhang Y, Lin D. The COX-2-selective antagonist (NS-398) inhibits choroidal neovascularization and subretinal fibrosis. PLoS One. 2016;**11**:e0146808. DOI: 10.1371/journal.pone.0146808

[193] Rizzolo LJ. Barrier properties of cultured retinal pigment epithelium. Experimental Eye Research. 2014;**126**:16-26. DOI: 10.1016/j.exer.2013.12.018

[194] Del Priore LV, Kuo YH, Tezel TH. Age-related changes in human RPE cell density and apoptosis proportion *in situ*. Investigative Ophthalmology and Visual Science. 2002;**43**:3312-3318. Available from: https://iovs.arvojournals.org/article.aspx?articleid=2123280 [Accessed: December 25, 2020]

[195] Cano M, Wang L, Wan J, Barnett BP, Ebrahimi K, Qian J, et al. Oxidative stress induces mitochondrial dysfunction and a protective unfolded protein response in RPE cells. Free Radical Biology & Medicine. 2014;**69**:1-14. DOI: 10.1038/jid.2014.371

[196] Angulo Daniela F. Intracellular redox status and cell death induced by H_2O_2 in a human retinal epithelial cell line (ARPE-19). American Journal of BioScience. 2015;**3**:93. DOI: 10.11648/j.ajbio.20150303.15

[197] Bakall B, Folk JC, Boldt HC, Sohn EH, Stone EM, Russell SR, et al. Aflibercept therapy for exudative age-related macular degeneration resistant to bevacizumab and ranibizumab. American Journal of Ophthalmology. 2013;**156**:15-22.e1. DOI: 10.1016/j.ajo.2013.02.017

[198] Ishikawa K, Kannan R, Hinton DR. Molecular mechanisms of subretinal fibrosis in age-related macular degeneration. Experimental Eye Research. 2014;**142**:19-25. DOI: 10.1016/j.exer.2015.03.009

Chapter 4

Early Macular Involvement in Non-syndromic Retinitis Pigmentosa

Alessia Amato, Nida Wongchaisuwat, Andrew Lamborn, Lesley Everett, Paul Yang and Mark E. Pennesi

Abstract

Retinitis pigmentosa (RP) is the most common inherited retinal disease (IRD), with a worldwide prevalence of about 1:4000. Functionally, RP is a rod-cone dystrophy (RCD), where rod photoreceptors are affected earlier and more severely than cone photoreceptors. As a consequence, RP typically manifests with night blindness beginning in adolescence followed by concentric constriction of visual field, while central visual loss usually occurs later in life. The molecular bases of this disorder, however, are highly heterogeneous, with over 100 genes implicated, and in some RP subtypes macular manifestations occur relatively early in the disease course. The subsequent rapid decline in visual acuity in such patients blurs the line between RP and other IRDs, namely cone-rod dystrophies (CORDs), and increases the difficulty in narrowing down the differential diagnosis. This chapter aims to review the features of non-syndromic RP caused by mutations in genes that have been commonly associated with early macular involvement and to provide an updated overview on recent preclinical or clinical studies addressing these rare diseases.

Keywords: retinitis pigmentosa, macular involvement, *RPGR*, *RP1*, *C2orf71*, *PCARE*, *MERTK*, *CERKL*, *PROM1*, *IMPG2*

1. Introduction

Retinitis pigmentosa (RP) is an inherited retinal disease (IRD) that causes progressive vision impairment commonly leading to legal blindness, with an estimated worldwide prevalence of about 1:4000 [1], but highly variable based on geographic area. The highest frequency of occurrence has been reported among the Navajo Indians (1:1878), from Northern China (1:1000), and from southern and central India (1:600–750), while countries, such as Switzerland (1:7000) and England (1:4800), have a lower prevalence.

Non-syndromic RP, which accounts for approximately 70–80% of all RP cases [2], can be classified according to its inheritance pattern in: autosomal dominant (AD) RP (20–25%), autosomal recessive (AR) RP (15–20%), and X-linked (XL) RP (5–15%). The remaining 40–50% of patients are designated as simplex RP, representing isolated cases with only one affected family member [3, 4]. In addition, 20–30%

of patients present with syndromic forms of the disease, where the retinal disorder is accompanied by extraocular abnormalities [2].

RP is a rod-cone dystrophy (RCD) as there is a primary degeneration of rod photoreceptors, while cone photoreceptors are involved in more advanced diseases. Traditionally, the distinction between RCD and cone/cone-rod dystrophy (COD/CORD) has been established based on the pattern of generalized retinal dysfunction displayed on full-field electroretinograms (ERGs). In RCDs, scotopic dim flash (0.01 cd/m^2) ERGs show a decrease in amplitude and a delay in implicit time that exceed those measured on bright single flash (3.0 cd/m^2) or 30 Hz flicker ERGs, while the opposite occurs in CORDs. While this definition often allows to make an unequivocal diagnosis and to provide patients with accurate information on likely progression of symptoms, some cases are not as clear-cut. For example, since in RCDs and CORDs functional damage usually precedes structural change, patients can have no recordable scotopic and photopic ERGs at relatively early disease stages. In these circumstances, when ophthalmoscopy does not reveal obvious signs of RP, retinal imaging, such as optical coherence tomography (OCT) or fundus autofluorescence (FAF), can help identify biomarkers (e.g., subfoveal sparing of outer retinal layers on OCT or altered autofluorescence at the posterior pole) that are consistent with a certain pattern of dysfunction (rod versus cone-dominated). Similarly, psychophysical exams, such as microperimetry and chromatic full-field perimetry, can isolate rod and cone contributions and guide physicians in counseling their patients.

In classic RP, nyctalopia is often the initial symptom, followed by a progressive constriction of the visual field. Macular function and visual acuity (VA) are usually relatively preserved until later stages. However, in certain RP subtypes, the degeneration of central photoreceptors and retinal pigment epithelium (RPE) occurs earlier than one would expect based on the degree of visual field constriction. As discussed above, these subtypes are often characterized by extinguished scotopic and photopic ERGs which, in the presence of macular atrophy, can make differentiating the diagnosis with CORDs challenging.

RP with early macular involvement is a particularly debilitating as patients experience a rapid decline in best-corrected visual acuity (BCVA) in addition to the progressive visual field constriction that is typical in RP. These patients often meet both criteria for legal blindness as defined in the United States (i.e., BCVA of 20/200 or less in the better eye and visual field less than 20 degrees in the better eye) at a young age. Some genes have been more often associated with early macular atrophy and a more aggressive phenotype. In order to provide patients with accurate prognostic information, it is important for the IRD specialist to be aware of these genotype-phenotype correlations and up-to-date with current research.

In this chapter, we will review the molecular biology and clinical features of RP-associated genes that most often result in early macular involvement, and we will provide an overview of relevant research efforts.

2. Common causative genes of non-syndromic RP with early macular involvement

In this section, we will provide an overview of RP-associated genes that cause non-syndromic RP with early macular involvement, focusing on those that are being investigated in preclinical studies and clinical trials.

2.1 Non-syndromic retinal ciliopathies

Ciliopathies are defined as a group of disorders resulting from impaired function of the cilium, a highly specialized and evolutionarily conserved organelle in eukaryotes [5]. Cilia are classified into two subtypes: motile, mainly localized in epithelial cells of the lung, ventricles of the brain and spermatozoa, and nonmotile (or primary), which are ubiquitous [6]. While motile cilia have the main function of generating movement, primary cilia are involved in cell signaling and trafficking [7]. In photoreceptors, the primary cilium is responsible for connecting the outer segments (OS) to the inner segments (IS), where it plays a critical role in transport, and it is estimated that every minute approximately 2000 opsin molecules are delivered to the OS through the cilium [8–10].

Primary cilia dysfunction may present as a single organ disorder, including an isolated retinal degeneration (e.g., XLRP), or it can affect multiple organs resulting in a syndromic ciliopathy, such as Bardet-Biedl syndrome (BBS) [5]. Although some ciliary gene-associated forms of RP, such as those caused by biallelic variants in *MAK*, are reported to spare central vision until well into adulthood [11], patients with mutations in connecting cilium genes are often reported to have a more severe RCD with early macular degeneration [12, 13].

Herein, we will review the molecular and clinical features of genes expressed in the primary cilium of photoreceptors that often cause non-syndromic RP with early macular involvement.

2.1.1 RPGR

RPGR is located on the X chromosome and is comprised of 19 exons encoding the retinitis pigmentosa GTPase regulator, a protein involved in photoreceptor ciliary function. Alternative splicing results in more than 10 different isoforms [14, 15]. The two major isoforms are $RPGR^{Ex1-19}$, the full-length variant and $RPGR^{ORF15}$, which encompasses the first 14 exons of the gene and the open reading frame (ORF) 15 region, derived from an alternatively spliced exon 15 with part of intron 15 (**Figure 1**). While $RPGR^{Ex1-19}$ is expressed throughout the body, $RPGR^{ORF15}$ is primarily expressed in the connecting cilia of retinal photoreceptors. Approximately 80% of pathogenic variants in *RPGR* are located in the ORF15 region [16], and the remaining 20% are found in exons 1–14. No disease-causing mutations have been reported in exons 16–19 [14].

RPGR pathogenic variants can manifest as a rod-cone dystrophy (RCD), which is the most common phenotype, a cone/cone-rod dystrophy (COD/CORD), and a macular dystrophy (MD) [17, 18]. Genotype-phenotype correlations are controversial. Some authors report that variants in exon 1–14 are characterized by a more severe disease than ORF15 variants [17, 19, 20], while others report the opposite [18, 21, 22]. There seems to be a broader agreement on the fact that patients with mutations in the ORF15 region exhibit greater phenotypic variability [17, 19, 23], and that variants at the 3′-end are more often responsible for CORD, while 5′ variants frequently cause RCD [24].

RPGR is responsible for approximately 80% of XLRP which, compared to other forms of RP, generally displays an earlier onset and a more rapidly progressive course (**Figure 2**). Macular abnormalities, including cystoid macular edema (CME), vitreomacular traction (VMT), epiretinal membrane (ERM), full-thickness macular hole (FTMH), and lamellar macular hole (LMH), are common. Early macular involvement in XLRP patients is also associated with a reduced sensitivity on microperimetry,

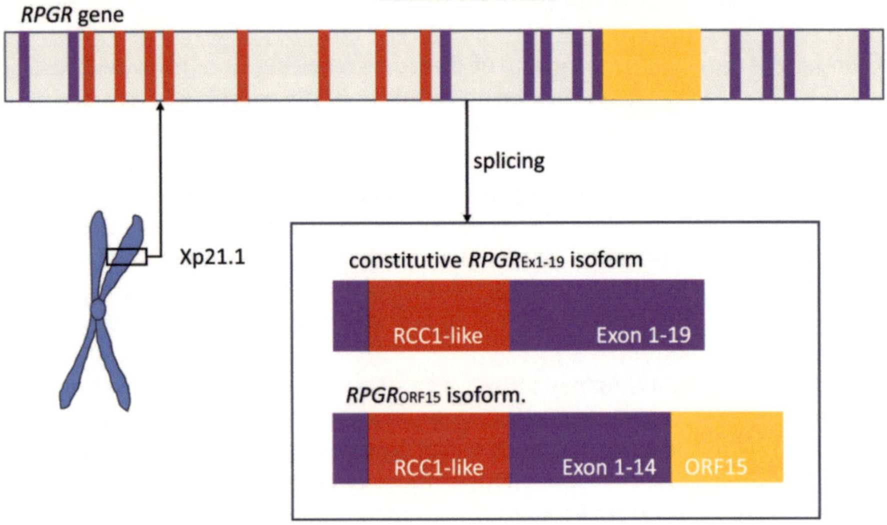

Figure 1.
Structural diagram of the retinitis pigmentosa GTPase regulator (RPGR) gene and two common splicing isoforms.

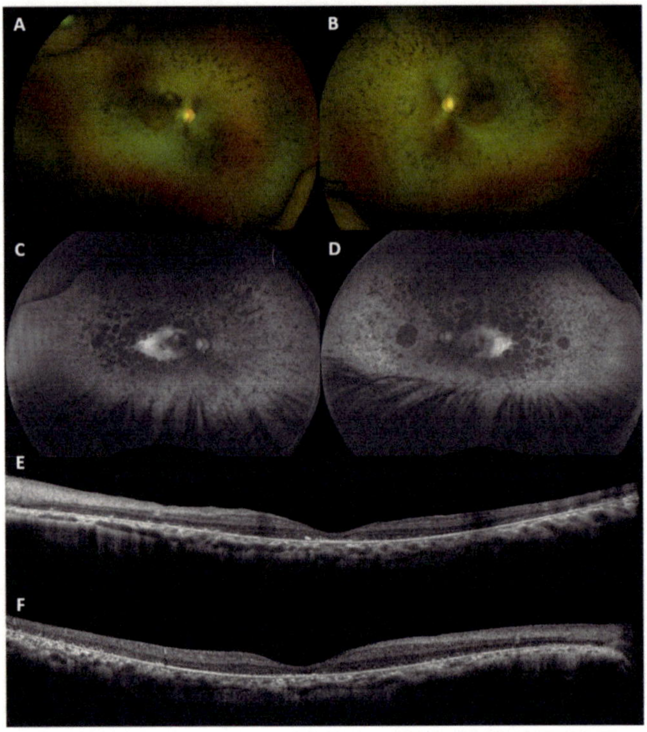

Figure 2.
Multimodal imaging of a 35-year-old male hemizygous for a pathogenic variant in RPGR. Pseudocolor fundus photos (A, B) show diffuse bone spicule pigmentation and macular RPE mottling, although the view of the posterior pole is partially obscured by the patient's posterior subcapsular cataract. FAF (C, D) better highlights the atrophic and dystrophic changes in the macular region. OCT (E, F) shows a severe attenuation of outer retinal structures, with a near complete loss of the EZ band, accounting for the patient's poor BCVA (20/400 OU) despite his young age. FAF = fundus autofluorescence; OCT = optical coherence tomography; EZ = ellipsoid zone; BCVA = best-corrected visual acuity.

which does not seem to correlate with older age [21]. High myopia is frequent with a prevalence of up to 80% and is associated with a more rapid decline in BCVA [18, 21].

Female carriers show high phenotypic variability and asymmetry between affected eyes [25]. The presentation can range from asymptomatic to severe disease indistinguishable from that seen in males [26]. Even in asymptomatic subjects, carrier status can often be detected with clinical examination and fundus autofluorescence (FAF), which sometimes show a typical radial tapetal reflex and radial pattern of hyperautofluorescence, respectively [27, 28].

There are a number or reasons why *RPGR* stands out as an optimal candidate for gene replacement therapy, including its small size fitting the cargo capacity of the common viral vectors, the loss-of-function (LOF) mechanism underlying its pathogenic variants, along with the relatively high prevalence and more severe disease burden in the IRD population. However, the repetitive purine-rich sequence of ORF15 is prone to spontaneous mutations, making it a challenge to produce a safe and effective therapeutic vector. Two main strategies have been adopted to address this problem. The first consists of using a truncated form of $RPGR^{ORF15}$ since moderate shortening of its length improves stability while preserving function [29]. The second strategy is through codon optimization, which aims to modify the codon composition to make it more stable without altering the amino acid sequence [29]. There are five ongoing clinical trials, each of which has adopted either of these two strategies, with promising results.

2.1.2 RP1

RP1 is a four-exon gene encoding oxygen-regulated protein 1, a photoreceptor-specific microtubule-associated protein, which is involved in photoreceptor development, organization of the OS, and regulation of ciliary trafficking [30]. The *RP1* locus was first identified in 1982 in a large family with AD RP [31], and the gene linked to the disease was named retinitis pigmentosa 1 (RP1, OMIM 603937) [32], which is now known to be one of the most frequent causative genes in AD RP, with a prevalence as high as 10% [33]. Later publications revealed that variants in *RP1* can also cause AR RP [34–36], and a recent study depicted that mutations in this gene are a relatively common cause of AR RCD [37].

Generally, AD RP tends to have a milder presentation, and *RP1*-associated AD RCD is no exception, with patients typically being diagnosed in their 20s and exhibiting classical signs of RP with relatively preserved central vision and visual field [33], as shown in **Figure 3**. Incomplete penetrance and variable expressivity have also been reported in families with dominantly inherited *RP1* mutations [33, 38]. Biallelic pathogenic variants lead to more severe disease (**Figure 4**), with early onset and frequent central involvement, which has been variably described in previous reports as macular RPE degeneration [36], macular stippling [34], and macular atrophy [39]. BCVA often declines in the second decade of life, sometimes progressing to hand motion (HM) or light perception (LP) by the third or fourth decade [39].

RP1 mutations responsible for both AD and AR forms are mostly truncating (i.e., nonsense and frameshift) and result in premature termination codons, while missense mutations are rare [33]. Variants near the 5′ end tend to generate transcripts that are sensitive to nonsense-mediated decay (NMD), an mRNA surveillance mechanism that leads to degradation of the transcripts with introns in the 3′ untranslated region [40]. These mutations create a null allele causing LOF and have been associated with recessive RP, suggesting that haploinsufficiency of *RP1* protein does not cause RP in humans [39]. AD *RP1*-related RCD is typically caused by pathogenic variants located

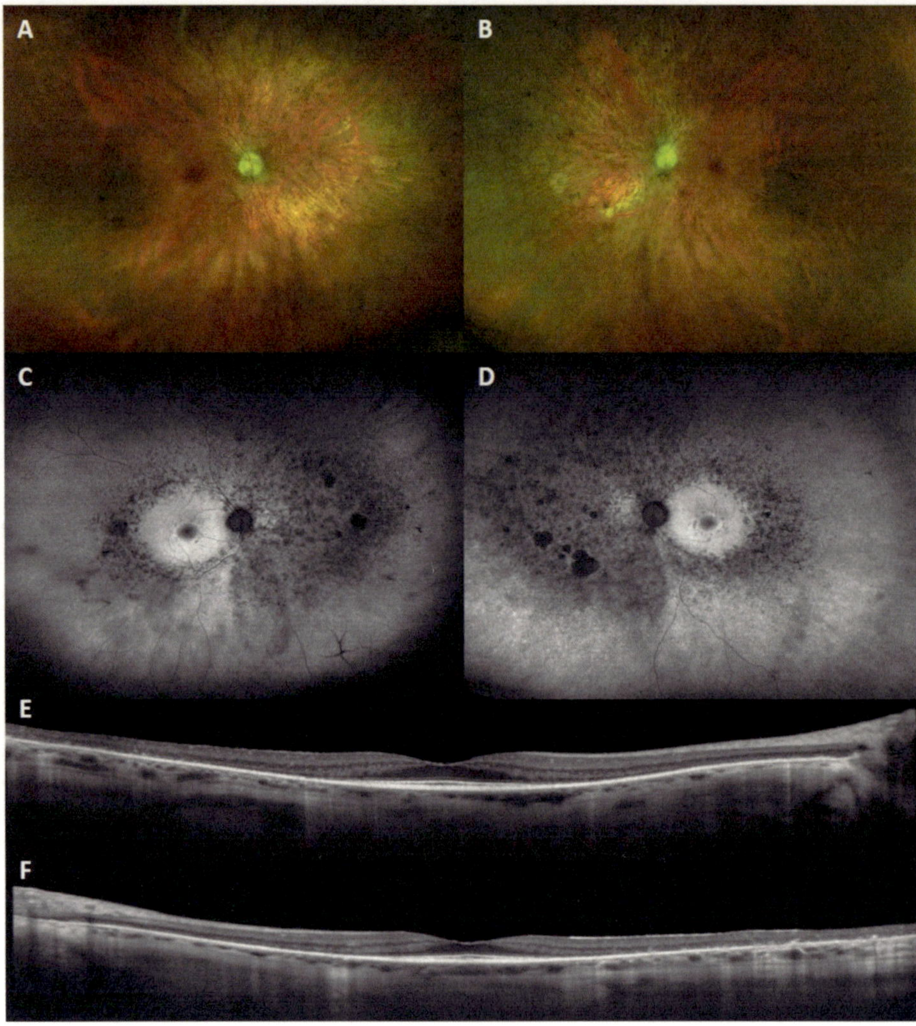

Figure 3.
Multimodal imaging of a 65-year-old female heterozygous for a pathogenic variant in RP1. Compared to AR forms of RP1-retinopathy, AD forms are less severe. Pseudocolor fundus photos (A, B) show the classic clinical triad of optic disc pallor, vessel attenuation, and bone spicule pigmentation. FAF (C, D) shows a perifoveal hyperautofluorescent ring, speckled midperipheral hypoautofluorescent changes, and some peripheral patches of deep hypoautofluorescence, especially nasally. OCT (E, F) shows relatively preserved outer retinal layers, including ONL, EZ, and IZ, subfoveally and parafoveally. BCVA is 20/25 OU. FAF = fundus autofluorescence; OCT = optical coherence tomography; ONL = outer nuclear layer; EZ = ellipsoid zone; IZ = interdigitation zone; BCVA = best-corrected visual acuity.

within a hot spot (spanning approximately p.500 to p.1053) in exon 4 [33], which tend to escape NMD due to the lack of intronic structure downstream [39]. Mutations in this region are the vast majority and mutant proteins are expected to cause a deleterious effect on photoreceptors [39], either through gain-of-function (GOF) or a dominant negative effect (DNE). In mouse models, it has been shown that when nonsense variants are located within the hot spot, then photoreceptor degeneration can be delayed or prevented by adding wild-type Rp1 protein, suggesting a DNE rather than a GOF for at least some variants [41, 42].

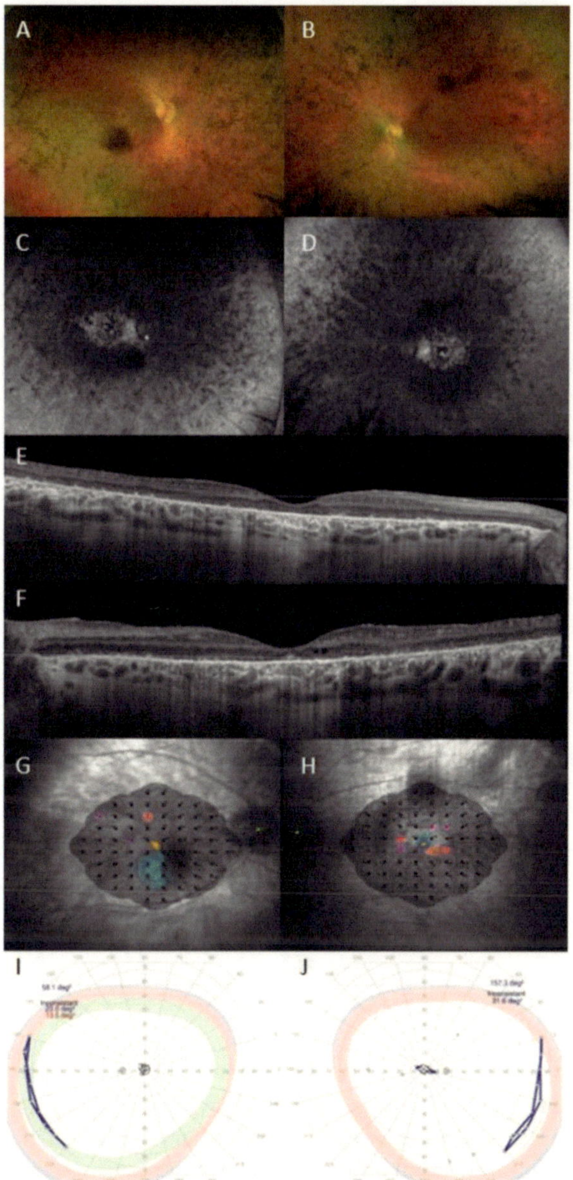

Figure 4.
Multimodal imaging and psychophysical assessment of a 27-year-old male, harboring two frameshift variants in the RP1 gene. Pseudocolor fundus photos (A, B) show extensive bone spicule pigmentation, as well as atrophic changes in the macula, which appear as hypoautofluorescent lesions on FAF (C, D). OCT B-scan through the fovea (E, F) shows outer retinal atrophy OU and some parafoveal hyporeflective cysts in the INL OS. Microperimetry (G, H) reveals an unstable eccentric fixation OD, which is fairly stable OS. Macular sensitivity is severely depressed in both eyes, with no measurable threshold at most loci. On KVF (I, J) only target size V4e could be detected in a small (<5°) central island, as well as in a temporal crescent in the far periphery. FAF = fundus autofluorescence; OCT = optical coherence tomography; INL = inner nuclear layer; KVF = kinetic visual field.

These observations are of translational interest as shedding light on the molecular mechanisms underlying *RP1*-related IRDs is crucial in selecting the most appropriate therapeutic strategies. GOF mutations are not amenable to gene replacement therapy alone, while LOF and, potentially, DNE variants are. However, the pathogenic mechanism of many dominant mutations is still unclear; thus, suppression of the mutant protein may be required in addition to delivery of a healthy gene. A recent study showed that a CRISPR-Cas9 approach successfully reduced *RP1* expression in Hap1-EF1a-RP1 cells, providing proof-of-concept of efficacy of gene editing in the treatment of patients with *RP1*-associated dominant IRDs [43].

2.1.3 PCARE

PCARE (previously known as *C2orf71*) encodes the photoreceptor cilium actin regulator protein (PCARE), an intracellular protein exclusively expressed in the retina, specifically at the initiation site of OS discs [44]. Although its function is not fully understood, it has been proposed that PCARE acts as an actin-associated protein and interacts with other molecular complexes, such as WASF3, to regulate the actin-driven expansion of the ciliary membrane during the development of new OS in photoreceptors [44].

Biallelic pathogenic variants in *PCARE* cause RP54 (OMIM #613428) [45–47] and, less frequently, CORD [48, 49]. Moreover, a digenic inheritance has been proposed, although evidence for this is confined to case reports suggesting a possible pathogenic effect in combination with other genes, such as *CEP250* [50] and *RP1L1* [51].

RP54 is more prevalent in Swiss [52] and Chinese [53] subjects, in whom *PCARE* is responsible for 15 and 8% of RP cases, respectively. This form of RCD is characterized by early age of onset and cone involvement with frequent macular degeneration [45–47], as shown in **Figure 5**. Recently, two animal models of *PCARE*-retinopathy have been developed, including the zebrafish *PCARE* [54] and a knockout of the mouse *PCARE* homolog, *BC027072* (*BC-/-*) [55]. Zebrafish, such as humans, are diurnal animals with a cone-rich retina, but they have duplicated genes (*pcare1* and *pcare2*), so decreasing or abolishing the function of *pcare1* does not entirely mimic the retinal phenotype of *PCARE*-related retinopathy. Mice share 79% of the amino acid sequence identity of proteins coded by IRD-causing genes, but they are nocturnal animals without a cone-rich region comparable to the fovea. Despite these shortcomings, loss of function of both the zebrafish and mouse orthologs has been shown to lead to outer nuclear layer (ONL) thinning and OS disorganization, resulting in early-onset alterations in visual behavior, suggesting that *PCARE* is likely implicated in outer retinal development. Moreover, there are six dog breeds whose AR rod-cone dysplasia type 4 has been linked to the c.3149_3150insC variation in *C17H2orf71* (*PCARE* human homolog), which could represent a feasible natural-occurring model to help develop new treatments [44]. *PCARE* is a two-exon gene spanning a 12.5 kb region (with one of the exons containing 95% of the coding sequence) [55] and therefore exceeds the cargo capacity of adeno-associated viral (AAV) vectors. However, limitations related to size are likely to be overcome in the near future as dual vector strategies are currently being developed to allow the delivery of large genes through a standard AAV gene therapy approach.

2.2 *MERTK*

MERTK encodes the widely expressed MER receptor tyrosine kinase, a transmembrane protein involved in a signal transduction pathway that regulates numerous

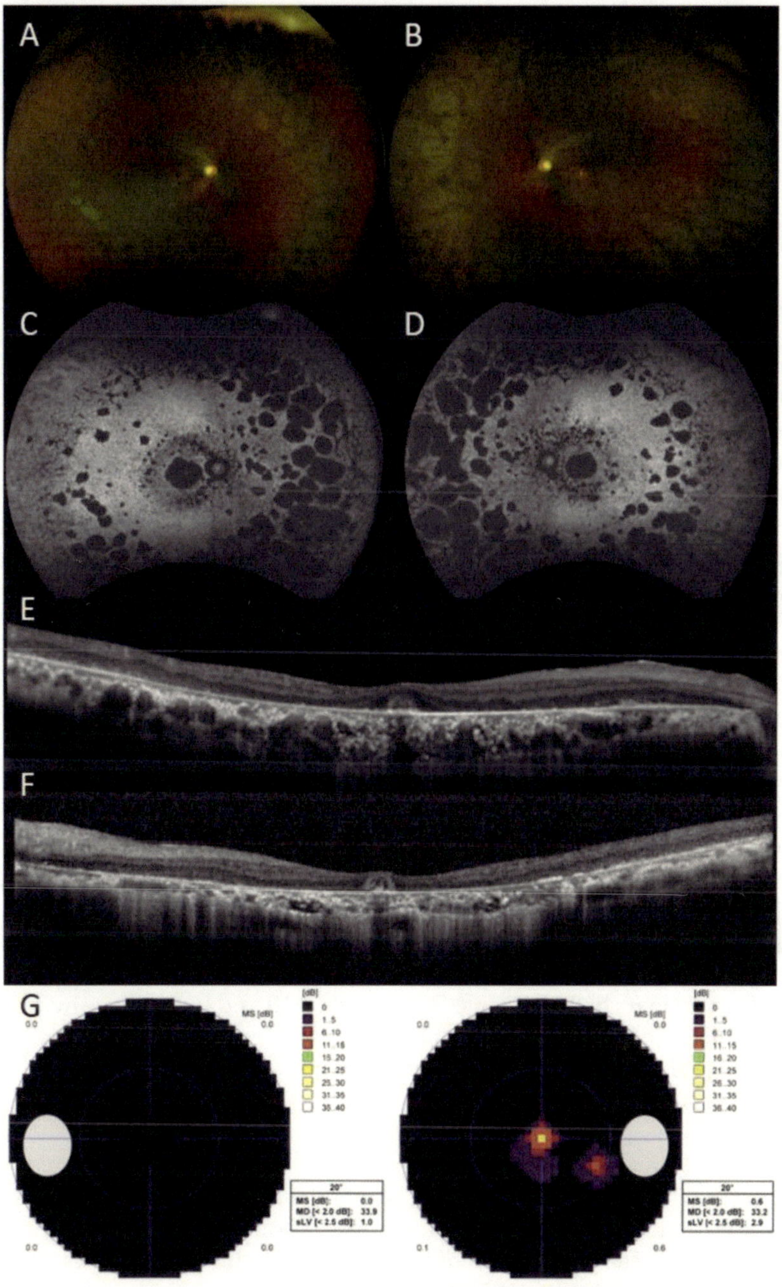

Figure 5.
Multimodal imaging and psychophysical assessment of a 46-year-old female with two pathogenic variants in PCARE. Pseudocolor fundus photos (A, B) show extensive regions of atrophy and dots of hypopigmentation with large peripheral areas of nummular punched-out atrophy 360 degrees OU. FAF (C, D) reveals a large central zone of hypoautofluorescence sparing a very small island, as well as large mid and far peripheral patches of hypoautofluorescence OU. OCT (E, F) displays extensive loss of outer retinal structures with minimal foveal sparing, hyperreflective granular deposits in the outer retina, along Bruch's membrane and inner choroid. Static perimetry (G) shows a severely decreased sensitivity. BCVA of this patient is 20/50 OD and light perception OS. FAF = fundus autofluorescence; OCT = optical coherence tomography; BCVA = best-corrected visual acuity.

cellular processes. In the retina, *MERTK* is expressed in the apical membrane of RPE cells and plays a role in the initiation steps of OS phagocytosis [56]. Failure of the RPE-mediated phagocytic pathway leads to accumulation of toxic debris in the subretinal space and to subsequent photoreceptor degeneration. To date, more than 90 *MERTK* variants have been identified in patients with AR RCD, Leber congenital amaurosis (LCA), and, more rarely, CORD [57]. *MERTK*-related RP or RP38 (OMIM #613862) accounts for approximately 2% of all RP cases and is generally characterized by childhood-onset nyctalopia and early macular involvement with decrease in BCVA often occurring after 2 years of age [58]. Clinically, RP38 can present, most notably in young patients, with discrete whitish dots on fundoscopy that are hyperautofluorescent on FAF consistently with impaired RPE phagocytosis [58]. Optical coherence tomography (OCT) displays a severe retinal thinning with loss of outer retinal layers and debris-like material in the subretinal space [59]. Foveal hyperautofluorescence in the absence of peripheral bone-spicule pigmentation, even when ERGs show a clear rod-cone pattern of dysfunction, is a common finding (**Figure 6**) and highlights the importance of a combined structural and functional assessment [57].

MERTK has several features that make it an appealing target for gene therapy, including expression in the RPE, which is efficiently targeted by AAV vectors, small size of the cDNA sequence, and availability of preclinical models for vector validation. AAV-mediated retinal gene therapy was first tested in the Royal College of Surgeons (RCS) rat, which has recessive mutations in the *Mertk* gene, with promising results [60–62].

A gene augmentation therapy phase one trial in six patients with biallelic *MERTK* mutations was conducted in Saudi Arabia, and the results were published in 2016 [63]. The primary end point was safety at the 2-year follow-up, while secondary outcome measures included BCVA, full-field stimulus test (FST), and central macular thickness (CMT) on OCT. Subretinal injection of the vector was not associated with major side effects, and 50% of patients demonstrated increased BCVA though only one of them maintained these results [64]. In one patient, BCVA improved from <20/6400 at baseline to 20/40 90 days posttreatment but was 20/800 2 years after surgery. Although there was limited functional improvement, it should be noted that four out of six patients had a baseline BCVA <20/6400 and foveal atrophy, a scenario in which an increase in BCVA is not to be expected. A long-term follow-up to assess safety will be performed up to 15 years after treatment.

2.3 *CERKL*

CERKL encodes ceramide kinase-like protein, which has many isoforms due to extensive alternative splicing and multiple translational start sites [65]. Although the pathophysiology of this protein has yet to be fully elucidated, it has been shown that overexpression of *CERKL* protects cells from oxidative stress-induced apoptosis [66]. Biallelic pathogenic variants in *CERKL* have been associated with isolated MD, CORD, and RCD or RP26 (OMIM #608380), the latter representing a major cause of AR RP in the Spanish [67], Finnish [68], and Yemenite Jewish [69] populations.

However, unlike the majority of other IRDs, in *CERKL*-retinopathy the boundaries between these categories are not clearly cut. Many patients have a similar degree of rod and cone dysfunction on ERG, and even those with an electrophysiological pattern of RCD or CORD present overlapping features, an early drop in BCVA with

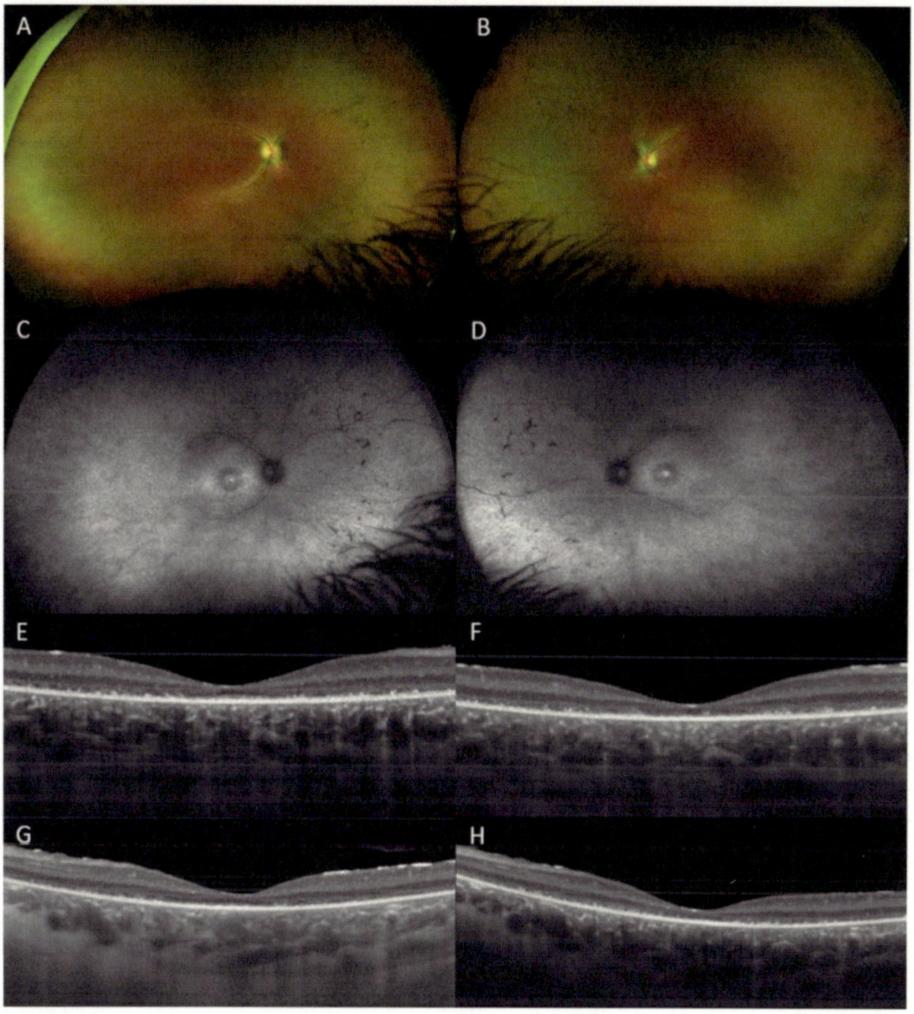

Figure 6.
Multimodal imaging of a 13-year-old female with two variants in MERTK. Although the macular abnormalities are not evident on pseudocolor fundus photos (A, B), FAF (C, D) shows foveal hyperautofluorescence, which is a common finding in MERTK-retinopathy. OCT (E-H) shows rapid progression over time: Compared to baseline scans (E and G), acquired when patient was 11 years old, the 2-year follow-up imaging (F and H) reveals loss of the small subfoveal island of preserved EZ, corresponding to a significant decrease in BCVA (from 20/30 OD and 20/40 OS to 20/300 OD and 20/100 OS). FAF = fundus autofluorescence; OCT = optical coherence tomography; EZ = ellipsoid zone.

central scotomas in patients functionally classified as RCD, as well as nyctalopia and progressive constriction of visual field in those with a diagnosis of CORD [70]. Although the rate of BCVA decline is extremely variable, this was found to be higher than other genotypes and especially faster in the 25–40 age group, suggesting preserved BCVA until the third decade of life, followed by a more rapid decline [70]. Indeed, a common finding in early stages is the presence of foveal atrophy with sparing of a small central island and a relatively retained BCVA, which severely diminishes once the atrophy encompasses the foveola in more advanced disease (**Figure** 7) [68, 70, 71].

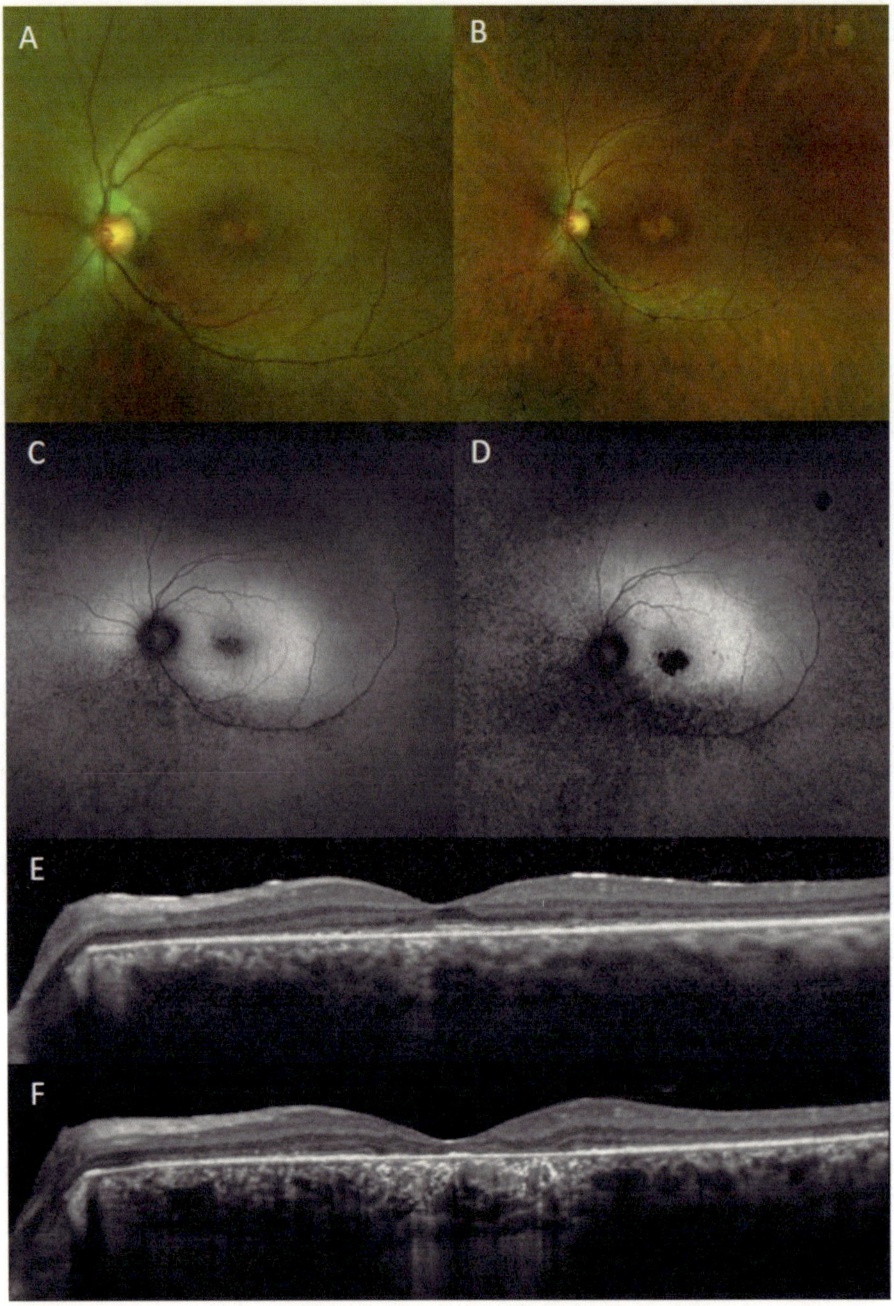

Figure 7.
Multimodal imaging of a male harboring two variants in CERKL with a 6-year follow-up. Only OS is shown. OD had similar findings. At baseline (A, C, E), patient was 32 years old and displayed mild RPE mottling on pseudocolor fundus photos (A), while FAF (C) showed diffuse hyperautofluorescence around the fovea and speckled hypoautofluorescent changes in the midperiphery. OCT (E) revealed a relatively large area of EZ sparing. At this time, BCVA in OS was 20/20. Six years later (B, D, F), imaging shows a dramatic progression of the disease. Foveal atrophy is now evident on fundus photo (B), corresponding to a dense hypoautofluorescent lesion on FAF (D), which also shows tiny midperipheral hyperautofluorescent dots. OCT displays severe subfoveal outer retinal atrophy, with no detectable EZ (F). Functionally, these anatomic changes corresponded to a drop in BCVA OS from 20/20 to 20/100. FAF = fundus autofluorescence; OCT = optical coherence tomography; EZ = ellipsoid zone; BCVA = best-corrected visual acuity.

Other typical retinal changes include peripheral punched-out areas of chorioretinal atrophy with little to no pigment deposits and fine macular dots, which are hyperautofluorescent on blue autofluorescence (BAF) [70]. The FAF pattern suggests that these lesions are at least partially composed by lipofuscin-like material and that they may correspond to photoreceptor debris resultant from impaired RPE phagocytosis, similar to what is observed in *MERTK*-retinopathy [70]. These findings can help distinguish between *CERKL*-retinopathy and *ABCA4*-retinopathy, the latter being one of the most common initial diagnoses for macula-involving IRDs before genetic testing is performed [68, 70]. Given the link between *CERKL* and oxidative stress, antioxidants—which are generally recommended to all IRD patients—might be particularly beneficial in these cases. On the other hand, although presenting with a relatively favorable window of opportunity, gene therapy is hampered by the size of the cDNA, which would not fit into a regular AAV vector and will require more complex editing strategies. Recently, a new *Cerkl* mouse model was generated to provide insights into the molecular pathways downstream of this gene and to help design effective treatments [72].

2.4 *PROM1*

PROM1 encodes prominin-1, a 5-transmembrane domain glycoprotein [73], which is expressed ubiquitously in plasma membrane protrusions. Seven alternative splice variants have been reported [74], two of which are highly expressed in the retina [75]. In photoreceptors, prominin-1 localizes at the base of rod and cone OS, where it is involved in disc membrane morphogenesis [74], and subsequent photopigment sorting [76]. More recently, *PROM1* has also been associated with the regulation of photoreceptor autophagy in RPE cells [77]. It has also been shown that *PROM1* is required for the maintenance of physiological levels of ABCA4 and RDH12 [78], which is consistent with the assumption that this gene is also involved in the regulation of the visual cycle, and that it may play a role on lipofuscin accumulation indirectly through *ABCA4* dysfunction [79].

PROM1-retinopathy encompasses a broad spectrum of phenotypes, including MD, cone dystrophy (COD), CORD, and, more rarely, RCD and LCA [80–87]. This preferential cone involvement can be explained by the fact that cone opsins are more prone to mislocalization than rhodopsin [88] together with the wider distribution of prominin-1 in the cone OS [73, 89].

Regardless of the pattern of dysfunction on electrophysiological testing, *PROM1*-retinopathy is generally characterized by macular degeneration, which tends to be mild and isolated (i.e., normal ERG) in dominant forms, or severe with associated with panretinal involvement (manifesting as COD, CORD or RCD) in recessive forms [80, 81]. Other genotype-phenotype correlations, for example, with the type of variant, have proven less meaningful since similar phenotypes have been observed in patients with homozygous missense and splice variants compared with age-matched patients with truncating variants [80].

The vast majority of RP cases caused by pathogenic variants in *PROM1* is AR [81, 84, 90], although AD inheritance has also been reported [81, 87]. AR *PROM1*-related RP is often difficult to distinguish from CORD because of the severely reduced photopic responses on ERG, the virtually constant macular involvement, and the possible absence of the typical ophthalmoscopic features (optic disc pallor, attenuated retinal vessels, peripheral bone spicules) [84]. Data on AD forms is scant in the literature (**Figure 8**). The largest series of AD *PROM1*-related RP describes the phenotype

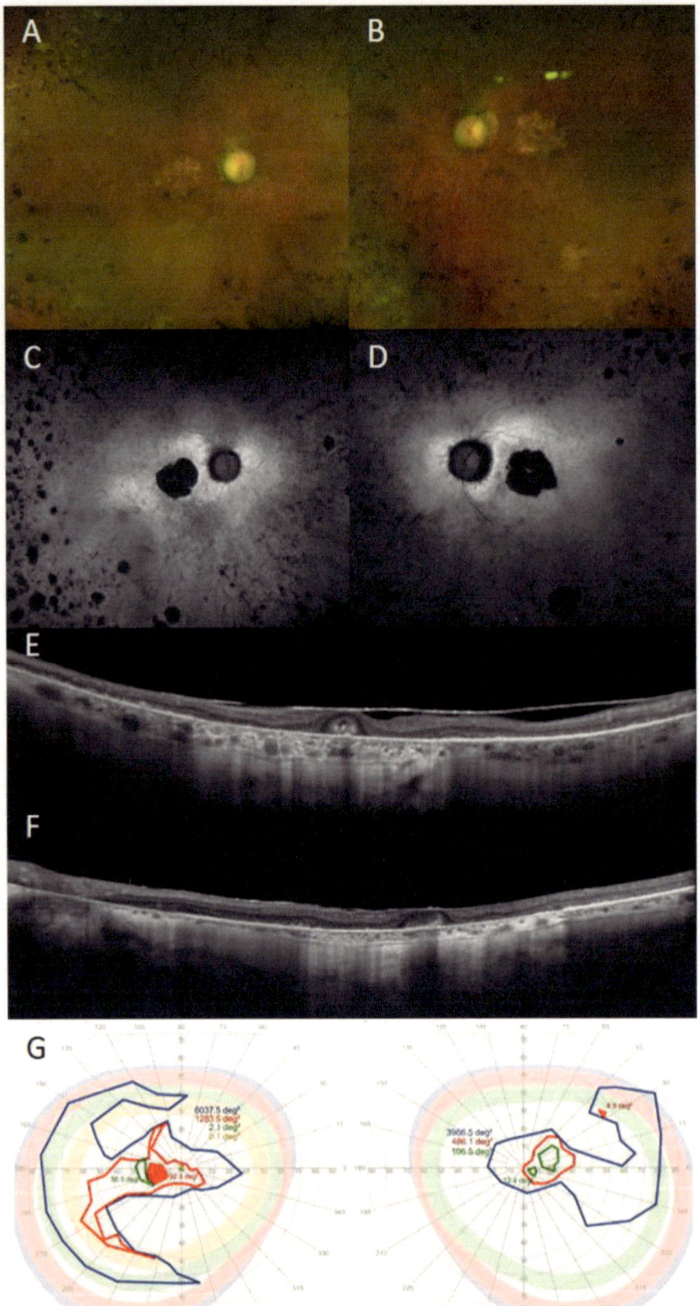

Figure 8.
Multimodal imaging and psychophysical assessment of a 60-year-old female heterozygous for a pathogenic variant in PROM1. Pseudocolor fundus photos (A, B) show a large area of central atrophy, with sparing of a tiny foveal island, as better highlighted on FAF (C, D). OCT scans show an ERM (more prominent OD) and a severe loss of outer retinal layers, with a more preserved subfoveal region. On KVF (G), all isopters are constricted, and patient was not able to detect targets smaller than III4e (red line) centrally OD, while I4e (green) and I3e (yellow) could still be seen OS in a small central area of 2.1 deg2 and 0.7 deg2, respectively, likely due to the larger preserved foveal island. Patient had a BCVA of 20/200 OD and 20/50 OS. FAF = fundus autofluorescence; OCT = optical coherence tomography; ERM = epiretinal membrane; KVF = kinetic visual field; BCVA = best-corrected visual acuity.

of eight members of an Italian family harboring the R373C mutation, a variant that generally results in isolated maculopathy [83, 87]. Reduced BCVA was the most common presenting symptom, with night blindness being noticed increasingly over time, reversed from the typical sequence for RP. Moreover, all patients displayed bull's eye maculopathy (BEM) that gradually progressed into macular atrophy. A variable combination of the hallmark fundus abnormalities seen in RP was also observed [87].

Although there are no ongoing clinical trials, *PROM1* is a gene that holds potential for future development of novel treatments. *PROM1* is a small gene (2.5 kb) that mostly causes disease through recessive truncating variants, resulting in LOF or missense variants acting through a DNE [80], both mechanisms amenable to gene replacement therapy. Moreover, there is a natural occurring mouse model [91] that can further investigate *PROM1's* pathophysiology, in addition to transgenic [74] and *Prom1* knock-out models [78].

2.5 *IMPG2*

IMPG2 encodes the interphotoreceptor matrix proteoglycan-2 (IMPG2), formerly known as IPM 200 or SPACRCAN [92], which is localized in the interphotoreceptor matrix (IPM). The IPM, composed of glycoproteins and proteoglycans, fills the space between individual photoreceptors, as well as between photoreceptors and the RPE [93]. The IPM regulates multiple functions, including intercellular communication, neovascularization, cell survival, membrane turnover, photoreceptor differentiation and maintenance, retinoid transport, matrix turnover, and the precise alignment of the photoreceptors to the optical light path [92, 94]. Rods and cones synthesize IMPG2 and secrete it in the IPM [95], where it binds to polysaccharides, such as hyaluronan, and it anchors in the plasma membrane of photoreceptors, thereby fixating these cells to the retinal extracellular matrix [96]. Additionally, IMPG2 has calcium-binding potential, which suggests it plays a role in sequestering extracellular calcium released by photoreceptors in response to light [96].

Pathogenic variants in *IMPG2* are responsible for RP [97–99] and MD, the latter often displaying a vitelliform phenotype [97, 100–102]. *IMPG2*-related maculopathy is generally caused by heterozygous missense variants, with only one previous report of an adult patient who harbored a homozygous missense *IMPG2* variant with a mild MD [97]. *IMPG2*-associated RP presents as a recessive retinal dystrophy with early macular involvement (**Figure 9**). The two largest published series on *IMPG2*-related RP report some form of macular damage in the majority of patients [97, 98]. Macular abnormalities ranged from subtle RPE mottling, to a BEM, to macular chorioretinal atrophy, often with subsequent severely decreased BCVA. Longitudinal data is available for one patient, who showed progression of BEM to atrophy covering the entire fovea [98]. In most patients, the onset of the disease is either during childhood or during the early teens [97–99]. Of note, a recent publication showed that all [3] tested heterozygotes from families with AR *IMPG2*-related RP showed carrier signs in the form of macular focal thickening detected by OCT [99].

Despite the current lack of trials, preclinical research is being conducted on retinal organoids (ROs) generated from patient-derived induced pluripotent stem cells (iPSCs) and gene-edited embryonic stem cells to model human *IMPG2*-RP *in vitro* [103]. All ROs harboring *IMPG2* mutations exhibited lacked an OS layers, in contrast to isogenic control, providing a model for advanced RP and a robust platform to study *IMPG2*-retinopathy [103].

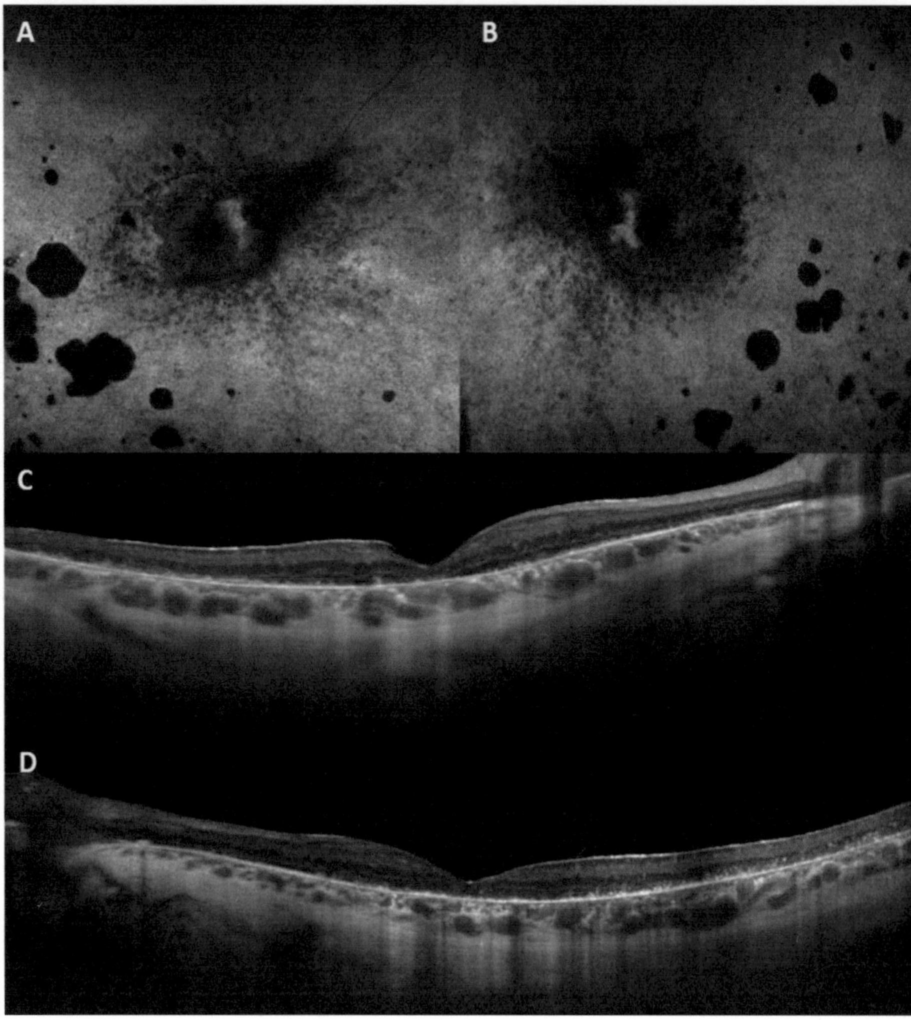

Figure 9.
Multimodal imaging of a 49-year-old male with two pathogenic variants in the IMPG2 gene. FAF (A, B) shows dense central hypoautofluorescence surrounded by mottled hyperautofluorescence, as well as large nummular areas of hypoautofluorescence in the mid and far periphery. OCT (C, D) displays in both eyes and ERM and severe thinning of outer retinal structures, including foveal loss of EZ line. BCVA is 20/1000 OD and 20/150 OS. FAF = fundus autofluorescence; OCT = optical coherence tomography; EZ = ellipsoid zone; BCVA = best-corrected visual acuity.

3. Conclusions

In conclusion, we provided a thorough description of RP genotypes associated with severe phenotypes characterized by childhood-onset and early macular involvement. These subtypes of RP are rare, difficult to manage, and challenging to treat; therefore, biotechnology and pharmaceutical companies are often unwilling to invest in research on them. In this chapter, we summarized the features, expected course, and recent preclinical or clinical studies addressing these orphan diseases and discussed relevant prognostic and therapeutic implications.

Author details

Alessia Amato*, Nida Wongchaisuwat, Andrew Lamborn, Lesley Everett, Paul Yang and Mark E. Pennesi
Department of Ophthalmic Genetics, Casey Eye Institute, Oregon Health and Science University, Portland, OR, USA

*Address all correspondence to: alessia.amato1894@gmail.com

References

[1] Hamel C. Retinitis pigmentosa. Orphanet Journal of Rare Diseases. 2006;**1**:40

[2] Verbakel SK, van Huet RAC, Boon CJF, den Hollander AI, Collin RWJ, Klaver CCW, et al. Non-syndromic retinitis pigmentosa. Progress in Retinal and Eye Research. 2018;**66**:157-186

[3] Ferrari S, Di Iorio E, Barbaro V, Ponzin D, Sorrentino FS, Parmeggiani F. Retinitis pigmentosa: Genes and disease mechanisms. Current Genomics. 2011;**12**(4):238-249

[4] Branham K, Othman M, Brumm M, Karoukis AJ, Atmaca-Sonmez P, Yashar BM, et al. Mutations in RPGR and RP2 account for 15% of males with simplex retinal degenerative disease. Investigative Ophthalmology & Visual Science. 2012;**53**(13):8232-8237

[5] Chandra B, Tung ML, Hsu Y, Scheetz T, Sheffield VC. Retinal ciliopathies through the lens of Bardet-Biedl syndrome: Past, present and future. Progress in Retinal and Eye Research. 2022;**89**:101035

[6] Wallmeier J, Nielsen KG, Kuehni CE, Lucas JS, Leigh MW, Zariwala MA, et al. Motile ciliopathies. Nature Reviews. Disease Primers. 2020;**6**(1):77

[7] Fliegauf M, Benzing T, Omran H. When cilia go bad: Cilia defects and ciliopathies. Nature Reviews. Molecular Cell Biology. 2007;**8**(11):880-893

[8] Mykytyn K, Sheffield VC. Establishing a connection between cilia and Bardet-Biedl syndrome. Trends in Molecular Medicine. 2004;**10**(3):106-109

[9] Pazour GJ, Baker SA, Deane JA, Cole DG, Dickert BL, Rosenbaum JL, et al. The intraflagellar transport protein, IFT88, is essential for vertebrate photoreceptor assembly and maintenance. The Journal of Cell Biology. 2002;**157**(1):103-113

[10] Wolfrum U, Schmitt A. Rhodopsin transport in the membrane of the connecting cilium of mammalian photoreceptor cells. Cell Motility and the Cytoskeleton. 2000;**46**(2):95-107

[11] Stone EM, Luo X, Heon E, Lam BL, Weleber RG, Halder JA, et al. Autosomal recessive retinitis pigmentosa caused by mutations in the MAK gene. Investigative Ophthalmology & Visual Science. 2011;**52**(13):9665-9673

[12] Bocquet B, Marzouka NA, Hebrard M, Manes G, Senechal A, Meunier I, et al. Homozygosity mapping in autosomal recessive retinitis pigmentosa families detects novel mutations. Molecular Vision. 2013;**19**:2487-2500

[13] Takahashi VKL, Xu CL, Takiuti JT, Apatoff MBL, Duong JK, Mahajan VB, et al. Comparison of structural progression between ciliopathy and non-ciliopathy associated with autosomal recessive retinitis pigmentosa. Orphanet Journal of Rare Diseases. 2019;**14**(1):187

[14] He S, Parapuram SK, Hurd TW, Behnam B, Margolis B, Swaroop A, et al. Retinitis Pigmentosa GTPase regulator (RPGR) protein isoforms in mammalian retina: Insights into X-linked retinitis Pigmentosa and associated ciliopathies. Vision Research. 2008;**48**(3):366-376

[15] Hong DH, Li T. Complex expression pattern of RPGR reveals a role for

purine-rich exonic splicing enhancers. Investigative Ophthalmology & Visual Science. 2002;**43**(11):3373-3382

[16] Vervoort R, Lennon A, Bird AC, Tulloch B, Axton R, Miano MG, et al. Mutational hot spot within a new RPGR exon in X-linked retinitis pigmentosa. Nature Genetics. 2000;**25**(4):462-466

[17] Sharon D, Sandberg MA, Rabe VW, Stillberger M, Dryja TP, Berson EL. RP2 and RPGR mutations and clinical correlations in patients with X-linked retinitis pigmentosa. American Journal of Human Genetics. 2003;**73**(5):1131-1146

[18] Talib M, van Schooneveld MJ, Thiadens AA, Fiocco M, Wijnholds J, Florijn RJ, et al. Clinical and genetic characteristics of male patients with rpgr-associated retinal dystrophies: A long-term follow-up study. Retina. 2019;**39**(6):1186-1199

[19] Fahim AT, Bowne SJ, Sullivan LS, Webb KD, Williams JT, Wheaton DK, et al. Allelic heterogeneity and genetic modifier loci contribute to clinical variation in males with X-linked retinitis pigmentosa due to RPGR mutations. PLoS One. 2011;**6**(8):e23021

[20] Yang L, Yin X, Feng L, You D, Wu L, Chen N, et al. Novel mutations of RPGR in Chinese retinitis pigmentosa patients and the genotype-phenotype correlation. PLoS One. 2014;**9**(1):e85752

[21] Di Iorio V, Karali M, Melillo P, Testa F, Brunetti-Pierri R, Musacchia F, et al. Spectrum of disease severity in patients with X-linked retinitis pigmentosa due to RPGR mutations. Investigative Ophthalmology & Visual Science. 2020;**61**(14):36

[22] Andréasson S, Breuer DK, Eksandh L, Ponjavic V, Frennesson C, Hiriyanna S, et al. Clinical studies of X-linked retinitis pigmentosa in three Swedish families with newly identified mutations in the RP2 and RPGR-ORF15 genes. Ophthalmic Genetics. 2003;**24**(4):215-223

[23] Sandberg MA, Rosner B, Weigel-DiFranco C, Dryja TP, Berson EL. Disease course of patients with X-linked retinitis pigmentosa due to RPGR gene mutations. Investigative Ophthalmology & Visual Science. 2007;**48**(3):1298-1304

[24] Demirci FY, Rigatti BW, Wen G, Radak AL, Mah TS, Baic CL, et al. X-linked cone-rod dystrophy (locus COD1): Identification of mutations in RPGR exon ORF15. American Journal of Human Genetics. 2002;**70**(4):1049-1053

[25] Nanda A, Salvetti AP, Clouston P, Downes SM, MacLaren RE. Exploring the variable phenotypes of RPGR carrier females in assessing their potential for retinal gene therapy. Genes (Basel). 2018;**9**(12)

[26] Kousal B, Skalicka P, Valesova L, Fletcher T, Hart-Holden N, O'Grady A, et al. Severe retinal degeneration in women with a c.2543del mutation in ORF15 of the RPGR gene. Molecular Vision. 2014;**20**:1307-1317

[27] Wegscheider E, Preising MN, Lorenz B. Fundus autofluorescence in carriers of X-linked recessive retinitis pigmentosa associated with mutations in RPGR, and correlation with electrophysiological and psychophysical data. Graefe's Archive for Clinical and Experimental Ophthalmology. 2004;**242**(6):501-511

[28] Acton JH, Greenberg JP, Greenstein VC, Marsiglia M, Tabacaru M, Theodore Smith R, et al. Evaluation of multimodal imaging in carriers of X-linked retinitis pigmentosa. Experimental Eye Research. 2013;**113**:41-48

[29] Cehajic, Kapetanovic J, McClements ME, Martinez-Fernandez de la Camara C, MacLaren RE. Molecular strategies for RPGR gene therapy. Genes (Basel). 2019;**10**(9)

[30] Liu Q, Zuo J, Pierce EA. The retinitis pigmentosa 1 protein is a photoreceptor microtubule-associated protein. The Journal of Neuroscience. 2004;**24**(29):6427-6436

[31] Field LL, Heckenlively JR, Sparkes RS, Garcia CA, Farson C, Zedalis D, et al. Linkage analysis of five pedigrees affected with typical autosomal dominant retinitis pigmentosa. Journal of Medical Genetics. 1982;**19**(4):266-270

[32] Blanton SH, Heckenlively JR, Cottingham AW, Friedman J, Sadler LA, Wagner M, et al. Linkage mapping of autosomal dominant retinitis pigmentosa (RP1) to the pericentric region of human chromosome 8. Genomics. 1991;**11**(4):857-869

[33] Audo I, Mohand-Said S, Dhaenens CM, Germain A, Orhan E, Antonio A, et al. RP1 and autosomal dominant rod-cone dystrophy: Novel mutations, a review of published variants, and genotype-phenotype correlation. Human Mutation. 2012;**33**(1):73-80

[34] Khaliq S, Abid A, Ismail M, Hameed A, Mohyuddin A, Lall P, et al. Novel association of RP1 gene mutations with autosomal recessive retinitis pigmentosa. Journal of Medical Genetics. 2005;**42**(5):436-438

[35] Riazuddin SA, Zulfiqar F, Zhang Q, Sergeev YV, Qazi ZA, Husnain T, et al. Autosomal recessive retinitis pigmentosa is associated with mutations in RP1 in three consanguineous Pakistani families. Investigative Ophthalmology & Visual Science. 2005;**46**(7):2264-2270

[36] Singh HP, Jalali S, Narayanan R, Kannabiran C. Genetic analysis of Indian families with autosomal recessive retinitis pigmentosa by homozygosity screening. Investigative Ophthalmology & Visual Science. 2009;**50**(9):4065-4071

[37] El Shamieh S, Boulanger-Scemama E, Lancelot ME, Antonio A, Demontant V, Condroyer C, et al. Targeted next generation sequencing identifies novel mutations in RP1 as a relatively common cause of autosomal recessive rod-cone dystrophy. BioMed Research International. 2015;**2015**:485624

[38] Berson EL, Grimsby JL, Adams SM, McGee TL, Sweklo E, Pierce EA, et al. Clinical features and mutations in patients with dominant retinitis pigmentosa-1 (RP1). Investigative Ophthalmology & Visual Science. 2001;**42**(10):2217-2224

[39] Chen LJ, Lai TY, Tam PO, Chiang SW, Zhang X, Lam S, et al. Compound heterozygosity of two novel truncation mutations in RP1 causing autosomal recessive retinitis pigmentosa. Investigative Ophthalmology & Visual Science. 2010;**51**(4):2236-2242

[40] Brogna S, Wen J. Nonsense-mediated mRNA decay (NMD) mechanisms. Nature Structural & Molecular Biology. 2009;**16**(2):107-113

[41] Liu Q SA, Hu J, Cao H, Auricchio A, Pierce EA. The degeneration of photoreceptor cells in the rp1 form of retinitis pigmentosa is caused by a dominant mechanism. Investigative Ophthalmology & Visual Science, ARVO abstract. 2009;**50**:2285

[42] Won J, Shi LY, Hicks W, Wang J, Hurd R, Naggert JK, et al. Mouse model resources for vision research. Journal of Ophthalmology. 2011;**2011**:391384

[43] Collin C, Liu Q. CRISPR/Cas9-based genome editing approaches for RP1 associated autosomal dominant retinitis Pigmentosa. In: ARVO Annual Meeting Abstract. Virtual; 2021

[44] Zufiaurre-Seijo M, Garcia-Arumi J, Duarri A. Clinical and molecular aspects of C2orf71/PCARE in retinal diseases. International Journal of Molecular Sciences. 2023;**24**(13)

[45] Audo I, Lancelot ME, Mohand-Said S, Antonio A, Germain A, Sahel JA, et al. Novel C2orf71 mutations account for approximately 1% of cases in a large French arRP cohort. Human Mutation. 2011;**32**(4):E2091-E2103

[46] Collin RW, Safieh C, Littink KW, Shalev SA, Garzozi HJ, Rizel L, et al. Mutations in C2ORF71 cause autosomal-recessive retinitis pigmentosa. American Journal of Human Genetics. 2010;**86**(5):783-788

[47] Nishimura DY, Baye LM, Perveen R, Searby CC, Avila-Fernandez A, Pereiro I, et al. Discovery and functional analysis of a retinitis pigmentosa gene, C2ORF71. American Journal of Human Genetics. 2010;**86**(5):686-695

[48] Boulanger-Scemama E, Mohand-Said S, El Shamieh S, Demontant V, Condroyer C, Antonio A, et al. Phenotype analysis of retinal dystrophies in light of the underlying genetic defects: Application to cone and cone-rod dystrophies. International Journal of Molecular Sciences. 2019;**20**(19)

[49] Serra R, Floris M, Pinna A, Boscia F, Cucca F, Angius A. Novel mutations in c2orf71 causing an early onset form of cone-rod dystrophy: A molecular diagnosis after 20 years of clinical follow-up. Molecular Vision. 2019;**25**:814-820

[50] Khateb S, Zelinger L, Mizrahi-Meissonnier L, Ayuso C, Koenekoop RK, Laxer U, et al. A homozygous nonsense CEP250 mutation combined with a heterozygous nonsense C2orf71 mutation is associated with atypical usher syndrome. Journal of Medical Genetics. 2014;**51**(7):460-469

[51] Liu YP, Bosch DG, Siemiatkowska AM, Rendtorff ND, Boonstra FN, Moller C, et al. Putative digenic inheritance of heterozygous RP1L1 and C2orf71 null mutations in syndromic retinal dystrophy. Ophthalmic Genetics. 2017;**38**(2):127-132

[52] Tiwari A, Bahr A, Bahr L, Fleischhauer J, Zinkernagel MS, Winkler N, et al. Next generation sequencing based identification of disease-associated mutations in Swiss patients with retinal dystrophies. Scientific Reports. 2016;**6**:28755

[53] Yang L, Cui H, Yin X, Dou H, Zhao L, Chen N, et al. Dependable and efficient clinical molecular diagnosis of Chinese RP patient with targeted exon sequencing. PLoS One. 2015;**10**(10):e0140684

[54] Corral-Serrano JC, Messchaert M, Dona M, Peters TA, Kamminga LM, van Wijk E, et al. C2orf71a/pcare1 is important for photoreceptor outer segment morphogenesis and visual function in zebrafish. Scientific Reports. 2018;**8**(1):9675

[55] Kevany BM, Zhang N, Jastrzebska B, Palczewski K. Animals deficient in C2Orf71, an autosomal recessive retinitis pigmentosa-associated locus, develop severe early-onset retinal degeneration. Human Molecular Genetics. 2015;**24**(9):2627-2640

[56] Feng W, Yasumura D, Matthes MT, LaVail MM, Vollrath D. Mertk triggers

uptake of photoreceptor outer segments during phagocytosis by cultured retinal pigment epithelial cells. The Journal of Biological Chemistry. 2002;**277**(19):17016-17022

[57] Audo I, Mohand-Said S, Boulanger-Scemama E, Zanlonghi X, Condroyer C, Demontant V, et al. MERTK mutation update in inherited retinal diseases. Human Mutation. 2018;**39**(7):887-913

[58] Ksantini M, Lafont E, Bocquet B, Meunier I, Hamel CP. Homozygous mutation in MERTK causes severe autosomal recessive retinitis pigmentosa. European Journal of Ophthalmology. 2012;**22**(4):647-653

[59] Mackay DS, Henderson RH, Sergouniotis PI, Li Z, Moradi P, Holder GE, et al. Novel mutations in MERTK associated with childhood onset rod-cone dystrophy. Molecular Vision. 2010;**16**:369-377

[60] Smith AJ, Schlichtenbrede FC, Tschernutter M, Bainbridge JW, Thrasher AJ, Ali RR. AAV-mediated gene transfer slows photoreceptor loss in the RCS rat model of retinitis pigmentosa. Molecular Therapy. 2003;**8**(2):188-195

[61] Tschernutter M, Schlichtenbrede FC, Howe S, Balaggan KS, Munro PM, Bainbridge JW, et al. Long-term preservation of retinal function in the RCS rat model of retinitis pigmentosa following lentivirus-mediated gene therapy. Gene Therapy. 2005;**12**(8):694-701

[62] Vollrath D, Feng W, Duncan JL, Yasumura D, D'Cruz PM, Chappelow A, et al. Correction of the retinal dystrophy phenotype of the RCS rat by viral gene transfer of Mertk. Proceedings of the National Academy of Sciences of the United States of America. 2001;**98**(22):12584-12589

[63] Ghazi NG, Abboud EB, Nowilaty SR, Alkuraya H, Alhommadi A, Cai H, et al. Treatment of retinitis pigmentosa due to MERTK mutations by ocular subretinal injection of adeno-associated virus gene vector: Results of a phase I trial. Human Genetics. 2016;**135**(3):327-343

[64] Amato A, Arrigo A, Aragona E, Manitto MP, Saladino A, Bandello F, et al. Gene therapy in inherited retinal diseases: An update on current state of the art. Frontiers in Medicine (Lausanne). 2021;**8**:750586

[65] Garanto A, Riera M, Pomares E, Permanyer J, de Castro-Miro M, Sava F, et al. High transcriptional complexity of the retinitis pigmentosa CERKL gene in human and mouse. Investigative Ophthalmology & Visual Science. 2011;**52**(8):5202-5214

[66] Garcia-Arroyo R, Gavalda-Navarro A, Villarroya F, Marfany G, Mirra S. Overexpression of CERKL protects retinal pigment epithelium mitochondria from oxidative stress effects. Antioxidants (Basel). 2021;**10**(12)

[67] Avila-Fernandez A, Riveiro-Alvarez R, Vallespin E, Wilke R, Tapias I, Cantalapiedra D, et al. CERKL mutations and associated phenotypes in seven Spanish families with autosomal recessive retinitis pigmentosa. Investigative Ophthalmology & Visual Science. 2008;**49**(6):2709-2713

[68] Avela K, Sankila EM, Seitsonen S, Kuuluvainen L, Barton S, Gillies S, et al. A founder mutation in CERKL is a major cause of retinal dystrophy in Finland. Acta Ophthalmologica. 2018;**96**(2):183-191

[69] Auslender N, Sharon D, Abbasi AH, Garzozi HJ, Banin E, Ben-Yosef T. A common founder mutation of CERKL

underlies autosomal recessive retinal degeneration with early macular involvement among Yemenite Jews. Investigative Ophthalmology & Visual Science. 2007;**48**(12):5431-5438

[70] Daich, Varela M, Duignan ES, De SilvaSR,Ba-AbbadR,Fujinami-YokokawaY, Leo S, et al. CERKL-associated retinal dystrophy: Genetics, phenotype, and natural history. Ophthalmology Retina. Oct 2023;**7**(10):918-931

[71] Downes SM, Nguyen T, Tai V, Broadgate S, Shah M, Al-Khuzaei S, et al. Genetic and clinical findings in an ethnically diverse cohort with retinitis Pigmentosa associated with pathogenic variants in CERKL. Genes (Basel). 2020;**11**(12)

[72] Domenech EB, Andres R, Lopez-IniestaMJ,MirraS,Garcia-ArroyoR, Milla S, et al. A new Cerkl mouse model generated by CRISPR-Cas9 shows progressive retinal degeneration and altered morphological and electrophysiological phenotype. Investigative Ophthalmology & Visual Science. 2020;**61**(8):14

[73] Jaszai J, Fargeas CA, Florek M, Huttner WB, Corbeil D. Focus on molecules: Prominin-1 (CD133). Experimental Eye Research. 2007;**85**(5):585-586

[74] Yang Z, Chen Y, Lillo C, Chien J, Yu Z, Michaelides M, et al. Mutant prominin 1 found in patients with macular degeneration disrupts photoreceptor disk morphogenesis in mice. The Journal of Clinical Investigation. 2008;**118**(8):2908-2916

[75] Fargeas CA, Huttner WB, Corbeil D. Nomenclature of prominin-1 (CD133) splice variants - an update. Tissue Antigens. 2007;**69**(6):602-606

[76] Zacchigna S, Oh H, Wilsch-Brauninger M, Missol-Kolka E, Jaszai J, Jansen S, et al. Loss of the cholesterol-binding protein prominin-1/CD133 causes disk dysmorphogenesis and photoreceptor degeneration. The Journal of Neuroscience. 2009;**29**(7):2297-2308

[77] Bhattacharya S, Yin J, Winborn CS, Zhang Q, Yue J, Chaum E. Prominin-1 is a novel regulator of autophagy in the human retinal pigment epithelium. Investigative Ophthalmology & Visual Science. 2017;**58**(4):2366-2387

[78] Dellett M, Sasai N, Nishide K, Becker S, Papadaki V, Limb GA, et al. Genetic background and light-dependent progression of photoreceptor cell degeneration in Prominin-1 knockout mice. Investigative Ophthalmology & Visual Science. 2014;**56**(1):164-176

[79] Gliem M, Muller PL, Birtel J, Herrmann P, McGuinness MB, Holz FG, et al. Quantitative fundus autofluorescence and genetic associations in macular, cone, and cone-rod dystrophies. Ophthalmology Retina. 2020;**4**(7):737-749

[80] Cehajic-Kapetanovic J, Birtel J, McClements ME, Shanks ME, Clouston P, Downes SM, et al. Clinical and molecular characterization of PROM1-related retinal degeneration. JAMA Network Open. 2019;**2**(6):e195752

[81] Del Pozo-Valero M, Martin-Merida I, Jimenez-Rolando B, Arteche A, Avila-Fernandez A, Blanco-Kelly F, et al. Expanded phenotypic Spectrum of retinopathies associated with autosomal recessive and dominant mutations in PROM1. American Journal of Ophthalmology. 2019;**207**:204-214

[82] Fujinami K, Oishi A, Yang L, Arno G, Pontikos N, Yoshitake K, et al. Clinical and genetic characteristics of 10 Japanese

patients with PROM1-associated retinal disorder: A report of the phenotype spectrum and a literature review in the Japanese population. American Journal of Medical Genetics. Part C, Seminars in Medical Genetics. 2020;**184**(3):656-674

[83] Lee IJ, Abbey C, Leys M. Clinical characterization of autosomal dominant and autosomal recessive PROM1 mutation with a report of novel mutation. Ophthalmic Surgery, Lasers & Imaging Retina. 2022;**53**(8):422-428

[84] Liang J, She X, Chen J, Zhai Y, Liu Y, Zheng K, et al. Identification of novel PROM1 mutations responsible for autosomal recessive maculopathy with rod-cone dystrophy. Graefe's Archive for Clinical and Experimental Ophthalmology. 2019;**257**(3):619-628

[85] Schließleder G, Kalitzeos A, Kasilian M, et al. Deep phenotyping of PROM1-associated retinal degeneration. British Journal of Ophthalmology. 20 Apr 2023. DOI: 10.1136/bjo-2022-322036

[86] Ragi SD, Lima de Carvalho JR Jr, Tanaka AJ, Park KS, Mahajan VB, Maumenee IH, et al. Compound heterozygous novel frameshift variants in the PROM1 gene result in Leber congenital amaurosis. Cold Spring Harbor Molecular Case Studies. 2019;**5**(6)

[87] Michaelides M, Gaillard MC, Escher P, Tiab L, Bedell M, Borruat FX, et al. The PROM1 mutation p.R373C causes an autosomal dominant bull's eye maculopathy associated with rod, rod-cone, and macular dystrophy. Investigative Ophthalmology & Visual Science. 2010;**51**(9):4771-4780

[88] Zhang T, Zhang N, Baehr W, Fu Y. Cone opsin determines the time course of cone photoreceptor degeneration in Leber congenital amaurosis. Proceedings of the National Academy of Sciences of the United States of America. 2011;**108**(21):8879-8884

[89] Han Z, Anderson DW, Papermaster DS. Prominin-1 localizes to the open rims of outer segment lamellae in Xenopus laevis rod and cone photoreceptors. Investigative Ophthalmology & Visual Science. 2012;**53**(1):361-373

[90] Permanyer J, Navarro R, Friedman J, Pomares E, Castro-Navarro J, Marfany G, et al. Autosomal recessive retinitis pigmentosa with early macular affectation caused by premature truncation in PROM1. Investigative Ophthalmology & Visual Science. 2010;**51**(5):2656-2663

[91] Piotter E, McClements ME, MacLaren RE. Therapy approaches for Stargardt disease. Biomolecules. 2021;**11**:8

[92] Inatani M, Tanihara H. Proteoglycans in retina. Progress in Retinal and Eye Research. 2002;**21**(5):429-447

[93] Adler AJ, Klucznik KM. Proteins and glycoproteins of the bovine interphotoreceptor matrix: Composition and fractionation. Experimental Eye Research. 1982;**34**(3):423-434

[94] Enoch JM, Laties AM. An analysis of retinal receptor orientation. II. Predictions for psychophysical tests. Investigative Ophthalmology. 1971;**10**(12):959-970

[95] Acharya S, Foletta VC, Lee JW, Rayborn ME, Rodriguez IR, Young WS 3rd, et al. SPACRCAN, a novel human interphotoreceptor matrix hyaluronan-binding proteoglycan synthesized by photoreceptors and pinealocytes. The Journal of Biological Chemistry. 2000;**275**(10):6945-6955

[96] Chen Q, Cai S, Shadrach KG, Prestwich GD, Hollyfield JG. Spacrcan binding to hyaluronan and other glycosaminoglycans. Molecular and biochemical studies. The Journal of Biological Chemistry. 2004;**279**(22):23142-23150

[97] Bandah-Rozenfeld D, Collin RW, Banin E, van den Born LI, Coene KL, Siemiatkowska AM, et al. Mutations in IMPG2, encoding interphotoreceptor matrix proteoglycan 2, cause autosomal-recessive retinitis pigmentosa. American Journal of Human Genetics. 2010;**87**(2):199-208

[98] van Huet RA, Collin RW, Siemiatkowska AM, Klaver CC, Hoyng CB, Simonelli F, et al. IMPG2-associated retinitis pigmentosa displays relatively early macular involvement. Investigative Ophthalmology & Visual Science. 2014;**55**(6):3939-3953

[99] Khan AO, Al Teneiji AM. Homozygous and heterozygous retinal phenotypes in families harbouring IMPG2 mutations. Ophthalmic Genetics. 2019;**40**(3):247-251

[100] Brandl C, Schulz HL, Charbel Issa P, Birtel J, Bergholz R, Lange C, et al. Mutations in the genes for Interphotoreceptor matrix proteoglycans, IMPG1 and IMPG2, in patients with Vitelliform macular lesions. Genes (Basel). 2017;**8**(7)

[101] Meunier I, Manes G, Bocquet B, Marquette V, Baudoin C, Puech B, et al. Frequency and clinical pattern of vitelliform macular dystrophy caused by mutations of interphotoreceptor matrix IMPG1 and IMPG2 genes. Ophthalmology. 2014;**121**(12):2406-2414

[102] Vazquez-Dominguez I, Li CHZ, Fadaie Z, Haer-Wigman L, Cremers FPM, Garanto A, et al. Identification of a complex allele in IMPG2 as a cause of adult-onset Vitelliform macular dystrophy. Investigative Ophthalmology & Visual Science. 2022;**63**(5):27

[103] Mayerl SJ, Bajgai S, Ludwig AL, Jager LD, Williams BN, Bacig C, et al. Human retinal organoids harboring IMPG2 mutations exhibit a photoreceptor outer segment phenotype that models advanced retinitis pigmentosa. Stem Cell Reports. 2022;**17**(11):2409-2420

Chapter 5

Macular Imaging

Ogugua Ndubuisi Okonkwo, Chineze Thelma Agweye, Toyin Akanbi and Utam Ashibel Utam

Abstract

Since its inception, retinal imaging has been vital in documenting and understanding macular diseases. The early thinking was to document retinal pathology as it became possible to visualize the retina using an ophthalmoscope. This reasoning quickly evolved into the need to monitor disease evolution and treatment changes using digital images. With further rapid advancement in imaging technology, it has become possible to visualize and image at a subcellular level, the macula, in health and disease. Technological advances have resulted in the scanning laser ophthalmoscope, optical coherence tomography, and adaptive optics incorporation into imaging. The "dye" and "non-dye" based evaluation of retinal vasculature has improved our understanding of various macula and retinovascular diseases. The fundus photograph and optical coherence tomography are the most utilized technologies for imaging the macula. With an expected increase in diabetic retinopathy and macular degeneration patients, more macular imaging will be done in years to come. Consequently, more macula image data will be available for data analysis using artificial intelligence, improving our predictive ability and personalization. Therefore, macular imaging will assume increasing significance and imaging techniques for the macula should be known and understood. This chapter provides an exhaustive list of common and less-known imaging techniques for macular imaging and an overview of their use in evaluating the macula in clinical practice and research.

Keywords: macula, macular imaging, color fundus photography, optical coherence tomography, optical coherence tomography angiography, scan laser ophthalmoscopy, adaptive optics, multimodal imaging, artificial intelligence

1. Introduction

Retina and macula imaging have come a long way. From the early years after the invention of the ophthalmoscope in 1850, through the introduction of the slit-lamp biomicroscope in 1921, combined with the use of Leonhard Koeppe's contact lens affording the stereoscopic examination of the vitreous and retina with X40 magnification, several outstanding contributions have been made by clinicians and scientist [1, 2]. This effort is driven by a desire to see more, understand the retina's anatomy and physiology, and document the disease's evolution. After ophthalmoscopy, the first photograph of the animal eye was in 1886. The first clinical use of the fundus camera was born by a collaboration between Swedish Dr. Johan Wilhelm Nordenson and the German Zeiss company. This collaboration led to the Zeiss-Nordenson camera, which became the prototype for subsequent retinal cameras [3, 4].

Since the introduction of the early retina camera, digitizing images in the 1980s, and incorporating cutting-edge technologies, including improvements in lighting (such as monochromatic light), vital stains, fluorescent dyes, filters, image resolution, have significantly improved retina and macular imaging [2, 5]. The introduction of these technologies has made retinal imaging invaluable in the clinical assessment of diverse retina and macula pathologies, understanding and documentation of retinal pathoanatomy and physiology, teaching, and research. Advances in macular imaging in the past two decades have been phenomenal. Macular imaging has witnessed the development of high-impact and high-resolution imaging, including optical coherence tomography (OCT). Because of the development of OCT into faster scanning speed equipment, OCT Angiography (OCTA) has become a reality. OCTA will evolve into wide-field imaging with a further increase in scanning speed. More recently, analytics of retinal imaging have become faster and more dynamic, resulting in the ability to prognosticate. Artificial intelligence (AI) incorporation into image analytics means more robust data reviews utilizing large amounts of image data, which can show trends, prognosticate outcomes, and guide management. Personalization of patient care is the ultimate goal of image analytics. This review focuses on macular imaging, intending to provide a comprehensive, updated review of the technology used for imaging macular diseases, including commonly encountered diseases like age-related macular degeneration (AMD), diabetic macular edema (DME), retinal vein occlusion (RVO), central serous chorioretinopathy (CSCR), polypoidal choroidal vasculopathy (PCV), and disorders characterized by macular ischemia and others. OCT and OCTA feature prominently, including their biomarkers, which have become a focus of AI analytics. Functional imaging of the macula and less-known imaging modalities, including macula pigment optical density (MPOD), photoacoustic microscopy (PAM), and fluorescence lifetime imaging ophthalmoscopy (FLIO), are also discussed in this chapter.

2. Color fundus photography

Fundus images obtained by fundus cameras date to the late nineteenth century, and modern fundus photographs were reported by Friedrich Dimmer in the early twentieth century [6]. Dimmer is credited with the first reflex-free photographs of the fundus in 1905. The quality of fundus images and the ease of photography have significantly improved over the years, producing digitized images with computer-based storage. Fundus imaging generates a two-dimensional image of the interior three-dimensional surface of the eye. Fundus imaging uses a specialized low-power microscope and an attached camera [7].

Standard fundus photography provides a 30- to 50-degree image that includes the macula and peripheral retina. Ultrawide field (UWF) imaging can produce a 200-degree retinal view extending beyond the macula to the peripheral retina [8]. In some cases, evaluation of the retina periphery through retina imaging can have significant implications for macular diseases, such as the clinical scenario of persistent or recurrent diabetic macular edema. UWF imaging using fluorescein dye evaluation could reveal peripheral nonperfusion as the cause of lingering macular edema. The retina examination is done in full color with white light illumination. The white light can be filtered, removing the red component, and in this way, a red-free image can be created. This red-free image results in improved contrast of retinal and choroidal blood vessels [9].

Fundus photography helps diagnose and monitor macular diseases, for example, AMD, polypoidal choroidal vasculopathy, and diabetic maculopathy; it is also helpful in educating and counseling patients [10]. There are some disadvantages, including the image created being in 2D, lack of depth, visualizing small details may be problematic, and abnormalities in the refractive media, such as cataracts, resulting in lower image clarity [11]. **Figures 1** and **2** illustrate the resolution of subretinal

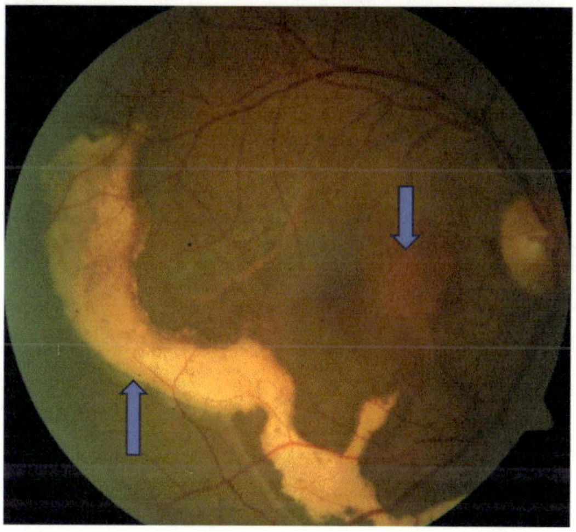

Figure 1.
Right eye fundus photograph showing temporal macular subretinal exudates and reddish-orange polypoidal lesion nasal to the fovea in an eye diagnosed with polypoidal choroidal vasculopathy.

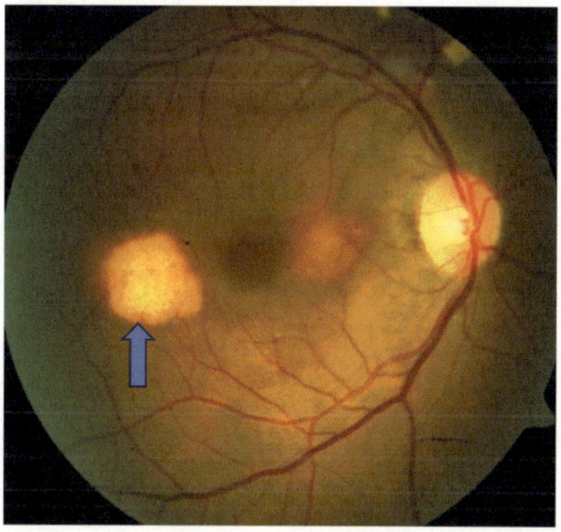

Figure 2.
*Same eye as in **Figure 1**, after treatment with six doses of intravitreal Aflibercept. Showing marked resolution of subretinal exudates (blue arrow), but persistent reddish-orange polyp. Fundus photographs can be used to monitor the response to treatment of exudative maculopathy from retinal diseases that respond to medical therapy.*

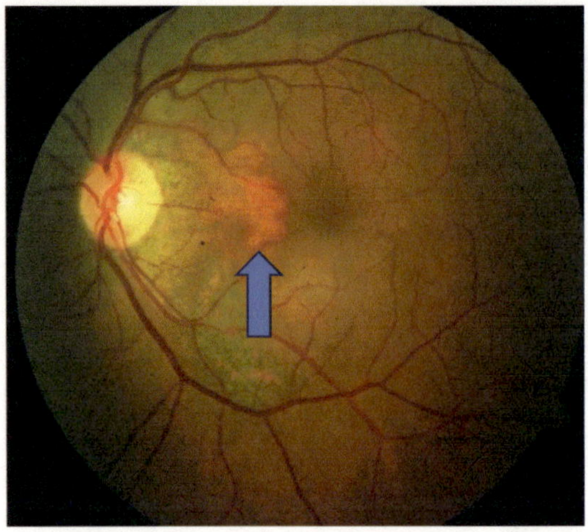

Figure 3.
The fellow left eye of the image in ***Figures 1*** *and* ***2****, shows a similar reddish-orange polyp (blue arrow) nasal to the fovea and an adjoining area of chorioretinal atrophy along the inferonasal arcade.*

exudates after intravitreal injection of anti-vascular endothelial growth factors in a PCV right eye. The fellow eye (**Figure 3**) shows a similar reddish-orange subretinal PCV lesion.

Drusen often changes in size and number over time; computer image analysis of fundus photographs is used to measure the drusen area and monitor the changes in drusen pattern over time [12]. The fundus photograph helps monitor changes in the degree of a disease over time or in response to therapy. Progression of clinical retina

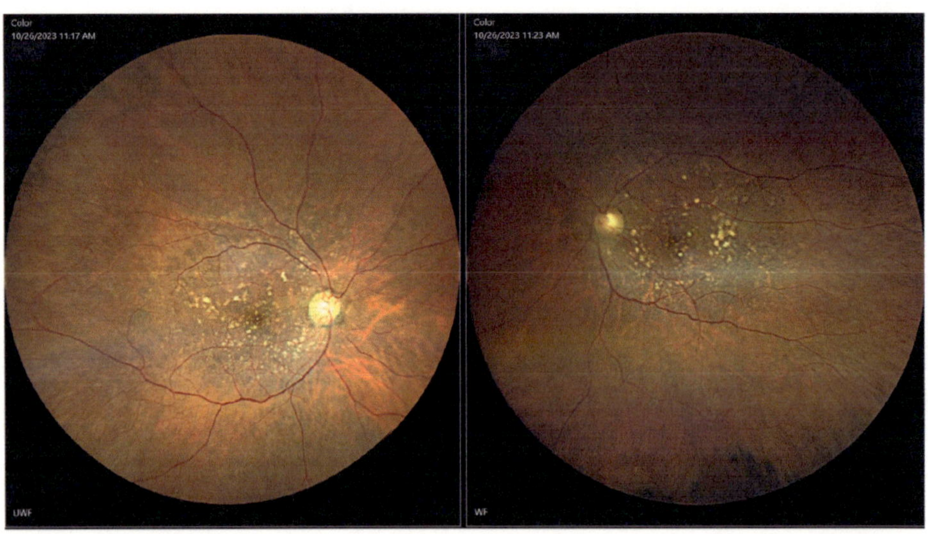

Figure 4.
The right and left fundus images of an 81-year-old female, with characteristic discrete yellowish flecks in the macula, which are macular drusen deposits.

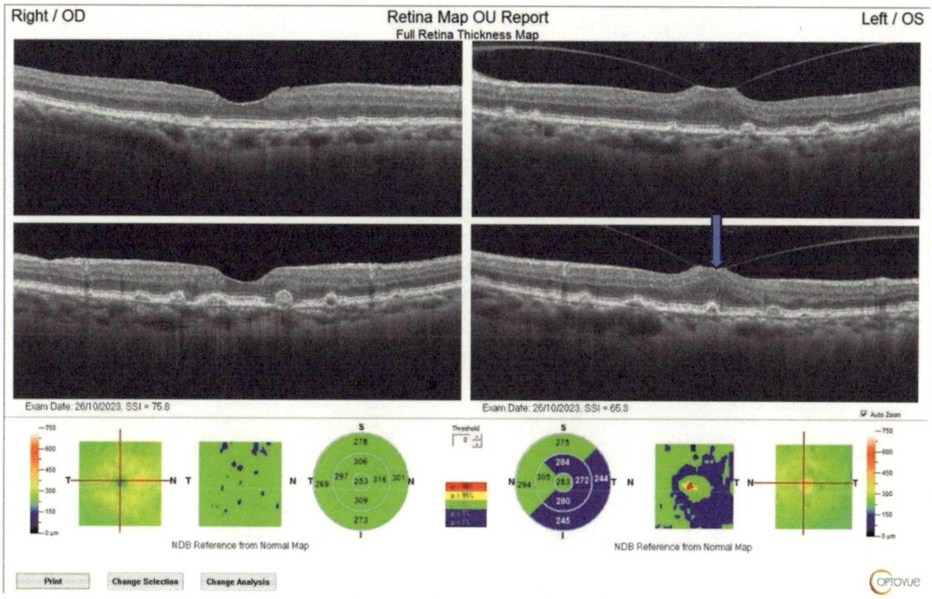

Figure 5.
Optical coherence tomography images of the same patient in ***Figure 4****. Note the appearance of the outer retina irregularity and pigment epithelial detachment characteristic of drusenoid deposits. There is a presence of vitreomacular traction in the left eye (blue arrow).*

findings can be easily determined. **Figure 4** illustrates the accumulation of drusenoid deposits in the macula of an elderly female. Fundus photographs are used with optical coherence tomography, seen in **Figure 5**, to assess Drusen.

In 2010, the first report on the use of smartphones for retinal imaging was published [13]. The principles of the indirect ophthalmoscope apply to smartphone fundus photography using a 20D condensing lens. Smartphone photography is convenient because of its portability and cost-effectiveness [14]. It is utilized for documentation, screening, and monitoring the progression of macular diseases, for example, diabetic macular edema and age-related macular degeneration [15]. Other portable, handheld photographic devices have been used for imaging the macula and are helpful in remote screening of diabetic retinopathy eyes. The Welch Allyn iExaminer System can be attached to an Apple iPhone 4/4S and has gained FDA approval as an ophthalmoscope for mobile phones [16]. The disadvantages of handheld devices to conventional color photographs include a narrower field of view, reduced image quality, lower illumination, and reduced image contrast.

Advancements in electronic media have increased the importance of macular imaging using fundus photographs, which can aid disease evaluation and diagnosis through "teleophthalmology" [15]. In the future, patients will be able to send macular images to control centers without the need for physical attendance at a screening venue.

Biomarkers can be identified from macular imaging. These could be biomarkers of systemic or more generalized disease and ocular disease. For example, arterial width, arterial angle, venous angle, and fractal dimensions, reflective of arteriosclerosis present in the retinal vasculature, could be a potential biomarker for atherosclerosis in the coronary artery [17]. Deep learning algorithms have been developed for

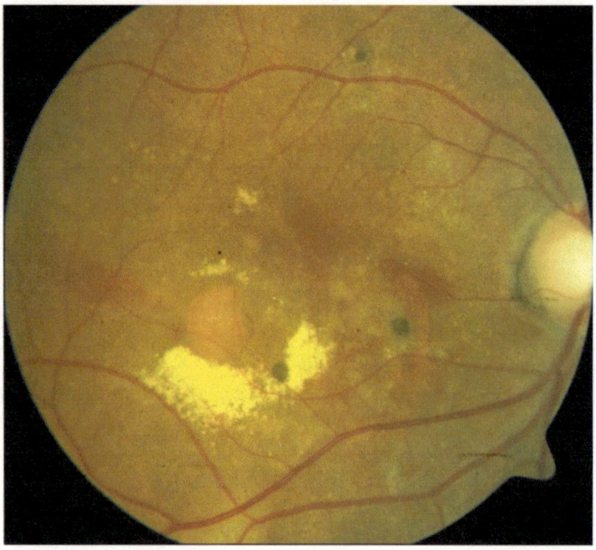

Figure 6.
Hard exudates and hemorrhage in the right eye macula of an eye diagnosed with exudative age-related macular degeneration. There are pigmentary changes with hyper- and hypo-pigmented spots spread over the macula.

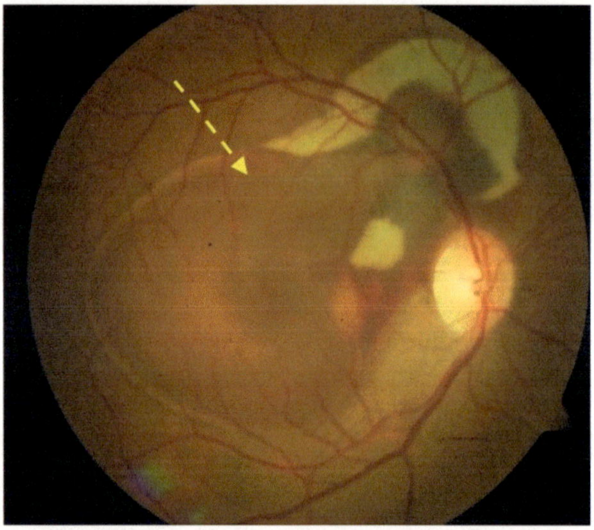

Figure 7.
Large area of serosanguinous leakage into the macula (yellow dash arrow).

predicting age, sex, and cardiovascular disease using retinal biomarkers [18, 19]. In the case of ocular diseases, the findings of microaneurysm, retinal hemorrhage, hard exudates, and cotton-wool spots are biomarkers of retinovascular disease, which can be imaged, segmented, and analyzed using computer analytics for disease management [16]. **Figures 6** and 7 are representative fundus images that contain leakage of hard exudates and serosanguinous material into the retina. **Figure 8** depicts features of non-proliferative diabetic retinopathy, including macular hemorrhages, hard

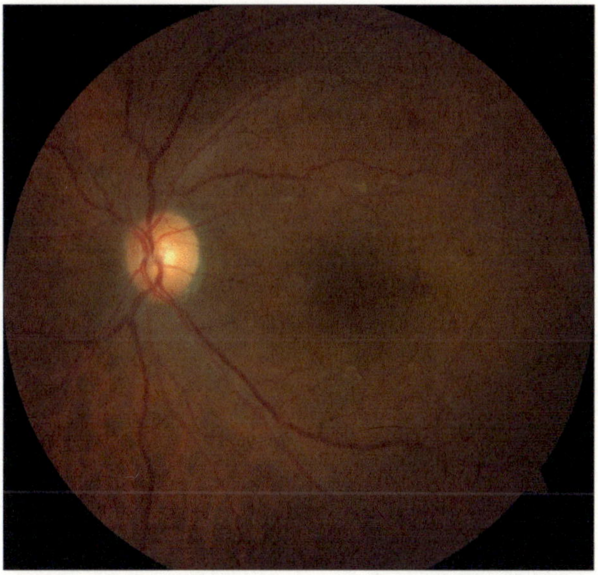

Figure 8.
Left eye macula hemorrhages, microaneurysms, and hard exudates in an eye diagnosed with non-proliferative diabetic retinopathy.

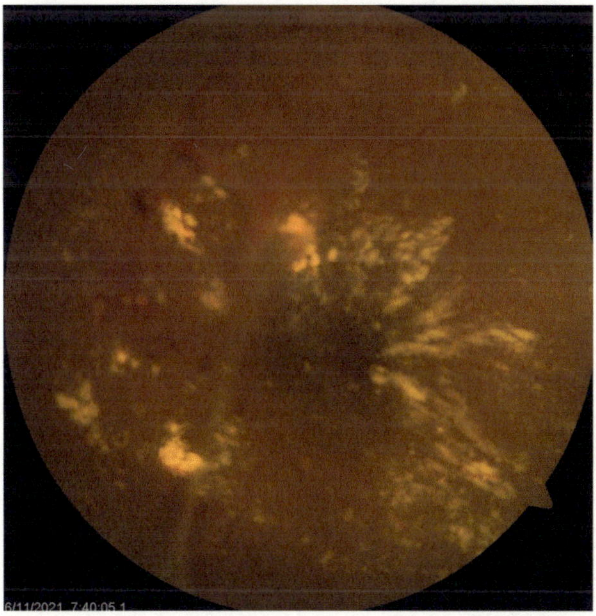

Figure 9.
Widespread macula hard exudates, hemorrhages, and vitreous opacities in diabetic macular edema.

exudates, and microaneurysms. **Figure 9** shows significant macular hard exudates and hemorrhages. In **Figures 10** and **11**, there is neovascularization of the disk and retina, respectively.

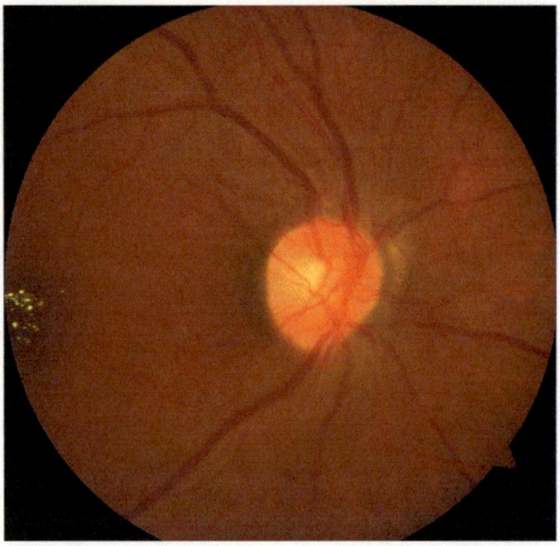

Figure 10.
Right eye disk neovascularization from proliferative diabetic retinopathy. Macular exudates are also seen.

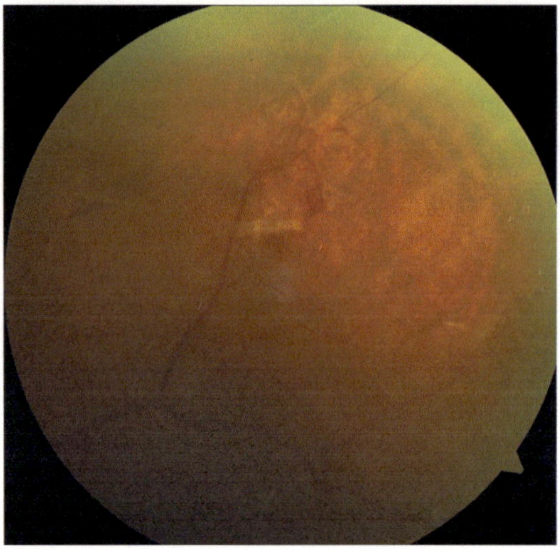

Figure 11.
Left eye retinal neovascularization along the superotemporal arcade secondary to proliferative diabetic retinopathy.

3. Stereoscopic photography

A stereo image is produced by taking photographs of the same scene from two slightly different positions so that the viewer fuses the images and obtains a three-dimensional reconstruction of the image. It is less practiced in the clinics [20]. Two photographs from slightly different viewpoints of the object are acquired to obtain any stereoscopic photography. Then, present these right and left images to the right and left eyes of the observer utilizing a stereo viewer. To obtain stereoscopic retina images, the retina camera begins in the same position used for single fundus photography. Then shifted, first to the left and then 3–4 mm to the right. Digital images are taken and saved, and the software incorporated into the camera enables viewing of the stereo pair. The right and left images are presented on the viewing monitor. A pair of viewing glasses should be used to merge the two images [21].

Stereoscopic fundus photography's advantage compared to conventional photography is its ability to image the depth of the retina. The usefulness of stereo viewing can be seen in diabetic retinopathy, where it can help differentiate raised retinal neovascularization from the typically flat intraretinal microvascular anomaly. **Figure 10** shows disk neovascularization and exudative maculopathy, and **Figure 11** neovascularization on the retina, using conventional photography, both occurring from proliferative diabetic retinopathy. Stereoscopic imaging better appreciates the raised nature of this neovascularization. However, a comparative study of monoscopic and stereoscopic fundus photography found no difference in the ability of an ophthalmologist to evaluate diabetic retinopathy's severity using the criteria established by the early treatment of diabetic retinopathy study (ETDRS) [22].

4. Fundus autofluorescence (FAF)

This noninvasive imaging technique relies on detecting fluorophores, which occur naturally and absorb and emit light of specific wavelengths [23]. Intravenously injected agents are not required for FAF imaging. It is dependent on intrinsic molecules present in the eye. FAF also differs from angiography in that the FAF signal intensity is much weaker at approximately two orders of magnitude lower than the fluorescein angiogram's background intensity during the most intense part of the dye transit [23].

To generate autofluorescence, a fluorophore will absorb a photon of the excitatory wavelength that elevates an electron to an excited, high-energy state. The electron then dissipates some energy through molecular collisions, emitting light with lower energy and longer wavelength as it transitions to the ground state [24]. FAF's image signal intensity depends on lipofuscin concentration and, to a minor degree, other fluorophores. Lesions can be categorized as hyper-auto, hypo-auto, or iso-auto fluorescent [24].

FAF can be used in the evaluation of age-related macular degeneration, diabetic macular edema, central serous chorioretinopathy, macular dystrophies, acute exudative polymorphous vitelliform choroidal dystrophy, macular telangiectasia, pentosan maculopathy, and hydroxychloroquine toxicity [24–26].

Several FAF patterns have been described in AMD. Drusen may have normal, hyper-, or hypo-autofluorescent patterns on fundus autofluorescence imaging [27]. A hyper-autofluorescent appearance can be seen due to lipofuscin within the drusen or in the RPE overlying the drusen, and a hypo-autofluorescent appearance is caused by regressed drusen or degenerated RPE cells. Large, soft drusen typically display relatively well-defined hyper-autofluorescence [27]. Drusenoid pigment epithelial detachments display a patchy pattern of hyper- and hypo-autofluorescence [28].

The International Fundus Autofluorescence Classification Group (IFAG) described a classification scheme for a range of distinct fundus autofluorescence patterns associated with early and intermediate AMD, including normal, minimal change, focal increased, patchy, linear, lace-like, reticular, or speckled [29].

FAF is especially valuable in detecting, evaluating, and monitoring geographic atrophy, used as an endpoint in clinical trials [29]. In neovascular AMD, FAF reveals distinct patterns of classic choroidal neovascularization noninvasively and may be especially useful for determining which eyes are likely to benefit from therapeutic intervention [29]. The spectrum of FAF imaging has been expanded with the increasing use of green in addition to blue FAF and the introduction of spectrally resolved FAF, near-infrared FAF, quantitative FAF imaging, and fluorescence lifetime imaging (FLIO) [30].

Figures 12–15 are the multimodal imaging of bilateral active peripapillary choroidal neovascular membrane with exudation and scarring involving the macula. **Figure 12** (fundus photography), **Figure 13** (fluorescein angiography), **Figure 14** (fundus autofluorescence-green), and **Figure 15** (optical coherence tomography angiography – montage) show the same pathology utilizing different imaging techniques.

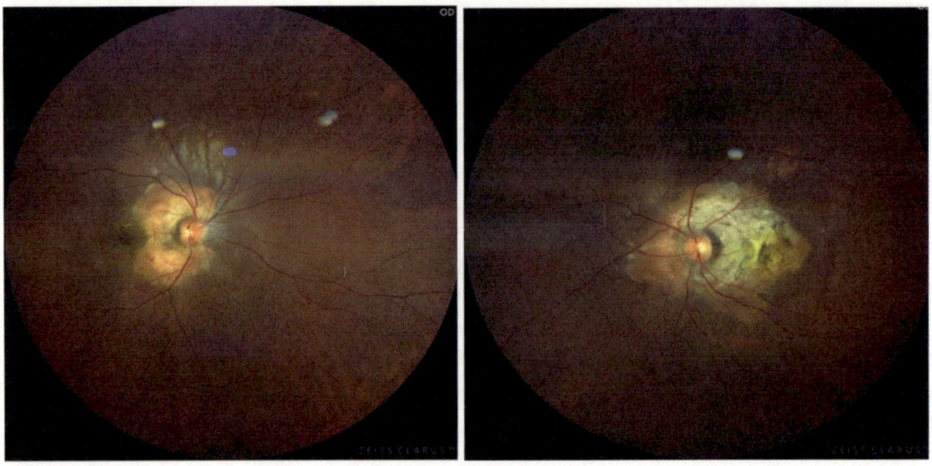

Figure 12.
Right eye and left eye fundus photograph of a middle-aged female. Macular imaging shows peripapillary neovascularization, with leakage and scarring, more pronounced and involving the fovea in the left eye.

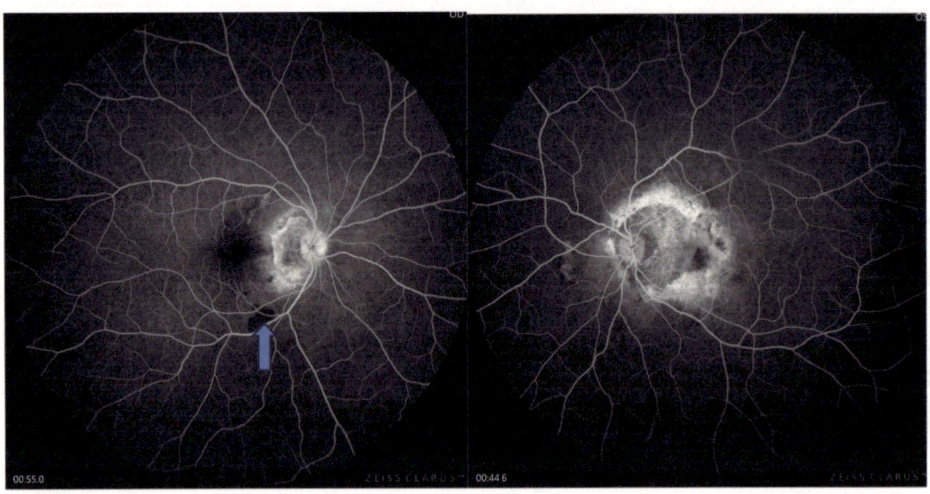

Figure 13.
*Fluorescein angiography of the same eyes in **Figure 12**. A normal appearing hypofluorescent right eye fovea suggests less involvement of the right eye and better vision. Notice focal hypofluorescence along the right eye infero temporal arcade, due to blocked fluorescence from retinal hemorrhage. Left eye macula hyperfluorescence resulting from dye leakage and staining of central scar tissue.*

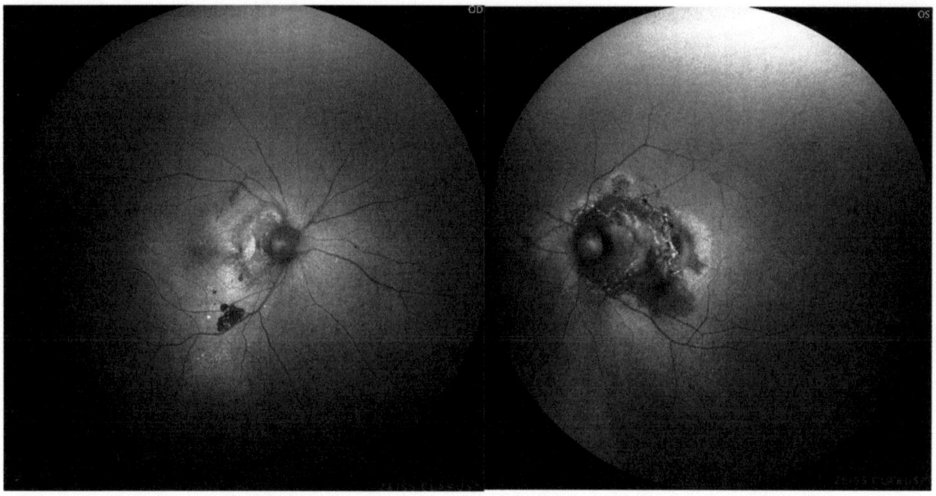

Figure 14.
*Fundus auto fluorescence of the same eye in **Figure 12** showing areas of hypo- and hyper-autofluorescence reflecting areas of subretinal leakage and scarring.*

5. Scanning laser ophthalmoscopy (SLO), including retromode imaging

The SLO gives high-quality retina images utilizing a small fraction of light used for conventional indirect ophthalmoscopy [31]. It is light, efficient imaging. The SLO utilizes the ophthalmoscopic principle in which a dim laser beam scans across the fundus, and reflected light is collected only from one retinal point at a time. Because the SLO illuminates only a single retinal point at a time, only 0.9 mm of the patient's pupil (the diameter of the laser beam) is used for illumination, and the rest is available for light collection. This makes the SLO a very light-efficient instrument. Because of SLO's light efficiency, illumination levels are comfortable for the patient, and fundus fluorescein angiography can be performed with about a tenth of the fluorescein dye dose [31]. The confocal scanning laser ophthalmoscopy (e.g., Heidelberg retina tomograph, HRT) is famous for examining macular structures in several macular diseases [32]. It offers a three-dimensional analysis of the macula and gives a retinal map. It has been used to evaluate diabetic macular edema and macular edema from branch retinal vein occlusion, age-related macular degeneration, and idiopathic macular holes [33].

SLO's clinical applications, image contrast, and axial resolution are determined by an aperture overlying its photodetector. In high contrast, reflectance images are produced using small-diameter, centered apertures (confocal apertures) that collect retroreflections and reject side-scattered veiling light returned from the fundus. Retro illumination images are obtained with annular on-axis or laterally displaced off-axis apertures that capture scattered light and reject the retroreflected light used for reflectance imaging. Retro illumination highlights and shades the boundaries of chorioretinal tissues and abnormalities, facilitating small drusen detection, subretinal drusenoid deposits, and subthreshold laser lesions. It also facilitates screening for large area chorioretinal irregularities not readily identified with other enface retinal imaging modalities [34–36].

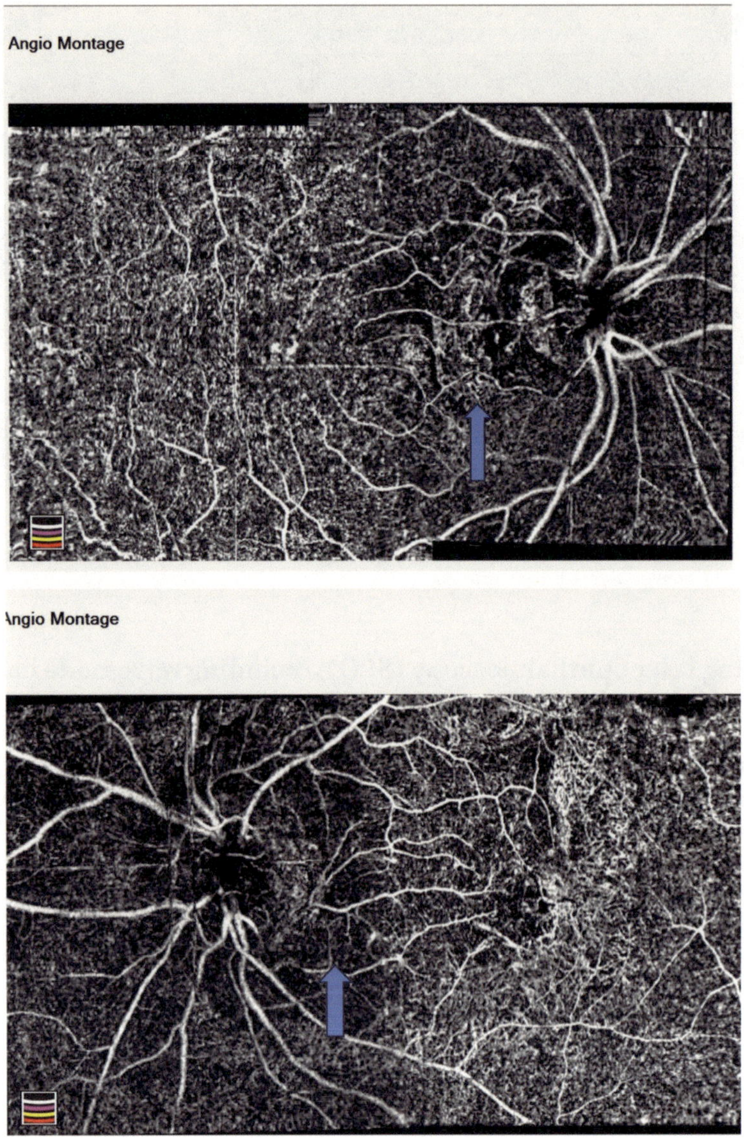

Figure 15.
Right and left eye optical coherence tomography angiography (OCTA). The right eye demonstrates a temporal peripapillary network of blood vessels (blue arrow), that is missing in the left eye (blue arrow) because access to the left eye temporal peripapillary area is restricted by the presence of scar tissue.

6. Multicolor imaging (MCI)

MCI uses the confocal scanning laser ophthalmoscopy (CSLO) to capture three simultaneous reflectance images using three monochromatic laser sources: (1) blue reflectance (BR; 488 nm), (2) green reflectance (GR; 515 nm), and (3) infrared reflectance (IR; 820 nm). These different wavelengths of light can penetrate the different retinal surfaces at diverse depths to show details of the retinal layers. The BR mainly enables the visualization of the inner retina and the vitreoretinal interface, including epiretinal membrane (ERM), retinal nerve fiber layer thinning, and macular pigment changes. GR images allow visualization of deeper details, such as retinal blood vessels and intraretinal lipid exudation. IR predominantly visualizes structures at the outer retina and choroid level, including drusen and retinal pigmentary epithelium alterations [34].

Compared to color fundus photography, which requires a bright flash of light to capture images, single-wavelength small laser spots are used in multicolor imaging, which may cause less photophobia. A disadvantage of multicolor imaging compared to conventional color fundus photography is that multicolor imaging may require a slightly more extended fixation period to take the three separate images compared to color fundus photography [37]. Multicolor imaging has been used to evaluate AMD, macular edema from retinal vein occlusion, central serous chorioretinopathy (CSCR), and inherited macular dystrophies [37].

7. Fundus fluorescein angiography (FFA)

FFA evaluates retinal and choroidal circulation's anatomy, physiology, and pathology [38]. It involves the intravenous injection of fluorescein sodium, a nonio-dinated contrast agent, followed by serial photographs to visualize the patency and permeability of the retinal vessels.

Sodium fluorescein molecules emit green light (wavelength of 520–530 nm) when stimulated by blue light (wavelength of 465–490 nm). Two filters are needed to perform FFA: a blue filter excites to produce fluorescence, and a green filter absorbs the green fluorescence and blocks the reflected blue light [38]. Sixty percent of sodium fluorescein is bound to plasma proteins, mainly to albumin. The free dye passes readily across systemic capillaries to the tissues. Retinal capillaries usually do not leak fluorescein dye. A loss of the blood-retinal barrier integrity (either of the retinal vessel endothelial cells or the RPE) allows free fluorescein leakage into the extracellular spaces of the surrounding neurosensory retina. Neovascularization in the retina, choroid, and iris leak fluorescein profusely [38].

There are five phases in FFA: choroidal, arterial, arteriovenous, venous, and recirculation [39]. Hypofluorescence appears as a reduction from the normal expected fluorescence, and hyperfluorescence implies an increased or abnormal fluorescence. Hyperfluorescence can be from dye leakage, staining, pooling, or transmission defects, and hypofluorescence is due to a blocking effect or a vascular filling defect [39]. **Figure 16a** and **b** show the fundus photograph and fluorescein angiography of central retinal vein occlusion with disk edema seen as hyperfluorescence from leakage on angiography and blocked fluorescence from the retina hemorrhages, respectively.

Geographic atrophy typically shows late, well-defined hyperfluorescence from the exposed deep choroid and sclera staining [40]. Classic choroidal neovascularization (CNV) is characterized by well-demarcated hyperfluorescence in the early phases of FA and late leakage that obscures the boundaries of the lesion [41]. Angiographically, the disciform scar shows late staining [40].

FFA is beneficial in evaluating macular edema, age-related macular degeneration, central serous chorioretinopathy, and inherited macular dystrophies [42, 43]. The standard fundus camera captures images of 30–50 degrees of the retina; however, wide-field imaging efficiently assesses peripheral vascular leakage, peripheral vascular loops, and capillary nonperfusion areas present in retinal vein occlusion, proliferative sickle cell retinopathy and diabetic retinopathy [44].

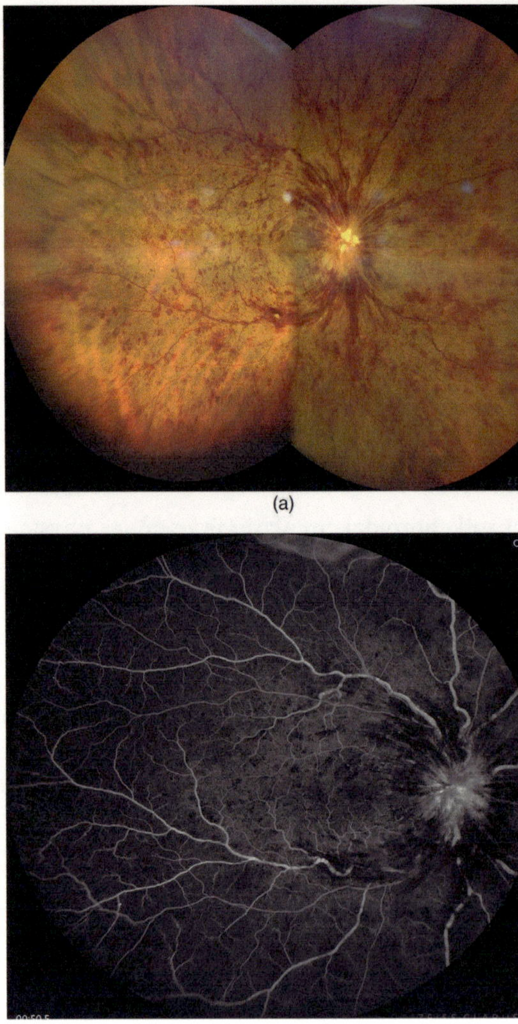

Figure 16.
a and b: Right eye central retinal vein occlusion; wide-field fundus photograph and corresponding fundus fluorescein angiography.

8. Indocyanine green angiography (ICGA)

Indocyanine green angiography (ICGA) is used to image choroidal circulation and its abnormalities [45]. ICGA uses indocyanine green dye, a high-molecular-weight contrast (775 kD), and projects 790 nm infrared light into the eye, allowing deep RPE penetration [46]. The dye used in ICGA binds to plasma proteins and thus leaks less compared to fluorescein dye used in FFA imaging. The ICGA leakage, then reabsorbed, produces hyper cyanescent in the late phase [47]. ICGA has three phases: early, mid, and late. Indications for ICGA include exudative age-related macular degeneration, idiopathic polypoidal choroidal vasculopathy, and central serous chorioretinopathy [48].

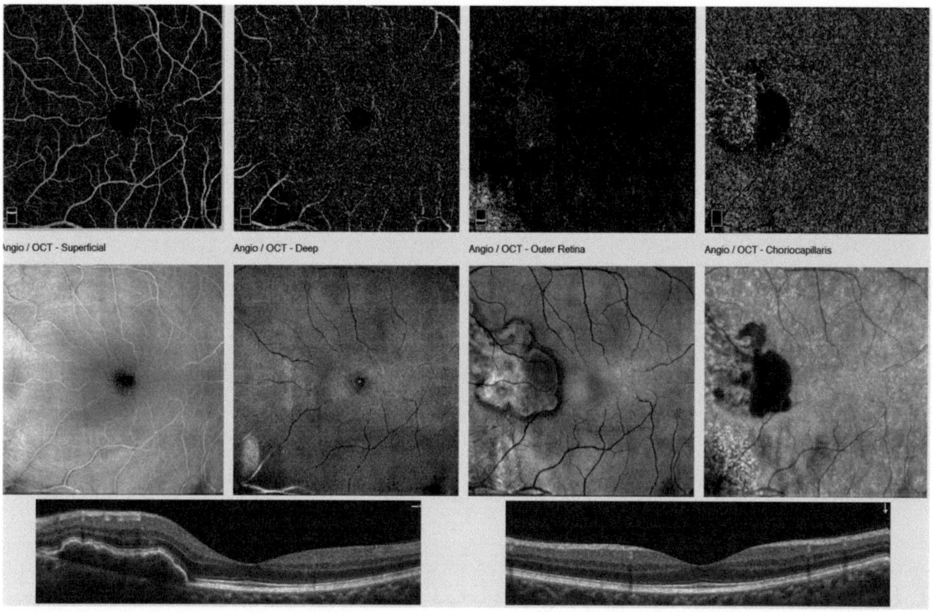

Figure 17.
*Optical coherence tomography angiography (OCTA) of the left eye (fundus photography shown in **Figure 3**), diagnosed with polypoidal choroidal vasculopathy (PCV). The cross-sectional OCT shows the broad pigment epithelial detachment in the area of the PCV lesion, which is also seen on the outer retina enface OCT. on OCTA, while the superficial and deep vascular plexi remain unperturbed, the outer retina and choriocapillaris layer feature a vascular network of capillaries associated with the PCV lesion.*

ICGA has been used to highlight the polyps and branching vascular network (BVN) present in polypoidal choroidal vasculopathy (PCV) and choroidal neovascular membrane present in exudative age-related macular degeneration, myopia, and other causes [49–51]. Often, ICGA is unavailable, so other imaging techniques, including the B-mode OCT scan, can be used as an alternative for polyp detection in PCV [50]. **Figure 17** shows the OCT angiography, enface, and cross-sectional OCT images of an eye diagnosed with polypoidal choroidal vasculopathy and polypoidal lesions. A broad pigment epithelial detachment can be seen on cross-sectional OCT of the polyp harboring area.

9. Retinal thickness analyzer (RTA)

The retinal thickness analyzer (RTA) is an automated, computerized slit-lamp biomicroscopic system. It utilizes a green (543 nm) He-Ne laser as a slit beam and provides optical cross sections of the retina. In the macula, the optical cross sections reveal retinal structural changes that are analyzed to generate two- and three-dimensional quantitative retinal thickness maps. The retinal thickness maps are obtained, like those obtained using the SLO and OCT. The RTA is error-prone, and the presence of retinopathy (edema) tends to cause false-positive readings [52]. RTA is not suitable for difficult reading situations since it is prone to erroneous or missing thickness readings under such conditions [53]. The OCT may be superior to the RTA in such situations.

10. B-mode ultrasonography

The ultrasound is a clinically useful imaging modality for the macula in conditions with a media opacity or unclear media. High-frequency ultrasound waves passing from the transducer to ocular tissue are transmitted back to the probe. Depending on the time and amplitude of the returning sound wave, which reflects the tissue density, the signal is summed to form a two-dimensional image of the eye. The more echogenic the appearance of the scanned image, the higher the amplitude of the detected signal and the higher the tissue density. A dense white appearance reflects echogenicity.

A B-scan has been used to detect macular thickening, and its sensitivity and specificity were determined. Ultrasonographic detection of macular thickening has been found to correlate with findings on retina examination using slit-lamp biomicroscopy, FFA, and OCT. B-scan ultrasonography has been described as a valuable technique for assessing macular thickness when biomicroscopy is impossible or when patients cannot tolerate alternatives, that is, FA or OCT [54].

11. Optical coherence tomography (OCT) and optical coherence tomography angiography (OCTA)

11.1 Optical coherence tomography (OCT)

Optical coherence tomography (OCT) is a non-contact, noninvasive ophthalmic imaging test [55]. The OCT uses the principle of light waves, which is based on the ability of ocular tissues to reflect and backscatter light involving low-coherence interferometry [56]. It provides a high-depth, resolution, cross-sectional image of the retina, enabling quantitative (mapping, volume, and thickness) evaluation of the retinal thickness and assessing qualitative (morphology and reflectivity) anatomic changes [56, 57].

OCT of the macular is used for the detection and monitoring of a diverse range of diseases affecting the macula, such as macular edema, macular holes, pseudo holes, epiretinal membranes (ERMs), vitreomacular adhesion (VMA), and vitreomacular traction (VMT) [55, 56]. **Figure 18** illustrates the usefulness of OCT in the evaluation of vitreomacular interface disorder. **Figure 18** is a full-thickness macular hole revealing basal and minimum diameters and a posterior vitreous detachment. Retinoschisis, as well as detachments of the neurosensory retina and pigment epithelium, diabetic retinopathy (DR), and drusen in age-related macular degeneration, can be detected by OCT [55, 56].

Macular OCT application can be broadly divided into localizing pathologies in the intraretinal, subretinal, and sub-RPE space. Intraretinal fluid collection is seen as retinal edema (focal or diffuse), cystoid edema, cysts, microcysts, and impending macular holes [56]. Subretinal fluid collection is typically seen in central serous chorioretinopathy (CSCR); here, the serous fluid causes elevation of the sensory retina [56].

Regular posterior segment ocular tissues are identified and localized due to their reflective properties [56]. Structures such as the internal limiting membrane, retinal nerve fiber layer, inner and outer plexiform layers are hyperreflective in nature; layers of the outer retina such as the external limiting membrane, the inner and

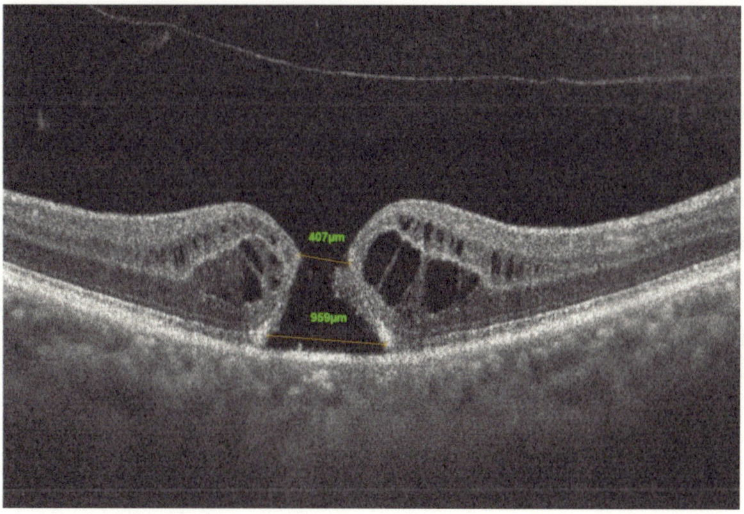

Figure 18.
A macular hole seen as full-thickness macular defect with detachment of the posterior hyaloid. There are intraretinal cystic spaces in the perifoveal retina. It is possible to measure the outer diameter and inner (minimum) diameter of the macular hole accurately. Macular holes can be closed effectively using surgical techniques. The choice of surgical technique to use and prognosis can be determined by the measurement of the macular hole size (diameter), provided by the OCT.

outer segments junction of the photoreceptor, and the retinal pigment epithelium-Bruch's membrane-choriocapillaris complex also exhibits high reflectivity [56]. Hyperreflectivity is also a feature of reduced retinal thickness (as in retinal atrophy) and scar tissue. Normal retinal tissues that are hyporeflective include the ganglion cell layer and the outer and inner nuclear layers. Retinal lesions that cause low or hyporeflectivity include cystic or pseudo cystic areas containing a serous fluid, atrophic RPE (loss of pigment), cystoid edema, serous neural retinal detachment, and RPE detachment. Such lesions appear as black, optically empty spaces.

In clinical practice, retino-vascular diseases and AMD biomarkers are sought to correlate visual function, predict treatment response, and forecast prognosis. These are useful in the decision to commence treatment or during treatment [55, 58, 59].

A biomarker is a measurable biological parameter evaluated and measured to indicate processes that can be normal biological processes, pathogenic processes, or some pharmacologic responses to a therapeutic intervention [55, 60]. Retinal OCT biomarkers are classified into seven categories, which are susceptibility or risk, diagnostic, monitoring, prognostic, predictive, pharmacodynamic or response, and safety [55]. Commonly used retinal OCT imaging biomarkers include central subfield thickness (CST) (which is the most popular), the junction in between the photoreceptor inner and outer segments (IS/OS) or ellipsoid zone (EZ), intraretinal fluid (IRF), subretinal fluid (SRF), subretinal hyperreflective material (SHRM), disorganization of retinal inner layers (DRIL), pigment epithelial detachment (PED), retinal pigmental epithelial (RPE) atrophy, outer retinal tubulation (ORT), hyperreflective foci (HRF), drusen type, subretinal drusenoid deposits (SDD), double-layer sign (DLS), incomplete retinal pigment epithelium (RPE) and outer retinal atrophy (iRORA), complete retinal pigment epithelium (RPE), and outer retinal atrophy (cRORA) [55].

11.2 Macular OCT biomarkers indicative of disease

11.2.1 Central subfield thickness (CST)

The OCT immediately measures the circular 1 mm diameter area surrounding the fovea's center point, taking its reading from the internal limiting membrane to the RPE [58, 59]. The CST is provided as a quantifiable value on OCT software [58]. This measurement gives an unbiased reading of the macular thickness. An increase in CST plays a significant role in macular edema, commonly seen in diseases such as diabetic macular edema (DME), retinal vein occlusion (RVO), nAMD, and non-infectious uveitis (NIU) [55, 58]. CST became one of the earliest OCT biomarkers implemented as an outcome measure in clinical trials of nAMD. CST measurement has been used to evaluate treatment outcomes, retreatment time, and overall clinical decision-making [59]. Fluid in the retina reflects disease activity and manifests as increased CST on OCT. Nevertheless, increased CST seen on OCT does not indicate the location of the fluid within the retina, which can be of visual prognostic value [55]. Various studies on DME, RVO-related macular edema, and macular edema in NIU have shown that there is only a modest or negative correlation between best-corrected visual acuity (BCVA) and CST [58]. However, large nAMD clinical trials, such as the PrONTO and SUSTAIN studies, showed that BCVA improvement correlated with the decreases in the mean CST [59]. Fluid located within the substance of the retina is referred to as intraretinal fluid (IRF); when the fluid is located between the neurosensory retina and RPE, it is termed subretinal fluid (SRF), while fluid located underneath the retinal pigment epithelium is referred to as sub-RPE, this is seen as pigment epithelial detachment (PED) [55]. Intraretinal cysts (IRC)/intraretinal fluid (IRF) at baseline and during anti-VEGF treatment are associated with poor visual outcomes [61]. SRF is more tolerated, described as being protective of vision, and is associated with better visual outcomes [55]. SRF may protect the retina from atrophy. For the above reason, CST is not a good predictor of baseline or final vision after anti-VEGF treatment, as this depends on the compartmentalization of the fluid rather than the overall central retina thickness [55].

11.2.2 Retinal structural alterations

1. The outer retina has four layers, which include the external limiting membrane (ELM), ellipsoid zone (EZ), [ELM and EZ represents the photoreceptor layer], interdigitation zone (IZ), and RPE. Damage to any of the outer retinal layers (ORL) has been correlated with worsening vision due to the associated photoreceptor defects [62]. Outer retinal layer integrity and presence on initial OCT evaluation for several retinal diseases, including nAMD, is associated with better pretreatment vision [55]. Likewise, the reconstitution of the outer retina after treating these retinal diseases has been correlated with improved visual outcomes [55]. Early treatment of retinal fluid with intravitreal anti-VEGF often results in the return or preservation of the ORL following fluid resolution. Ellipsoid zone alterations severely reduce retinal function. At the same time, IS/OS status has been reported to improve in response to anti-VEGF treatment, but ELM may show less improvement following treatment [55].

2. Malformations of the ORL are identified as outer retinal tubulations (ORT) and outer retinal corrugations. They are used to predict the clinical outcome of patients with nAMD [59]. Outer retinal tubulations (ORTs) can be found in nAMD

and many retinal diseases. ORT is a circular, tube-like structural reconfiguration of disrupted, damaged photoreceptors [63]. They are often found in advanced nAMD and rarely disappear with regular anti-VEGF injections. Since ORT involves the loss of photoreceptor function, it is highly predictive of a worsening BCVA over time [59]. Outer retinal corrugations are groups of wavy hyperreflective materials above the Bruchs membrane found on OCT imaging of AMD that are often associated with basal laminar deposits (BLamD) [59]. They are generally limited to areas in eyes with significant GA or choroidal neovascularization (CNV) and are correlated with late nAMD. Outer retinal corrugations do not have a strong predictive value of visual outcomes, as they do not indicate leakage [59].

11.2.2.1 Hyperreflective material (HRM) and hyperreflective foci (HRF)

Hyperreflective material: Any hyperdense, reflective deposits found between the retina and the RPE are referred to as subretinal hyperreflective material (SHRM) [59]. The contents of SHRM vary and can evolve. These include blood, fibrin, choroidal neovascularization, and scar tissue. SHRM presence, especially in the fovea at baseline, is strongly linked to poorer visual prognosis compared with eyes without SHRM due to the disruption of the photoreceptors [55, 59, 61].

Hyperreflective foci (HRF): On OCT imaging, HRF appears as hyperreflective roundish lesions or small-sized, well-defined dots across the neurosensory retina; it is seen around the intraretinal cystoid spaces or near the drusen edge [55, 59]. They occur in several retina diseases, including DME and nAMD. HRF is believed to be a strong risk factor for the progression of dry AMD to nAMD [59, 61]. When found at an inner location of the retina and in a cluster, distribution is associated with nAMD. The persistence of HRF after anti-VEGF treatment has been correlated with a poorer VA at baseline [59]. Further, the persistence of HRF in patients had been noted in non-responders to anti-VEGF, compared to a decline in HRF in patients responsive to treatment. Thus, it serves as a good prognostic sign. The presence of HRF has likewise been significantly connected with the presence of other key biomarkers [61]. In a retrospective study, the presence of IRF was substantially associated with the presence of HRF in the inner retina, SRF layer, and outer retina; the presence of PED was noticeably associated with HRF in the inner retina, and the presence of SRF was significantly associated with HRF in the SRF layer [64]. Tuerksever et al. reported that eyes with more HRF at baseline showed a significant decrease in CNV leakage area in the 12th month, with a rapid reduction in HRF in the second week associated with lower CST at month 12 [65]. HRF quantity was also significantly correlated with drusen volume at baseline and after 1 year [61].

11.2.2.2 Double-layer sign (DLS)

Is an OCT finding suggestive of early-stage macular neovascularization of choroidal origin (type 1 macular neovascularization (MNV)) [55, 66]. It consists of two hyperreflective bands, one on top of the other with a small hyperreflective space in between; the lower band is the Bruch's membrane, the upper band is the RPE and the space in between corresponds to the type 1 MNV that is referred to as "double-layer sign" (DLS) [55, 66]. Shallow, irregular RPE elevation (SIRE) has been used to describe the characteristic features of DLS in eyes with non-exudative MNV [55]; SIRE has been found to have a sensitivity of 100% for non-exudative MNV [55].

11.2.2.3 Retinal pigment epithelial (RPE) atrophy

A loss of retinal layers, RPE, and choriocapillaris characterize retinal pigment epithelial (RPE) atrophy [61]. There are two stages of atrophy in AMD, named according to the affected anatomic layers on OCT: cRORA (complete retinal pigment epithelium and outer retinal atrophy) and iRORA (incomplete RPE and outer retinal atrophy) [60]. The stage named cRORA is defined on OCT by a region of choroidal hypertransmission of diameter of at least 250 mm, a zone of attenuation or disruption of the RPE of 250 mm or more in diameter, and evidence of degeneration of the overlying photoreceptor, all of which occur in the absence of an RPE tear or scrolled RPE [60, 61]. The term iRORA is defined on OCT as evidence of some transmission but is discontinuous; the RPE band is present but irregular or interrupted; interrupted ELM and EZ is evidence of photoreceptor degeneration; the INL and OPL exhibit subsidence [61]. The finding of iRORA predates progression to cRORA in non-neovascular AMD; of multiple factors investigated, drusen collapse was the OCT feature most strongly correlated to progression to iRORA/cRORA [55].

11.2.2.4 Disorganization of retinal inner layers (DRIL)

The normal retina is an orderly, layered structure recognized by the hypo- and hyper-reflectivity patterns on OCT [55]. When there is a lack of demarcation in the inner retinal layers situated in the central fovea between the ganglion cell layer-inner plexiform layer complex (GCL-IPL), inner nuclear layer (INL), outer plexiform layer (OPL), and outer nuclear layer (ONL), this is described as DRIL [55, 58]. DRIL is a potentially important biomarker of reduced VA [58]. A large area of DRIL at baseline is correlated with worse baseline VA [55]. Regarding the measurement of DRIL on OCT, the central 1 mm retinal zone is the area considered. Disorganization of greater than 50% or > 500 μm of this area is considered significant and related to poorer visual prognosis [55]. A correlation has been found between DRIL, the foveal avascular zone (FAZ) size, and macular capillary nonperfusion [67]. Retinovascular diseases such as DME and retinal vein occlusions (RVO) studies have shown DRIL to be a marker for poor visual prognosis as these eyes have a worse baseline and final VA despite anti-VEGF treatment [67, 68].

11.2.2.5 Pigment epithelium detachment

Retinal pigment epithelium detachment (PED) is the separation between RPE's basal lamina layer and the inner collagenous layer of Bruch's membrane [59, 69, 70]. PEDs are seen as a prominent feature in AMD as well as in idiopathic polypoidal choroidal vasculopathy (IPCV) [69]. Various large treatment trials have shown that PEDs develop in 30–80% of eyes with nAMD [59, 69]. Cheong et al. provided a review of PED's effect on VA in nAMD and IPCV [71]. Numerous studies have focused on VA's association with the presence or absence of PED and its association with its morphological features, such as height, width, linear diameter, area, volume, reflectivity, and content of PED [59]. Despite several prospective and retrospective studies and randomized control trials, there is no clear agreement on the influence of these factors on the VA [59, 61]. Though some studies reported that the presence of PEDs may portend a slightly worse VA and hence a need for more regular retreatment, other studies counterintuitively report better vision in eyes with PEDs. There is evidence, however, that fibrovascular PED carries an inferior visual prognosis [59]. There are various types of PEDs, namely serous, drusenoid, fibrovascular, and mixed detachments [59, 70].

11.2.2.6 OCT imaging characteristics of types of PED

The OCT findings of a serous PED will appear as a dome-shaped elevation of the RPE over a hyporeflective space, with Bruch's membrane commonly visible as a straight, thin hyperreflective line at the base of the elevation [69]. The occurrence of IRF/SRF or hyperreflective structures within the PED implies the presence of CNV.

In drusenoid PEDs, OCT will reveal RPE elevations over homogeneous mildly hyperreflective spaces. Bruch's membrane is often seen at its base. CNV should be suspected in cases where significant heterogeneous optical reflectivity is seen within the PED and/or with the presence of IRF/SRF [69].

On OCT, fibrovascular PEDs usually appear as irregular elevations of the RPE with an interior that is not optically empty. It is seen as a non-uniform interior with hyper- and hypo-reflective layers [69].

11.2.2.7 Drusen

Drusen, a clinical hallmark of AMD, is a focal deposit of extracellular debris that could spontaneously appear, disappear, or change over time [72, 73]. Routine quantification of total drusen area and volume in the clinic is possible using the spectral domain OCT (SD-OCT) algorithms. The measurement of drusen load can accurately predict the development of advanced AMD [72].

Drusen associated with the development of advanced AMD, with baseline drusen volume greater than 0.03 mm^2 in the central 3 mm diameter circle of the macula occurring in up to 25% of intermediate AMD eyes was a significant prognosticator for developing advanced AMD in fellow eyes, [61, 72] with a greater than four-fold increase in risk at 1 and 2 years [61, 72]. Increased drusen volume and drusen area have also been linked to developing occult CNV, with baseline drusen volume significantly greater in eyes demonstrating CNV than in eyes without CNV [61]. Increased drusen height that is "taller" drusen disrupting or compressing the outer nuclear layer, external limiting membrane, and ellipsoid zone on OCT are likely to carry an unfavorable prognosis [72]. The AREDS - age-related eye disease study - research group reported that of 95 eyes that went on to develop geographic atrophy (GA), the following features were observed: large drusen ($\geq$ 125 μm in 96%, very large or $\geq$ 250 μm in 83%), confluent drusen (94%) and focal hyperpigmentation (96%), followed by drusen regression/fading and hypopigmentary changes (82%) occasionally accompanied by the deposition of refractile deposits (23%) [74]. Drusen is, therefore, an important biomarker of disease conversion to advanced AMD [61].

11.3 Optical coherence tomography angiography (OCTA)

OCT angiography (OCTA) is a non-dye, noninvasive technique that allows the in-depth visualization of the retinal plexuses layer by layer, quantifying microvascular parameters and comparing them with functional and morphological data [75, 76]. It has been evaluated as a complement or an alternative to fluorescein angiography (FA) and indocyanine green angiography (ICG-A) [76]. In **Figure 17** OCTA and OCT are used to illustrate imaging of polypoidal choroidal vascular lesions in a PCV eye.

OCTA has several comparative advantages over FA and ICG-A. OCTA does not require the administration of exogenous contrast; hence, it can be performed at any patient visit when FA or ICGA is contraindicated [77]. It can be used to achieve capillary scale resolution; this means that pathology affecting the capillaries, such as capillary dropout, is best imaged with OCTA [78]. OCTA acquires higher microvascular contrast and well-defined images than FA, as its images are not masked by hyperfluorescence from dye leakage that can obscure vessels [77, 78]. This high-quality image data is adaptable to software-based image processing, which can provide quantitative markers for vascular pathology [77].

OCTA volumetric data can be segmented with different retinal layers projected to enable separate visualization of retinal capillary plexus and the choriocapillaris, as well as visualizing vascular pathologies, including alterations in retinal capillary and choriocapillaris structure as well as neovascularization [77]. Additionally, OCTA is distinctively capable of providing depth-resolved biomarkers [78].

11.4 OCT angiography biomarkers

11.4.1 Perfusion

OCTA can detect blood flow in the retina and choriocapillaris by assessing perfusion through proxy measurements that are ultimately different means of assessing vascular anatomy [78]. Some of these proxy measurements are listed below:

i. Macular area vessel density (VD): Vessel density is a biomarker parameter in OCTA that can be used to observe the movement and perfusion of retinal blood flow [79]. VD measurement is achieved by segmenting vessels in enface images, which is measured as a percent area [78]. Vascular density can be divided into superficial capillary plexus (SCP), deep capillary plexus (DCP), the outer retina, and choriocapillaris [79, 80]. It is helpful in staging and diagnosing prevalent diseases, including age-related macular degeneration and diabetic retinopathy [78]. In dry AMD, it has been shown that the vascular density of the choriocapillaris decreases with increased drusen density [80]. A similar feature is seen in geographic atrophy, the advanced form of dry AMD. There are reports of significant loss of choriocapillaris flow under the RPE atrophy area and flow abnormalities observed at the borders of the atrophy. AttaAllah et al. reported that eyes with DME had significantly lower vessel densities at the deep capillary plexus (DCP) level compared to diabetic eyes without macular edema and controls [81]. The study concluded that VD was one of the biomarkers that could be used to predict the progression of visual acuity and to monitor the response to anti-VEGF treatment.

ii. Nonperfusion area: This refers to areas of impaired capillary perfusion [57]. Nonperfusion areas are localized regions of vessel loss and capillary dropout. They are identified as regions where the distance to the nearest vessel is larger than a physiologically determined threshold [78]. The most widely documented use of this OCTA capability has been to evaluate the shape, size enlargement, and remodeling of the fovea avascular zone (FAZ) among patients with diabetes of varying severity, RVO, and normal subjects [57, 78]. FAZ is quantified using the OCTA to gauge its development and progression using several metrics divided into size and shape categories. For size, these would include FAZ area, horizontal and vertical diameter, and Feret's diameter for shape, circularity, and aspect ratio [82–84]. Feret's diameter is the maximum diameter of the FAZ and is also known as the maximum caliper.

iii. Choriocapillaris flow deficits: In some retinovascular diseases such as AMD and DR, perfusion can be lost in the choriocapillaris [78]. Imaging the choriocapillaris with OCTA is more complex than imaging superficial retinal layers because the choriocapillaris is located beneath the RPE, a strongly reflecting layer that attenuates the reflectance signal [78]. Choriocapillaris imaging is consequently susceptible to both projection artifacts and signal attenuation, as well as the density of the choriocapillaris vasculature, meaning that individual capillaries may not be resolvable. To ensure the challenges of imaging in this region are met, it is essential to consider the anatomic slab boundaries used, the projection method employed, the effect of scan size, sample beam wavelength, and comparisons with other imaging modalities for validation.

11.4.2 Neovascularization

In neovascular lesions such as nAMD, polypoidal choroidal vasculopathy (PCV), and pathologic myopia, neovascularization creates pathology, which commonly leads to a severe threat to vision [78]. In contrast to conventional dye angiographies, OCTA provides an image of the exact boundaries and intrinsic details of neovascular membranes [80]. Three types of neovascularization in wet AMD have been described based on the location of abnormal vessels [57]. Visualized on OCTA, Type 1 macular neovascularization (MNV) refers to a network of vessels lying underneath the RPE, between it and the Bruch's membrane, often in the setting of a fibrovascular pigment epithelial detachment (PED) [57, 77, 78]. Type 2 MNV occurs as a network of vessels situated above the RPE but underneath the neurosensory retina, usually seen as a smaller but sharper vascular structure than type 1 MNV in the outer retinal section of OCTA [80]. Type 3 MNV originates from the deep capillary plexus within the retina and, on OCTA, is visualized as a discrete high-flow linear structure extending from the middle retinal layers into the deep retina and infrequently past the RPE [77, 80]. Various OCTA imaging features, such as the pattern of MNV (lacy wheel, sea fan, medusa, glomerular), the loop formation, branching characteristics, anastomosis, and the dark halo appearance around the lesion, have been previously described [80]. Studies have attempted to use the aforementioned OCTA features as biomarkers to determine MNV lesion activity criteria as either active or inactive [77, 80]. A recent biomarker termed "dark halo" is defined as a hypofluorescent choriocapillaris area surrounding the MNV, characterized by a flow deficit detected by OCTA [85]. Rispoli et al. have quantified dark halo (i.e., choriocapillaris vascular density changes) around MNV before and after anti-vascular endothelial growth factor (VEGF) injections using OCTA [70].

12. Functional imaging of the macula

Tests for potential vision assess the integrity of the retina and neural integrity of the visual system. Macular function tests are an essential part of evaluating potential vision [86]. A macular function test is vital for diagnosing and following up macula diseases. Imaging of the macular function includes the following:

12.1 Microperimetry

Microperimetry (MP), also known as macular perimetry, fundus perimetry, or fundus-related perimetry, is a functional test for the screening and follow-up of macular diseases [87, 88]. Conventionally, the Humphrey field analyzer (HFA) could be used to evaluate central macular sensitivity, but its role in monitoring macular disease has been limited by its inability to quantify retinal thresholds accurately over small, distinct retinal lesions and to retest these areas precisely over time [89]. Traditional visual field (VF) testing is not valuable for most patients with macular disease because central fixation is impacted, and VF tests need to be more reliable [90].

MP assesses retinal sensitivity *via* a VF test integrating perimetry and retinal imaging [91, 92]. It allows for the direct mapping of the stimulus in the region of interest, thus connecting functional information (visual field testing) with structural/anatomical data (retinal imaging) [91]. The characteristics of MP direct mapping of the stimulus and its independence from eye movements ensure that the VF sensitivities it measures have better spatial localization [92]. Microperimetry examination of the macula is a tool to assess the retinal sensitivity, scotoma size, and fixation behavior in patients with macular diseases [93].

Microperimetry is a method of choice for residual visual function assessment. Some macular diseases, including age-related macular degeneration (AMD), diabetic macular edema (DME), Stargardt disease, macular hole, idiopathic macular telangiectasia, and central serous chorioretinopathy, are studied using microperimetry [85, 88]. Visual rehabilitation training benefits from microperimetry. Identifying eccentric fixation locations, known as preferred retinal loci (PRL), and fixation-stability estimates at those sites allow the practitioner to use the best residual visual function available for rehabilitation [91].

12.2 Multifocal electroretinography

Multifocal electroretinography (mfERG) represents an objective, noninvasive retina examination to assess visual function [94]. mfERG produces a retinal function map reflecting cone-mediated responses from the photoreceptor and bipolar cells [95]. It is a diagnostic test that measures electrical activity in the retina when stimulated by light [96]. It is also valuable in distinguishing between retinal and optic nerve disease [97]. An abnormal mfERG indicates that the foveal cones and bipolar cell layers are dysfunctional and are the source of vision loss. mfERG also indicates the precise distribution of the retinal dysfunction [97]. mfERG is most applicable to patients with focal deficits in visual function and an otherwise normal appearing fundus, as commonly seen in macular dystrophies such as retinitis pigmentosa (RP), hydroxychloroquine retinopathy, bull's eye maculopathy, Stargardt's macular dystrophy, occult macular dystrophy [98]. Macular diseases, such as AMD and hereditary macular conditions, have reduced mfERG findings. A multifocal electroretinography test is recommended for patients on Plaquenil therapy, as it can detect subtle changes in the early stages of toxicity. The most specific waveform pattern observed with Plaquenil toxicity is paracentral amplitude loss, indicative of decreased retinal function in the susceptible perifovea [95].

12.3 Oxygen saturation of the macula

Human retina metabolism is supported by oxygen supply, and abnormality in oxygen perfusion is linked to various ischemic and degenerative retinopathies, leading to visual impairment and blindness [99, 100]. Oxygenation of the human retina is an energy-dependent process in which different mechanisms maintain the regulation [100]. Both hypoxia and hyperoxia are destructive for the retina; therefore, adequate blood supply and oxygen metabolism are necessary to maintain proper visual function. Anatomically, the inner retina is primarily supplied by the retinal arterial vessels and the superficial retinal capillaries. In contrast, the outer retina is primarily supplied by the choroidal vessels and, to a lesser degree, by the deep retinal capillaries. Notably, while the retinal blood flow is auto-regulated, the choroidal blood flow is not [100, 101]. In the presence of photoreceptor degeneration, the oxygen delivery to the outer retina remains unchanged, whereas the intraretinal oxygen level increases progressively. With disease progression, a measured increase of superoxide radicals in the cytoplasm of the cones and the mitochondria follows [101]. Furthermore, excess superoxide radicals generate other reactive oxygen species, resulting in even more significant oxidative damage to the cones [101]. Ischemic retinopathies show topographical patterns, and the macula is particularly affected in many cases, such as in vascular occlusions, diabetic macular edema, and age-related macular degeneration [102]. Consequently, the measurement of blood oxygen saturation within the retinal circulation is not only crucial to understanding the pathophysiology of retinal diseases, but it also plays a vital role in detection and monitoring [99].

12.4 Fundus autofluorescence (FAF)

FAF is a noninvasive imaging technique that predominantly highlights fluorophores such as lipofuscin, rhodopsin, melanin, and N-retinylidene-N-retinylethanolamine (A2E) present in the retinal pigment epithelium (RPE). Fluorophores are naturally occurring molecules that both absorb and emit light of specified wavelengths [103, 104]. To produce autofluorescence, FAF relies on the property of the RPE to emit specific wavelengths in response to excitation by short-wavelength light, with the dominant fluorophore being RPE lipofuscin, which contains the fluorescent pigment A2E. A photon of the excitation wavelength is absorbed by fluorophores, raising an electron to an excited, high-energy state [26]. This electron then dissipates some energy through molecular collisions. It emits a quantum of light at a lower energy and a longer wavelength as it transitions back to the ground state [103, 105]. FAF reveals RPE defects with reduced fluorescence and can show areas of photoreceptor damage, which appear as increased fluorescence from an accumulation of lipofuscin [95]. FAF imaging detects lipofuscin, a metabolic biomarker of the photoreceptor/RPE complex that indicates AMD, inherited retinal disorders, toxic maculopathy, and other macular diseases. Thus, it is useful diagnostically and prognostically [95, 105].

12.5 Automated 10-2 visual field

Automated 10-2 visual field testing is a valuable tool for functional assessment of macular damage. As the macular region ($\pm 8^0$) covers less than 2% of the retina, using other tests, such as the 24-2 visual field, misses damage to this area [106]. Visual field defects not respecting the vertical or horizontal midline are a feature of most macular diseases [107]. Macular diseases can cause central or paracentral scotomas depending on the location of the lesion.

Sometimes, patients with AMD may retain good visual acuity but experience distortion and other qualitative visual changes. Visual field assessment can detect the size and depth of the defects, leading to early detection and intervention [95].

Plaquenil (hydroxychloroquine-HCQ) screening guidelines mandate that a 10–2 white-stimulus visual field be performed on all patients taking this medication [95]. Other macular pathologies result in visual field defects that directly correlate with the retinal findings [107].

13. Multimodal imaging

Multimodal imaging of macular disease combines a series of imaging modalities, resulting in a better appreciation and understanding of the pathologic process, increased diagnostic sensitivity and specificity, and a clearer understanding of disease evolution [108]. The term multimodal imaging has been used in other medical disciplines, including cardiology, neurology, and oncology. In cardiology, multimodal imaging is "the efficient integration of various cardiovascular imaging methods to improve the ability to diagnose, guide therapy, or predict outcomes." [109]. Expertise in multiple imaging modalities is required for multimodal imaging [110].

The various imaging modalities already covered in this chapter can provide aspects of imaging information that complement each other for macular imaging. Various combinations of fundus photography, scanning laser ophthalmoscopy, fundus autofluorescence, fundus fluorescein angiography, indocyanine angiography, optical coherence tomography (OCT), and in recent times, addition of OCT angiography have been used in multimodal imaging of macular diseases. Because of the popularity, non-invasiveness, and three-dimensional imaging offered by the OCT (and, in recent times, OCTA), it is combined with the color fundus photograph in most multimodal imaging platforms. Macular diseases for which multimodal imaging has been utilized include diabetic macular edema, age-related macular degeneration, polypoidal choroidal vasculopathy, retinal vein, and choroidal vascular occlusion [111–113]. **Figures 12–15** utilize multimodal imaging to evaluate peripapillary choroidal neovascularization.

Yeung et al. observed a correlation between OCT and FFA findings in DME [114]. They noted a positive correlation between the severity of the outer retinal edema on OCT and the severity of leakage on FFA. Furthermore, inner and outer retina cystic changes also correlated with the severity of fluorescein dye leakage. Loss of inner retinal layers on OCT also correlated with capillary nonperfusion on FA, and large foveal cysts on SD-OCT corresponded to cystoid leakage patterns on FA. These findings suggest that diseased retinal structural changes highlighted by OCT can demonstrate patterns of leakage or non-perfusion, as seen on FA. On a case-by-case basis, multimodal imaging helps determine the appropriate diagnosis and extent of pathology, such as in polypoidal choroidal vasculopathy; OCT defines outer retina structure, including pigment epithelial detachment, and the thickened choroid, ICGA demonstrates the branching vascular network and choroidal polyps, which can also be demonstrated using OCTA. OCTA can image macular nonperfusion in diabetic macular ischemia or sickle cell maculopathy, while OCT images often present reduced temporal retina thickness, which can be associated with ischemic maculopathy.

14. Adaptive optics in macular imaging

Adaptive optics (AO) is an imaging modality that helps correct existing aberrations in the optical system, whose role in ophthalmology is emerging [115, 116]. It can significantly enhance visualization and assessment of the microstructure of retina cells, including ganglion cells (neurons), photoreceptors, and blood vessels (capillaries). The AO technique corrects for optical aberrations and was originally used to correct the blurring effect of atmospheric turbulence on images in ground-based telescopes. It is used in astronomy [117]. With AO's aid, the eye's imperfect optics can be corrected so that microscopic retinal changes can be visualized and imaged [117]. Because of its aberration correction, AO improves transverse resolution from 10 to 15 μm to approximately 2 μm, enabling the assessment of individual retinal cell types [118]. AO allows imaging of cellular and subcellular details of the macula and retina without histology [119]. Incorporation of AO into existing imaging technologies such as the fundus camera, scan laser ophthalmoscope, and OCT has greatly benefited the evaluation (including stratification of disease phenotypes), research, and treatment of several macular diseases [115]. In AO ophthalmoscopes, a synergy of AO with fundus photography, OCT, and scanning laser ophthalmoscopy (SLO) allows microscopic imaging. The AO ophthalmoscopes use a wavefront sensor to measure the ocular monochromatic aberrations and a deformable mirror to correct the detected aberrations [120].

AO retinal imaging is noninvasive and safe, used to study individual retinal cells' structure and function. Adaptive optics scanning laser ophthalmoscopy (AOSLO) systems have been used extensively [120]. It has been used to image cones, rods, retinal pigment epithelium, ganglion cells, and small retinal blood vessels and for studying cone function [121]. AO has been extensively used in the clinical evaluation and investigation of inherited retinal diseases (IRDs), including Stargardt disease, retinitis pigmentosa (RP), and achromatopsia [118–120]. Clinical trials on therapeutics for IRDs employ AO ophthalmoscopy for participant selection, stratification, and monitoring of treatment safety and efficacy. AO retina imaging has facilitated the study of photoreceptor distribution in the foveomacula area in healthy eyes and diseases, such as IRD. Cone density is the most used mosaic metric, with good reliability and repeatability shown in healthy controls [118]. Cone spacing is another metric that has found usage. Both cone density and spacing have been used successfully to determine treatment efficacy in patients with RP and Usher syndrome, treated with ciliary neurotrophic factor (CNF), resulting in a reduced rate of cone loss [122].

AO ophthalmoscopy has been used in AMD. Findings on macular imaging in AMD include the following observed by Paques et al.: improved drusen identification, limits of atrophy are better delineated, and the appreciation (visualization) of novel features, including punctate hyperreflectivity and mobile melanin-containing clumps [123]. AO retinal imaging has also been applied to study retinal vasculature. Retinal vascular biomarkers identified using AO flood illumination ophthalmoscopy (FLO) and AOSLO include inner diameter (ID), outer diameter (OD), parietal thickness (PT), wall cross-sectional area (WCSA), and wall-to-lumen ratio (WLR) [124].

15. Artificial intelligence in macular imaging

There has been much interest in incorporating artificial intelligence (AI) models to analyze retinal images. This interest is primarily because of the ability of AI to noninvasively, systematically, and rapidly analyze large amounts of data from digital images in a manner that is not humanly possible or would require a significant amount of time were it to be physically done by humans. Deep learning (DL) models have been commonly used in ophthalmology, and they can recognize, quantify, and describe several macular-related pathologic clinical features [125].

The expanding role of AI using different learning models includes screening, diagnostic grading, therapy guidance with automated detection of disease activity, recurrences, quantification of therapeutic effects, and identification of relevant targets for novel therapeutic approaches [126]. AI also offers the opportunity for personalized care for several macular diseases through its ability to predict and prognosticate outcomes since several biomarkers of macular diseases have been discovered and analyzed.

DL models have been applied to digital images from fundus photographs, mainly OCT, and are promising for the early detection of diabetic retinopathy and macular degeneration, two leading macular diseases. Of note, the increase in life expectancy and projected increase in the prevalence of diabetes suggest higher rates of AMD and DR, and by extension, more digital fundus photographs and OCT to train AI models [127]. Therefore, DL models will become valuable in rapidly, accurately, and efficiently analyzing such images.

DL has been validated for detecting diabetic retinopathy. Color fundus photography has been used for training AI models on DR. Shah et al. compared AI versus clinician examination for detecting diabetic retinopathy during screening of diabetic patients. Similarly, high sensitivity and specificity rates were demonstrated for any DR detection and prompt referral by AI and human screening [128]. In one study, AI was more sensitive than ophthalmologists in detecting DR [129]. Therefore, in situations of limited resources, the use of alternative AI models for the screening and early detection of DR, resulting in prompt referral for treatment, appears reasonable, given its performance in detecting vision-threatening DR and diabetic macular edema when used in population screening for DR [130]. In DR, DL algorithms diagnose microaneurysms, hemorrhages, hard exudates, cotton-wool spots, and neovascularization in people with DR [131].

AI has been used in AMD with reports of high detection rates of referable diseases. With success in using color fundus photographs, efforts have focused on utilizing OCT for volumetric quantification of intraretinal and subretinal fluid volumes [132]. Hwang et al. investigated the utility of AI- and cloud-based telemedicine interaction tools for diagnosis and proposed AMD treatment [132]. DL models used OCT images to diagnose AMD with a high degree of accuracy, and treatment recommendations were found to be similar to those of retina specialists [133]. The AI platform's detection accuracy was higher than 90%, superior rates to medical students, and equal to retinal specialists (92.7% and 91.9%) [133]. Yoo et al. investigated the diagnostic accuracy of DL using the combination of fundus photographs and OCT to diagnose AMD. They found this to be superior in accuracy to AI fundus photographs alone and AI OCT alone. DL using both OCT and fundus data outperformed DL using OCT alone and fundus image alone [134]. This finding supports the notion that DL using multimodal imaging could be more accurate than unimodal imaging.

DL models have been used for other novel applications, including OCT angiography images and biomarkers analysis [135, 136]. It has been used to accurately detect pathologies such as choroidal neovascularization, precise quantification of retinal perfusion, and more [135, 136]. Deep learning has been used to predict geographic atrophy areas and growth rates [137]. This study trained the DL network using multimodal imaging (baseline FAF images and OCT volumes) [137]. DL has also been used to accurately segment OCT images in different macular diseases, including GA, DR, and AMD [138–140]. DL has also been used to analyze different fundus photography and OCT biomarkers.

Despite the apparent usefulness of AI and DL models, significant challenges still need to be addressed to the adaptability of this platform to everyday use in clinical practice. Some of the challenges include the deskilling of physicians due to an increase in reliance on automation, the lack of AI programs to assume a comprehensive, holistic approach to clinical encounters with patients, the need for pre-existing robust datasets to train AI programs with, and lack of AI programs to incorporate the ambiguity and variability often encountered in clinical medicine [132]. Other reasons include security, privacy, poor pervasiveness, trust, and explainability concerns [141].

16. Other macular imaging techniques

There are other less-known macular imaging techniques. These include the following:

1. Macula pigment optical density (MPOD) measures the macular pigment, a dietary pigment thought to have a protective role in the retina. The estimated value of macular pigment is known to decrease in patients who suffer from AMD, and this pigment could be protective. Population studies suggest no significant differences in age after excluding patients with AMD. However, lower MPOD could be a risk factor for developing dry AMD [142]. MPOD is much lower in AMD patients than in age-matched healthy controls. Several methods have been proposed for measuring the degree of macular pigment. One of the methods is based on fundus reflectometry, which also features a photodetector for measuring reflectance at different wavelengths and retinal locations. The image of the pigment density can be spatially reconstructed, appearing as color codes [143].

2. Photoacoustic microscopy (PAM) and photoacoustic tomography (PAT) use acoustic detection to image optical absorption contrast with high-resolution deep into scattering tissue [144]. PAT is a three-dimensional (3-D) imaging modality based on the photoacoustic (PA) effect. PAM has been used as a non-contact technique for *in vivo* retina imaging and estimating the retinal vasculature's oxygen saturation [145]. An optical coherence photoacoustic microscopy (OC-PAM) system, which can accomplish optical coherence tomography (OCT) and photoacoustic microscopy (PAM) simultaneously, has also been developed [146]. The principle in PAM is that tissues undergo thermoelastic expansion with a nanosecond pulsed laser beam, releasing a wide-band acoustic wave that can be detected using a high-frequency ultrasound transducer [147]. In PAM, each laser pulse generates a one-dimensional (1-D) photoacoustic image (A-line) along the axial direction. Raster-scanning and piecing together all the A-lines provides a 3-D PA image. Image reconstruction is not required since each signal obtained by the transducer represents a 1-D image of a single line inside the object following minimal signal processing [145]. PAM can simultaneously image anatomical, functional, molecular, flow dynamic, and metabolic contrasts *in vivo* [148]. PAM has been used for macular blood flow imaging in retina vaso-occlusive diseases [149]. Of interest is that PAM has been integrated with adaptive optics for high-resolution retina imaging [150]. The AO-PAM system was used to image single RPE cells in *ex vivo* experiments [150]. The safety of PAM has been demonstrated using preclinical studies in which the laser energy from a PAM equivalent had no adverse effect on the retina [151].

3. Fluorescence lifetime imaging ophthalmoscopy (FLIO) is an emerging, noninvasive imaging modality to investigate the autofluorescence of the human fundus

in vivo. Lipofuscin is a fluorophore in the retinal pigment epithelium, strongly influencing macular autofluorescence. However, other endogenous retinal fluorophores exist. Fundus autofluorescence is characterized by the spatial distribution of the fluorescence intensity or emission spectrum and its characteristic fluorescence lifetime function. The average time a fluorophore remains excited following excitation is referred to as the fluorescence lifetime [152]. Different retinal and macular diseases can influence this FLIO. Diseases such as AMD, diabetic retinopathy, macular telangiectasia type 2, retinitis pigmentosa, and Stargardt disease affect FLIO [153]. In some normal eyes, FLIO changes already exist, suggesting a predisposition or increased risk of developing the disease, while changes in already diseased eyes may suggest progression. Because of its role in early disease detection, it holds promise as a tool for early diagnosis.

17. Conclusion

Imaging of the macula in health and disease has been revolutionized by technological advances and the need to understand disease pathophysiology and evolution, diagnosis, and monitoring outcome of treatment. This evolution in imaging has yielded significant benefits since macular imaging can now be accomplished at even subcellular levels, granting a better understanding of several macular diseases. The quest to integrate higher-resolution imaging and analytics of the macula into routine clinical practice and everyday patient decision-making will result in even more personalization of treatment and improvements in outcomes. Future goals to be accomplished with macular imaging include earlier detection and improved prognostication of disease, prediction of treatment outcome enhancement by imaging, and image-guided treatment for several untreatable inherited retinal diseases.

Already, breakthroughs in cellular imaging using adaptive optics have improved the understanding of inherited retinal diseases and have been used for patient selection in clinical trials, understanding inherited retinal disease natural history, and monitoring the response of genetic and other therapies in clinical trials. It is anticipated that newer and more robust macular imaging will continue to evolve. Multimodal imaging and artificial intelligence will play significant roles in clinical practice and research into macular diseases. As patient care moves from clinics to the comfort of homes, imaging devices such as the home OCT will gain popularity for screening and monitoring the evolution of macular diseases. Expanding the benefits of macular imaging will ultimately result in increased personalization of patient care, improved patient management decision-making, and better treatment outcomes for the patient.

Acknowledgements

We express our gratitude to Dr. Adekunle Hassan for his support in the writing of this manuscript and for contributing images.

Conflict of interest

There are no relevant conflicts of interest to be declared by any of the authors.

DOI: http://dx.doi.org/10.5772/intechopen.1004859

Author details

Ogugua Ndubuisi Okonkwo[1,2*], Chineze Thelma Agweye[3], Toyin Akanbi[2] and Utam Ashibel Utam[4]

1 Department of Ophthalmology, Eye Foundation Hospital and Eye Foundation Retina Institute, Lagos, Nigeria

2 Department of Ophthalmology, Eye Foundation Hospital, Abuja, Nigeria

3 Department of Ophthalmology, University Of Calabar and University of Calabar Teaching Hospital, Calabar, Nigeria

4 Department of Ophthalmology, Tulsi Chanri Foundation Eye Hospital, Abuja, Nigeria

*Address all correspondence to: o_okonkwo@yahoo.com

References

[1] Feibel RM. Looking back at ophthalmic imaging from the first century of the American Journal of Ophthalmology: Photography and ultrasonography. American Journal of Ophthalmology. 2018;**195**:xx-lv. DOI: 10.1016/j.ajo.2018.08.020. Epub 2018 Aug 22

[2] Hildred RB. A brief history on the development of ophthalmic retinal photography into digital imaging. The Journal of Audiovisual Media in Medicine. 1990;**13**(3):101-105. DOI: 10.3109/17453059009055111

[3] Hurtes R. Evolution of ophthalmic photography. International Ophthalmology Clinics. 1976;**16**:1-22

[4] Van Cader TC. History of ophthalmic photography. Journal of Ophthalmic Photography. 1978;**1**:7-9

[5] Bennett TJ, Barry CJ. Ophthalmic imaging today: An ophthalmic photographer's viewpoint - a review. Clinical & Experimental Ophthalmology. 2009;**37**(1):2-13. DOI: 10.1111/j.1442-9071.2008.01812.x. Epub 2009 Sep 23

[6] Meyer-Schwickerath GR. Ophthalmology and photography. American Journal of Ophthalmology. 1968;**66**:1011-1019. DOI: 10.1016/0002-9394(68)90809-X

[7] Saine PJ, Patrick J, Tyler ME. Ophthalmic photographers' society. Fundus Photography Overview. Available from: http://www.opsweb.org/?page5fundusphotography. [Accessed: November 28, 2013]

[8] Choudhry N, Duker JS, Freund KB, et al. Classification and guidelines for widefield imaging: Recommendations from the international widefield imaging study group. Ophthalmology Retina. 2019;**3**:843-849

[9] MacGillivray TJ, Trucco E, Cameron JR, Dhillon B, Houston JG, van Beek EJ. Retinal imaging as a source of biomarkers for diagnosis, characterization and prognosis of chronic illness or long-term conditions. The British Journal of Radiology. 2014;**87**(1040):20130832. DOI: 10.1259/bjr.20130832. Epub 2014 Jun 17

[10] Mishra C, Tripathy K. Fundus Camera. In: StatPearls [Internet]. Treasure Island (FL): StatPearls Publishing; 2023. Available from: https://www.ncbi.nlm.nih.gov/books/NBK585111/ [Accessed: Jul 31, 2023]

[11] Gobel AP, Fleckenstein M, Schmitz Valckenberg S, Brinkmann CK, Holz FG. Imaging geographic atrophy in age-related macular degeneration. Ophthalmologica. 2011;**226**(4):182-190

[12] Peli E, Lahav M. Drusen measurement from fundus photographs using computer image analysis. Ophthalmology. 1986;**93**(12):1575-1580. DOI: 10.1016/s0161-6420(86)33524-3

[13] Lord RK, Shah VA, San Filippo AN, Krishna RJO. Novel uses of smartphones in ophthalmology. Ophthalmology. 2010;**117**(6):1274-.e3

[14] Iqbal U. Smartphone fundus photography: A narrative review. International Journal of Retina and Vitreous. 2021;7:44. DOI: 10.1186/s40942-021-00313-9

[15] Patton N, Aslam TM, MacGillivray T, Deary IJ, Dhillon B, Eikelboom RH, et al. Retinal image analysis: Concepts,

applications and potential. Progress in Retinal and Eye Research. 2006;**25**(1):99-127

[16] Besenczi R, Tóth J, Hajdu A. A review on automatic analysis techniques for color fundus photographs. Computational and Structural Biotechnology Journal. 2016;**14**:371-384. DOI: 10.1016/j.csbj.2016.10.001

[17] Huang F, Lian J, Ng KS, Shih K, Vardhanabhuti V. Predicting CT-based coronary artery disease using vascular biomarkers derived from fundus photographs with a graph convolutional neural network. Diagnostics (Basel). 2022;**12**(6):1390. DOI: 10.3390/diagnostics12061390

[18] Chan YK, Cheng CY, Sabanayagam C. Eyes as the windows into cardiovascular disease in the era of big data. Taiwan Journal of Ophthalmology. 2023;**13**(2):151-167. DOI: 10.4103/tjo.TJO-D-23-00018

[19] Wu JH, Liu TYA. Application of deep learning to retinal-image-based Oculomics for evaluation of systemic health: A review. Journal of Clinical Medicine. 2022;**12**(1):152. DOI: 10.3390/jcm12010152

[20] Tyler ME. Stereo fundus photography: Principles and technique. Journal of Ophthalmic Photography. 1996;**18**:68-89

[21] Hancock R. Stereo imaging in ophthalmology. The Royal Photographic Society. 2020. Available from: https://rps.org/news/groups/medical/2020/stereo-imaging-in-ophthalmology/

[22] Li HK, Hubbard LD, Danis RP, Esquivel A, Florez-Arango JF, Krupinski EA. Monoscopic versus stereoscopic retinal photography for grading diabetic retinopathy severity. Investigative Ophthalmology & Visual Science. 2010;**51**:3184-3192

[23] Delori FC, Dorey CK, Staurenghi G, Arend O, Goger DG, Weiter JJ. In vivo fluorescence of the ocular fundus exhibits retinal pigment epithelium lipofuscin characteristics. Investigative Ophthalmology & Visual Science. 1995;**36**(3):718-729

[24] Yung M, Klufas MA, Sarraf D. Clinical applications of fundus autofluorescence in retinal disease. International Journal of Retina and Vitreous. 2016;**2**:12. DOI: 10.1186/s40942-016-0035-x

[25] Pole C, Ameri H. Fundus autofluorescence and clinical applications. Journal of Ophthalmic & Vision Research. 2021;**16**(3):432-461. DOI: 10.18502/jovr.v16i3.9439

[26] Calvo-Maroto AM, Cerviño A. Spotlight on fundus autofluorescence. Clinical Optometry (Auckl). 2018;**10**:25-32. DOI: 10.2147/OPTO.S134637

[27] Bindewald A, Bird AC, Dandekar SS, et al. Classification of fundus autofluorescence patterns in early age-related macular disease. Investigative Ophthalmology & Visual Science. 2005;**46**:3309Y14

[28] Forte R, Querques G, Querques L, et al. Multimodal imaging of dry age-related macular degeneration. Acta Ophthalmologica. 2012;**90**:e281Y7

[29] Ly A, Nivison-Smith L, Assaad N, Kalloniatis M. Fundus autofluorescence in age-related macular degeneration. Optometry and Vision Science. 2017;**94**(2):246-259. DOI: 10.1097/OPX.0000000000000997

[30] Schmitz-Valckenberg S, Pfau M, Fleckenstein M, Staurenghi G,

Sparrow JR, Bindewald-Wittich A, et al. Fundus autofluorescence imaging. Progress in Retinal and Eye Research. 2021;**81**:100893. DOI: 10.1016/j.preteyeres.2020.100893. Epub 2020 Aug 3

[31] Alten F, Clemens CR, Heiduschka P, Eter N. Characterisation of reticular pseudodrusen and their central target aspect in multi-spectral, confocal scanning laser ophthalmoscopy. Graefe's Archive for Clinical and Experimental Ophthalmology. 2014;**252**:715-721

[32] Tan ACS, Fleckenstein M, Schmitz-Valckenberg S, Holz FG. Clinical application of multicolor imaging technology. Ophthalmologica. 2016;**236**(1):8-18. DOI: 10.1159/000446857

[33] Laatikainen L. The fluorescein angiography revolution: A breakthrough with sustained impact. Acta Ophthalmologica Scandinavica. 2004;**82**(4):381-392. DOI: 10.1111/j.1395-3907.2004.00284.x

[34] Ruia S, Tripathy K. Fluorescein angiography. In: StatPearls [Internet]. Treasure Island (FL): StatPearls Publishing. 2023. Available from: https://www.ncbi.nlm.nih.gov/books/NBK576378/ [Accessed: Feb 22, 2023]

[35] Pieramici DJ, Bressler SB. Fluorescein angiography. In: Berger JW, Fine SL, Maguire MG, editors. Age-Related Macular Degeneration. St. Louis: Mosby; 2005. pp. 219-236

[36] Subfoveal neovascular lesions in age-related macular degeneration. Guidelines for evaluation and treatment in the macular photocoagulation study. Macular Photocoagulation Study Group. Archives of Ophthalmology. 1991;**109**(9):1242-1257

[37] Gass JDM. Stereoscopic Atlas of Macular Diseases: Diagnosis and Treatment. 4th ed. St. Louis: Mosby-Yearbook; 1997

[38] Tripathy K, Chawla R, Sharma YR, Gogia V. Ultrawide field fluorescein angiogram in a family with gyrate atrophy and foveoschisis. Oman Journal of Ophthalmology. 2016;**9**(2):104-106

[39] Yannuzzi LA. Indocyanine green angiography: A perspective on use in the clinical setting. American Journal of Ophthalmology. 2011;**151**(5):745-751.e1

[40] Talks SJ, Aftab AM, Ashfaq I, Soomro T. The role of new imaging methods in managing age-related macular degeneration. The Asia Pacific Journal of Ophthalmology. 2017;**6**(6):498-507

[41] Keane PA, Sim DA, Sadda SR. Advances in imaging in age-related macular degeneration. Current Ophthalmology Reports. 2013;**1**(1):1-11

[42] Muraleedharan S, Tripathy K. Indocyanine green (ICG) angiography. In: StatPearls [Internet]. Treasure Island (FL): StatPearls Publishing; 2023. Available from: https://www.ncbi.nlm.nih.gov/books/NBK580479/ [Accessed: Mar 27, 2023]

[43] Wong RL, Lai TY. Polypoidal choroidal vasculopathy: An update on therapeutic approaches. Journal of Ophthalmic & Vision Research. 2013;**8**(4):359-371

[44] Kokame GT, Omizo JN, Kokame KA, Yamane ML. Differentiating exudative macular degeneration and Polypoidal choroidal vasculopathy using OCT B-scan. Ophthalmology. Retina. 2021;**5**(10):954-961. DOI: 10.1016/j.oret.2021.05.009. Epub 2021 May 19

[45] Slakter JS, Yannuzzi LA, Guyer DR, Sorenson JA, Orlock DA.

Indocyanine-green angiography. Current Opinion in Ophthalmology. 1995;**6**(3):25-32. DOI: 10.1097/00055735-199506000-00005

[46] Mainster MA, Timberlake GT, Webb RH, Hughes GW. Scanning laser ophthalmoscopy. Clinical applications. Ophthalmology. 1982;**89**(7):852-857. DOI: 10.1016/s0161-6420(82)34714-4

[47] Yoshida A. New examination methods for macular disorders–Application of diagnosis and treatment. Nippon Ganka Gakkai Zasshi. 2000;**104**(12):899-942. Japanese

[48] Konno S, Takeda M, Yanagiya N, Akiba J, Yoshida A. Three-dimensional analysis of macular diseases with a scanning retinal thickness analyzer and a confocal scanning laser ophthalmoscope. Ophthalmic Surgery and Lasers. 2001;**32**(2):95-99

[49] MainsterMA, DesmettreT, QuerquesG, Turner PL, Ledesma-Gil G. Scanning laser ophthalmoscopy retroillumination: Applications and illusions. International Journal of Retina and Vitreous. 2022;**8**(1):71. DOI: 10.1186/s40942-022-00421-0

[50] Ranetti AE, Stanca HT, Tăbăcaru B, Teodoru A, Munteanu M, Stanca S. Retromode imaging in age-related macular degeneration. Medicina (Kaunas, Lithuania). 2023;**59**(4):647. DOI: 10.3390/medicina59040647

[51] Wylęgała A, Wozniak P, Sędziak-Marcinek B, Bolek B, Szkodny D, Wylęgała E. Retro-mode in NIDEK Mirante: A comparative analysis with other imaging modalities for AMD and CSR. Diagnostics (Basel). 2023;**13**(17):2846. DOI: 10.3390/diagnostics13172846

[52] Yang Y, Vitale S, Ding Y, O'Connell SR, Alexander J, Bressler NM, et al. A comparison of quantitative mapping and stereoscopic fundus photography grading of retinal thickness in diabetic eyes with macular edema. Ophthalmic Surgery, Lasers & Imaging. 2003;**34**(1):7-16

[53] Goebel W, Franke R. Retinal thickness in diabetic retinopathy: Comparison of optical coherence tomography, the retinal thickness analyzer, and fundus photography. Retina. 2006;**26**(1):49-57. DOI: 10.1097/00006982-200601000-00009

[54] Lai JC, Stinnett SS, Jaffe GJ. B-scan ultrasonography for the detection of macular thickening. American Journal of Ophthalmology. 2003;**136**(1):55-61. DOI: 10.1016/s0002-9394(02)02273-0

[55] Udoh M, Okudo A, Okonkwo ON. Optical coherence tomography and optical coherence tomography angiography biomarkers for age-related macular degeneration and retinovascular diseases. Nigerian Journal of Vitreoretinal Diseases. 2023;**6**(1):1-10. DOI: 10.4103/njvd.njvd_3_23

[56] Al-Mujaini A, Wali UK, Azeem S. Optical coherence tomography: Clinical applications in medical practice. Oman Medical Journal. 2013;**28**(2):86-91

[57] Kashani AH, Chen C, Gahm JK, Zheng F, Richter GM, Philip J. Review of current methods and clinical applications. Progress in Retinal and Eye Research. 2018;**60**:66-100

[58] Gemayel M, Ciulla T. Retinal OCT biomarkers for clinicians and clinical researchers. Retinal Physician. 2021;**18**:28-30

[59] Nawash B, Ong J, Driban M, Hwang J, Chen J, Selvam A, et al. Prognostic optical coherence tomography biomarkers in neovascular age-related macular

degeneration. Journal of Clinical Medicine. 22 Apr 2023;**12**(9):3049

[60] Goździewska E, Wichrowska M, Kocięcki J. Early optical coherence tomography biomarkers for selected retinal diseases—A review. Diagnostics. 2023;**13**(14):2444

[61] Hanson RLW, Airody A, Sivaprasad S, Gale RP. Optical coherence tomography imaging biomarkers associated with neovascular age-related macular degeneration: A systematic review. Eye. 2023;**37**(12):2438-2453

[62] Mitamura Y, Mitamura-Aizawa S, Katome T, Naito T, Hagiwara A, Kumagai K, et al. Photoreceptor impairment and restoration on optical coherence tomographic image. Journal of Ophthalmology. 2013;**2013**:518170

[63] Iaculli C, Barone A, Scudieri M, Palumbo MG, Noci ND. Outer retinal tubulation. Retina. 2015;**35**(10):1979-1984

[64] Huang CH, Yang CH, Hsieh YT, Yang CM, Ho TC, Lai TT. Hyperreflective foci in predicting the treatment outcomes of diabetic macular edema after anti-vascular endothelial growth factor therapy. Scientific Reports [Internet]. 2021;**11**(1):1-9. DOI: 10.1038/s41598-021-84553-7

[65] Tuerksever C, Pruente C, Hatz K. High-frequency SD-OCT follow-up leading to up to biweekly intravitreal ranibizumab treatment in neovascular age-related macular degeneration. Scientific Reports [Internet]. 2021;**11**(1):1-10. DOI: 10.1038/s41598-021-86348-2

[66] Berlin A, Chen L, Messinger J, Ferrara D, Freund KB, Curcio CA. Double-layer sign in neovascular age-related macular degeneration – Do we treat? Acta Ophthalmologica. 2022;**100**(3):348-349

[67] Markan A, Agarwal A, Arora A, Bazgain K, Rana V, Gupta V. Novel imaging biomarkers in diabetic retinopathy and diabetic macular edema. Therapeutic Advances in Ophthalmology. 2020;**12**:1-16

[68] Castro-Navarro V, Monferrer-Adsuara C, Navarro-Palop C, Montero-Hernández J, Cervera-Taulet E. Optical coherence tomography biomarkers in patients with macular edema secondary to retinal vein occlusion treated with dexamethasone implant. BMC Ophthalmology [Internet]. 2022;**22**(1):1-16. DOI: 10.1186/s12886-022-02415-w

[69] Karampelas M, Malamos P, Petrou P, Georgalas I, Papaconstantinou D, Brouzas D. Retinal pigment epithelial detachment in age-related macular degeneration. Ophthalmology and Therapy [Internet]. 2020;**9**(4):739-756. DOI: 10.1007/s40123-020-00291-5

[70] Rispoli M, Eandi CM, Di Antonio L, Kilian R, Montesel A, Savastano MC. Biomarkers in early response to brolucizumab on pigment epithelium detachment associated with exudative age-related macular degeneration. Biomedicines. 10 Jun 2021;**9**(6):668

[71] Cheong KX, Grewal DS, Teo KYC, Gan ATL, Jaffe GJ, Cheung GCM. The relationship between pigment epithelial detachment and visual outcome in neovascular age-related macular degeneration and polypoidal choroidal vasculopathy. Eye [Internet]. 2020;**34**(12):2257-2263. DOI: 10.1038/s41433-020-0803-6

[72] Ly A, Yapp M, Nivison-Smith L, Assaad N, Hennessy M, Kalloniatis M. Developing prognostic biomarkers

in intermediate age-related macular degeneration: Their clinical use in predicting progression. Clinical & Experimental Optometry. 2018;**101**(2):172-181

[73] Schlanitz F, Baumann B, Sacu S, Baumann L, Pircher M, Hitzenberger CK, et al. Impact of drusen and drusenoid retinal pigment epithelium elevation size and structure on the integrity of the retinal pigment epithelium layer. The British Journal of Ophthalmology. 2019;**103**(2):227-232

[74] Klein ML, Ferris FL, Armstrong J, Hwang TS, Chew EY, Bressler SB, et al. Retinal precursors and the development of geographic atrophy in age-related macular degeneration. Ophthalmology. 2008;**115**(6):1026-1031

[75] Suciu CI, Suciu VI, Nicoara SD. Optical coherence tomography (angiography) biomarkers in the assessment and monitoring of diabetic macular Edema. Journal Diabetes Research. 31 Dec 2020:6655021

[76] Coscas F, Cabral D, Pereira T, Geraldes C, Narotamo H, Miere A, et al. Quantitative optical coherence tomography angiography biomarkers for neovascular age-related macular degeneration in remission. PLoS One. 2018;**13**(10):1-13

[77] Spaide RF, Fujimoto JG, Waheed NK, Srinivas SR, Staurenghi G. Optical coherence tomography angiography. Progress in Retinal and Eye Research. Author manuscript; available PMC 2019. 2018;**64**:1-55

[78] Hormel TT, Jia Y. OCT angiography and its retinal biomarkers [invited]. Biomedical Optics Express. 2023;**14**(9):4542

[79] Lv M, Li T, Li Y. Clinical application of optical coherence tomography angiography in diabetic macular edema. African Health Sciences. 2023;**23**(2):484-489

[80] Batıoğlu F, Yanık Ö, Demirel S, Özmert E. Clinical use of optical coherence tomography angiography in retinal diseases. Diagnostics (Basel). 22 May 2023;**13**(10):1820

[81] AttaAllah H, Mohamed A, Ali M. Macular vessels density in diabetic retinopathy: Quantitative assessment using optical coherence tomography angiography. International Ophthalmology. 2019;**39**(8):1845-1859

[82] Krawitz BD, Mo S, Geyman LS, Agemy SA, Scripsema NK, Garcia PM, et al. A circularity index and axis ratio of the foveal avascular zone in diabetic eyes and healthy controls measured by optical coherence tomography angiography. Vision Research [Internet]. 2017;**139**:177-186. DOI: 10.1016/j.visres.2016.09.019

[83] Freiberg FJ, Pfau M, Wons J, Wirth MA, Becker MD, Michels S. Optical coherence tomography angiography of the foveal avascular zone in diabetic retinopathy. Graefe's Archive for Clinical and Experimental Ophthalmology [Internet]. 2016;**254**(6):1051-1058. DOI: 10.1007/s00417-015-3148-2

[84] Shiihara H, Terasaki H, Sonoda S, Kakiuchi N, Shinohara Y, Tomita M, et al. Objective evaluation of size and shape of the superficial foveal avascular zone in normal subjects by optical coherence tomography angiography. Scientific Reports [Internet]. 2018;**8**(1):1-9. DOI: 10.1038/s41598-018-28530-7

[85] Fossataro F, Cennamo G, Montorio D, Clemente L, Costagliola C. Dark halo, a new biomarker in macular neovascularization: Comparison between OCT angiography and

ICGA—A pilot prospective study. Graefe's Archive for Clinical and Experimental Ophthalmology [Internet]. 2022;**260**(10):3205-3211. DOI: 10.1007/s00417-022-05693-8

[86] Pooja P, Stokkermans TJ. Tests for potential vision. In: StatPearls [Internet]. Treasure Island (FL): NCBI Bookshelf; 2023. Available from: https://www.ncbi.nlm.nih.gov/books/NBK587444/

[87] Rodrigues Neto TDS, Silva Neto EDD, Higashi AH, Megnis BP, Haddad MAO, Monteiro MLR, Zacharias LC. Normative data for macular perimetry using the MP-3 microperimeter in healthy individuals. Arquivos Brasileiros de Oftalmologia. 2023;**87**(5):1-7

[88] Crossland M, Jackson M-L, Seiple WH. Microperimetry: A review of fundus-related perimetry. Optometry Reports. 2012;**2**(1):2

[89] Squirrell D, Ehrlich R. The use of macular microperimetry in the assessment and diagnosis of macular disease. Retinal Physician. 2012;**9**:53-57

[90] Huang L, Fields A, Ashimatey BS, Kashani AH. The evolving role of microperimetry. Retina Specialist. 2018;**4**:22-27

[91] Kim L, Madeira MF. Microperimetry. In: EyeWiki [Internet]. San Francisco (CA): EyeWiki; Aug 2023. Available from: https://eyewiki.aao.org/Microperimetry

[92] Rao HL, Hussain RSM, Januwada M, Pillutla LN, Begum VU, Chaitanya A, et al. Structural and functional assessment of macula to diagnose glaucoma. Eye. 2017;**31**:593-600

[93] Gella L, Nittala MG, Raman R. Retinal sensitivity in healthy Indians using microperimeter. Indian Journal of Ophthalmology. 2014;**62**(3):284-286

[94] Dettoraki M, Moschos MM. The role of multifocal electroretinography in the assessment of drug-induced retinopathy: A review of the literature. Ophthalmic Research. 2016;**56**(4):169-177

[95] Reynolds SA. Lesson_are you clear on your macular function screening responsibilities_

[96] Kumar UR, Ramkumar HL. Electroretinogram: EyeWiki [Internet]. American Academy of Ophthalmology. San Francisco (CA): EyeWiki; 2015. p. 1. Available from: https://eyewiki.aao.org/Electroretinogram

[97] Maluri K, Bleau L. Multifocal ERG in practice. Review of Ophtalmology. 2004;**XI**:42-43

[98] Asanad S, Karanjia R. Multifocal Electroretinogram. In: StatPearls [Internet]. Treasure Island (FL): NCBI Bookshelf; 2022. Available from: https://www.ncbi.nlm.nih.gov/books/NBK564322/

[99] Wang J, Song W, Sadlak N, Fiorello MG, Desai M, Yi J. A baseline study of oxygen saturation in Parafoveal vessels using visible light optical coherence tomography. Frontiers in Medicine. 2022;**9**(May):1-7

[100] Türksever C, López Torres LT, Valmaggia C, Todorova MG. Retinal oxygenation in inherited diseases of the retina. Genes (Basel). 2021;**12**(2):1-17

[101] Bojinova RI, Schorderet DF, Valmaggia C, Türksever C, Schoetzau A, Todorova MG. Higher retinal vessel oxygen saturation: Investigating its relationship with macular edema in retinitis pigmentosa patients. Eye [Internet]. 2018;**32**(7):1209-1219. DOI: 10.1038/s41433-018-0043-1

[102] Olafsdottir OB, Hardarson SH, Stefansson E. Retinal oxygen levels are

different in the macula compared to the periphery of the retina. Investigative Ophthalmology & Visual Science. 2018;**59**(9):4657

[103] Yung M, Klufas MA, Sarraf D. Clinical applications of fundus autofluorescence in retinal disease. International Journal of Retina and Vitreous. 2016;**2**(1):1-25

[104] Tsang SH, Sharma T. Fundus autofluorescence. Advances in Experimental Medicine and Biology. 2018;**1085**:15-16

[105] Jalalizadeh R, Durrani AK. Retinal physician - Fundus autofluorescence: An emerging window on the retina [Internet]. Available from: https://www.retinalphysician.com/issues/2013/april-2013/fundus-autofluorescence-an-emerging-window-on-the

[106] Grillo LM, Wang DL, Ramachandran R, Ehrlich AC, De Moraes CG, Ritch R, et al. Thc 24-2 visual field test misses central macular damage confirmed by the 10-2 visual field test and optical coherence tomography. Translational Vision Science & Technology. 2016;**5**(2):4-10

[107] Adelman RA, Pahk P. Visual field defects in Chorioretinal disorders. In: Thomas W, editor. Visual Fields. 3rd ed. New York: Oxford Academic; 2010. pp. 207-232

[108] Novais EA, Baumal CR, Sarraf D, Freund KB, Duker JS. Multimodal imaging in retinal disease: A consensus definition. Ophthalmic Surgery, Lasers & Imaging Retina. 2016;**47**(3):201-205. DOI: 10.3928/23258160-20160229-01

[109] Weissman NJ, Soman P, Shah DJ. Multimodality imaging: Opportunities and challenges. JACC: Cardiovascular Imaging. 2013;**6**(9):1022-1023. DOI: 10.1016/j.jcmg.2013.07.003

[110] Fox K, Achenbach S, Bax J, Cosyns B, Delgado V, Dweck MR, et al. Multimodality imaging in cardiology: A statement on behalf of the task force on multimodality imaging of the European association of cardiovascular imaging. European Heart Journal. 2019;**40**(6):553-558. DOI: 10.1093/eurheartj/ehy669

[111] Acón D, Wu L. Multimodal imaging in diabetic macular edema. Asia-Pacific Journal of Ophthalmology (Philadelphia, PA.). 2018;**7**(1):22-27. DOI: 10.22608/APO.2017504. Epub 2017 Jan 29

[112] Garrity ST, Sarraf D, Freund KB, Sadda SR. Multimodal imaging of non neovascular age-related macular degeneration. Investigative Ophthalmology & Visual Science. 20 Mar 2018;**59**(4):AMD48-AMD64. DOI: 10.1167/iovs.18-24158

[113] Nguyen VP, Zhu T, Henry J, Zhang W, Wang X, Paulus YM. Multimodal in vivo imaging of retinal and choroidal vascular occlusion. Photonics. 2022;**9**(3):201. DOI: 10.3390/photonics9030201. Epub 2022 Mar 21

[114] Yeung L, Lima VC, Garcia P, Landa G, Rosen RB. Correlation between spectral domain optical coherence tomography findings and fluorescein angiography patterns in diabetic macular edema. Ophthalmology. 2009;**116**(6):1158-1167. DOI: 10.1016/j.ophtha.2008.12.063. Epub 2009 Apr 23

[115] Ogbedo E, Chukwuebuka UV, Okonkwo ON. An introduction to adaptive optics. Nigerian Journal of Vitreoretinal Diseases. 2020;**3**(1):19-26. DOI: 10.4103/2222-2222.352613

[116] Morgan JIW, Chui TYP, Grieve K. Twenty-five years of clinical applications

using adaptive optics ophthalmoscopy [invited]. Biomedical Optics Express. 2022;**14**(1):387-428. DOI: 10.1364/BOE.472274

[117] Hampson KM, Turcotte R, Miller DT, Kurokawa K, Males JR, Ji N, et al. Adaptive optics for high-resolution imaging. Nature Reviews Methods Primers. 2021;**1**(1):1-26. DOI: 10.1038/s43586-021-00066-7

[118] Gill JS, Moosajee M, Dubis AM. Cellular imaging of inherited retinal diseases using adaptive optics. Eye (London, England). 2019;**33**(11):1683-1698. DOI: 10.1038/s41433-019-0474-3

[119] Burns SA, Elsner AE, Sapoznik KA, Warner RL, Gast TJ. Adaptive optics imaging of the human retina. Progress in Retinal and Eye Research. 2019;**68**:1-30. DOI: 10.1016/j.preteyeres.2018.08.002

[120] Georgiou M, Kalitzeos A, Patterson EJ, Dubra A, Carroll J, Michaelides M. Adaptive optics imaging of inherited retinal diseases. The British Journal of Ophthalmology. 2018;**102**(8):1028-1035. DOI: 10.1136/bjophthalmol-2017-311328

[121] Rossi EA, Chung M, Dubra A, Hunter JJ, Merigan WH, Williams DR. Imaging retinal mosaics in the living eye. Eye (London, England). 2011;**25**(3):301-308. DOI: 10.1038/eye.2010.221

[122] Talcott KE, Ratnam K, Sundquist SM, et al. Longitudinal study of cone photoreceptors during retinal degeneration and in response to ciliary neurotrophic factor treatment. Investigative Ophthalmology & Visual Science. 2011;**52**:2219-2226

[123] Paques M, Meimon S, Rossant F, Rosenbaum D, Mrejen S, Sennlaub F, et al. Adaptive optics ophthalmoscopy: Application to age-related macular degeneration and vascular diseases. Progress in Retinal and Eye Research. 2018;**66**:1-16. DOI: 10.1016/j.preteyeres.2018.07.001. Epub 2018 Jul 17

[124] Bakker E, Dikland FA, van Bakel R, Andrade De Jesus D, Sánchez Brea L, Klein S, et al. Adaptive optics ophthalmoscopy: A systematic review of vascular biomarkers. Survey of Ophthalmology. 2022;**67**(2):369-387. DOI: 10.1016/j.survophthal.2021.05.012

[125] Ferro Desideri L, Rutigliani C, Corazza P, Nastasi A, Roda M, Nicolo M, et al. The upcoming role of artificial intelligence (AI) for retinal and glaucomatous diseases. Journal of Optometry. 2022;**15**(Suppl. 1):S50-S57. DOI: 10.1016/j.optom.2022.08.001. Epub 2022 Oct 8

[126] Schmidt-Erfurth U, Sadeghipour A, Gerendas BS, Waldstein SM, Bogunović H. Artificial intelligence in retina. Progress in Retinal and Eye Research. 2018;**67**:1-29. DOI: 10.1016/j.preteyeres.2018.07.004. Epub 2018 Aug 1

[127] Balyen L, Peto T. Promising artificial intelligence-machine learning-deep learning algorithms in ophthalmology. Asia-Pacific Journal of Ophthalmology (Philadelphia, PA.). 2019;**8**(3):264-272. DOI: 10.22608/APO.2018479. Epub 2019 May 31

[128] Shah P, Mishra DK, Shanmugam MP, Doshi B, Jayaraj H, Ramanjulu R. Validation of deep convolutional neural network-based algorithm for detection of diabetic retinopathy - Artificial intelligence versus clinician for screening. Indian Journal of Ophthalmology. 2020;**68**(2):398-405. DOI: 10.4103/ijo.IJO_966_19

[129] Krause J, Gulshan V, Rahimy E, Karth P, Widner K, Corrado GS, et al. Grader variability and the importance of reference standards for evaluating

machine learning models for diabetic retinopathy. Ophthalmology. 2018;**125**(8):1264-1272

[130] Bellemo V, Lim ZW, Lim G, Nguyen QD, Xie Y, Yip MYT, et al. Artificial intelligence using deep learning to screen for referable and vision-threatening diabetic retinopathy in Africa: A clinical validation study. The Lancet. Digital Health. 2019;**1**(1):e35-e44. DOI: 10.1016/S2589-7500(19)30004-4. Epub 2019 May 2

[131] Dutt S, Sivaraman A, Savoy F, Rajalakshmi R. Insights into the growing popularity of artificial intelligence in ophthalmology. Indian Journal of Ophthalmology. 2020;**68**(7):1339-1346. DOI: 10.4103/ijo.IJO_1754_19

[132] Kapoor R, Whigham BT, Al-Aswad LA. Artificial intelligence and optical coherence tomography imaging. Asia-Pacific Journal of Ophthalmology (Philadelphia, PA.). 2019;**8**(2):187-194. DOI: 10.22608/APO.201904. Epub 2019 Apr 18

[133] Hwang DK, Hsu CC, Chang KJ, Chao D, Sun CH, Jheng YC, et al. Artificial intelligence-based decision-making for age-related macular degeneration. Theranostics. 2019;**9**(1):232

[134] Yoo TK, Choi JY, Seo JG, Ramasubramanian B, Selvaperumal S, Kim DW. The possibility of the combination of OCT and fundus images for improving the diagnostic accuracy of deep learning for age-related macular degeneration: A preliminary experiment. Medical & Biological Engineering & Computing. 2019;**57**(3):677-687. DOI: 10.1007/s11517-018-1915-z. Epub 2018 Oct 22

[135] Hormel TT, Hwang TS, Bailey ST, Wilson DJ, Huang D, Jia Y. Artificial intelligence in OCT angiography. Progress in Retinal and Eye Research. 2021;**85**:100965. DOI: 10.1016/j.preteyeres.2021.100965. Epub 2021 Mar 22

[136] Kalra G, Zarranz-Ventura J, Chahal R, Bernal-Morales C, Lupidi M, Chhablani J. Optical coherence tomography (OCT) angiolytics: A review of OCT angiography quantitative biomarkers. Survey of Ophthalmology. 2022;**67**(4):1118-1134. DOI: 10.1016/j.survophthal.2021.11.002. Epub 2021 Nov 5

[137] Anegondi N, Gao SS, Steffen V, Spaide RF, Sadda SR, Holz FG, et al. Deep learning to predict geographic atrophy area and growth rate from multimodal imaging. Ophthalmology. Retina. 2023;**7**(3):243-252. DOI: 10.1016/j.oret.2022.08.018. Epub 2022 Aug 28

[138] Spaide T, Jiang J, Patil J, Anegondi N, Steffen V, Kawczynski MG, et al. Geographic atrophy segmentation using multimodal deep learning. Translational Vision Science & Technology. 2023;**12**(7):10. DOI: 10.1167/tvst.12.7.10

[139] Pekala M, Joshi N, Liu TYA, Bressler NM, DeBuc DC, Burlina P. Deep learning based retinal OCT segmentation. Computers in Biology and Medicine. 2019;**114**:103445. DOI: 10.1016/j.compbiomed.2019.103445. Epub 2019 Sep 17

[140] Moraes G, Fu DJ, Wilson M, Khalid H, Wagner SK, Korot E, et al. Quantitative analysis of OCT for neovascular age-related macular degeneration using deep learning. Ophthalmology. 2021;**128**(5):693-705. DOI: 10.1016/j.ophtha.2020.09.025. Epub 2020 Sep 24

[141] Jin K, Ye J. Artificial intelligence and deep learning in ophthalmology: Current

status and future perspectives. Advances in Ophthalmology Practice and Research. 2022;**2**(3):100078. DOI: 10.1016/j.aopr.2022.100078

[142] Hong IH, Jung WH, Lee JH, Chang IB. Macular pigment optical density in the Korean population: A cross sectional study. Journal of Korean Medical Science. 2020;**35**(5):e30. DOI: 10.3346/jkms.2020.35.e30

[143] Christaras D, Ginis H, Pennos A, Mompean J, Artal P. Objective method for measuring the macular pigment optical density in the eye. Biomedical Optics Express. 2019;**10**(7):3572-3583. DOI: 10.1364/BOE.10.003572 [Accessed: November 11, 2023]

[144] Zhou Y, Yao J, Wang LV. Tutorial on photoacoustic tomography. Journal of Biomedical Optics. 2016;**21**(6):61007. DOI: 10.1117/1.JBO.21.6.061007

[145] Hosseinaee Z, Pellegrino N, Abbasi N, Amiri T, Simmons JAT, Fieguth P, et al. In-vivo functional and structural retinal imaging using multiwavelength photoacoustic remote sensing microscopy. Scientific Reports. 2022;**12**(1):4562. DOI: 10.1038/s41598-022-08508-2. Erratum in: Sci Rep. 2022 Mar 29;12(1):5318

[146] Liu X, Liu T, Wen R, Li Y, Puliafito CA, Zhang HF, et al. Optical coherence photoacoustic microscopy for in vivo multimodal retinal imaging. Optics Letters. 2015;**40**(7):1370-1373. DOI: 10.1364/OL.40.001370

[147] Zhang HF, Maslov K, Stoica G, Wang LV. Functional photoacoustic microscopy for high-resolution and noninvasive in vivo imaging. Nature Biotechnology. 2006;**24**(7):848-851. DOI: 10.1038/nbt1220. Epub 2006 Jun 25

[148] Yao J, Wang LV. Photoacoustic microscopy. Laser & Photonics Reviews. 1 Sep 2013;**7**(5). DOI: 10.1002/lpor.201200060

[149] Okonkwo ON, Agweye CT, Akanbi T. Neuroprotection for nonarteritic central retinal artery occlusion: Lessons from acute ischemic stroke. Clinical Ophthalmology. 2023;**17**:1531-1543. DOI: 10.2147/OPTH.S403433

[150] Jiang M, Zhang X, Puliafito CA, Zhang HF, Jiao S. Adaptive optics photoacoustic microscopy. Optics Express. 2010;**18**(21):21770-21776. DOI: 10.1364/OE.18.021770

[151] Li Y, Zhang W, Nguyen VP, Khan NW, Xia X, Wang X, et al. Retinal safety evaluation of photoacoustic microscopy. Experimental Eye Research. 2021;**202**:108368. DOI: 10.1016/j.exer.2020.108368. Epub 2020 Nov 24

[152] Dysli C, Wolf S, Berezin MY, Sauer L, Hammer M, Zinkernagel MS. Fluorescence lifetime imaging ophthalmoscopy. Progress in Retinal and Eye Research. 2017;**60**:120-143. DOI: 10.1016/j.preteyeres.2017.06.005. Epub 2017 Jun 30

[153] Sauer L, Andersen KM, Dysli C, Zinkernagel MS, Bernstein PS, Hammer M. Review of clinical approaches in fluorescence lifetime imaging ophthalmoscopy. Journal of Biomedical Optics. 2018;**23, 9**:1-20. DOI: 10.1117/1.JBO.23.9.091415. Erratum in: J Biomed Opt. 2018 Sep;23(9):1.

Chapter 6

Understanding the Biology in Current Cell and Gene Therapy for Treating Macular Diseases

Tina Guanting Qiu

Abstract

The 21st century ushers us into an information explosive era in modern medicine development. At the cusp of biology and technology convergence, significant advances are being made in the strategic approach toward preventing and treating retinal degeneration and neovascular diseases, in particular of a restoration of macular vision, from new surgical interventions to emerging pharmacotherapies through minimally invasive ocular drug delivery and genetic bio factory, and rapidly evolving retinal gene therapies and cell transplant, which are changing the landscape of retinal therapeutic horizon. Understanding disease physio pathological processes is becoming ever more important for developing and delivering these therapeutic modalities to individual patients with precision; in the light of cell & gene therapy, host-donor interplay is of strategic importance.

Keywords: macular degeneration, stem cell transplant, gene therapy, choroidal ischemia, Bruch's membrane, tissue restoration, stargardts macular degeneration, age-related macular degeneration

1. Introduction

The first retinal gene therapy product, Luxturna for Leber's congenital amaurosis –2 (LCA2) approved in 2017, was built upon the historical success of the human genome project (1990–2003) [1, 2]. Stem cell therapy is a younger cousin; the first creation of human embryonic stem cell (hESC) line in 1998 by James Thompson et al. revolutionized stem cell therapy with the promise of generating unlimited tissue lineage specific cells (donor) for retinal transplant [3, 4]. The eye is an excellent proof of concept (POC) model, for which subretinal space presents an immune privilege site for testing novel regenerative cell & genetic medicine in human conditions. Unlike pharmacotherapy (singular) that targets living cells by inhibiting or activating cell receptor signaling pathways to prevent neuronal cell loss, cell transplant or gene therapies are means to replace the cell loss (RPE or photoreceptor) or correct genetic defect in metabolically compromised cells in a complex diseased environment. In order to achieve clinical success, understanding the donor-host interplays is vital. This chapter will focus on current therapeutic advances in age-related macular degeneration

(AMD) and Stargardts macular degeneration and how the disease state impacts drug discovery and the future development of regenerative medicine.

2. Age-related macular degeneration (AMD)

2.1 Therapeutic advances

AMD is the leading cause of irreversible blindness in western countries in ages over 65-years. It is a multifactorial, slow progressive, and neural degenerative disease, clinically featured with drusen formation in the early stage; as the disease progresses, about 85% of patients progress toward geographic atrophy (GA), an advanced form of AMD (dry type), and 15% end up with choroidal neovascularization (CNV), leading to subretinal fluid or leakage (wet type), which accounts for 90% of vision loss in AMD [5]. In the past 15–20 years, the success of anti-VEGF therapies, from Macugen, Avastin (off-label) to Lucentis, Eylea, Beovu, and the recent approval of Vabysmo (bispecific Faricimab) [6], has revolutionized retinal specialty care for treating retinal angiogenesis pathologies by removing VEGF to prevent such devastating vision loss, caused by wet AMD, diabetic macular edema, retinal vein occlusion, and CNV secondary to other retinal diseases such as myopia and polypoidal choroidal vasculopathy (**Figure 1**). However, 1/3 to 2/3 of CNV lesions gradually evolve (switch) to

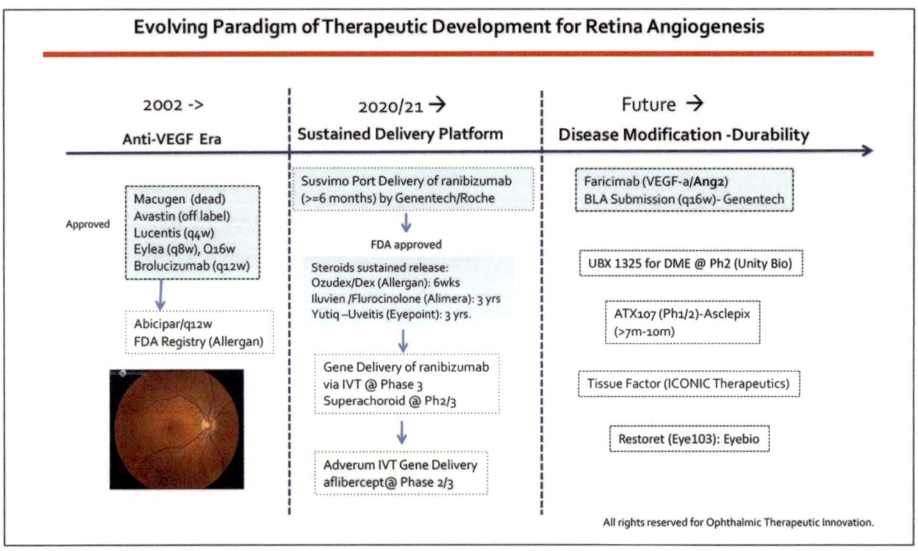

Figure 1.
Highlights anti-VEGF therapeutic development for treating retinal angiogenesis, from the first generation Macugen, Avastin (off-label) and Lucentis to current standard care of Eylea and Faricimab, which was recently approved by FDA for treating wAMD, DME and RVO. Brolucizumab is the smallest anti-VEGF drug approved by FDA in 2019, due to sight threatening vasculitis and endophthalmitis (rare cases), it did not become the market dominance as anticipated. The centra column represents sustained release drug delivery system, including Suvismo, ranibizumab in port delivery system, and Ozudex, Iluvien, and Yutiq which delivers steroid from 6 months to 3 years. Tyrosine kinase inhibitors (TKI) are being actively studied in sustained release delivery formula for treating wAMD and retinal angiogenesis. Due to the ceiling effect of anti-VEGF therapy, there is an unmet need for new pathway based therapies to address subretinal inflammatory scarring and prevent photoreceptor loss, such as UBX1325 (Unity bio), ATX 107 (Asclepix), Restoret (Eyebio) etc. FDA approved products are showed in blue box. All rights reserved @ 2023 Dr. Tina Guanting Qiu.

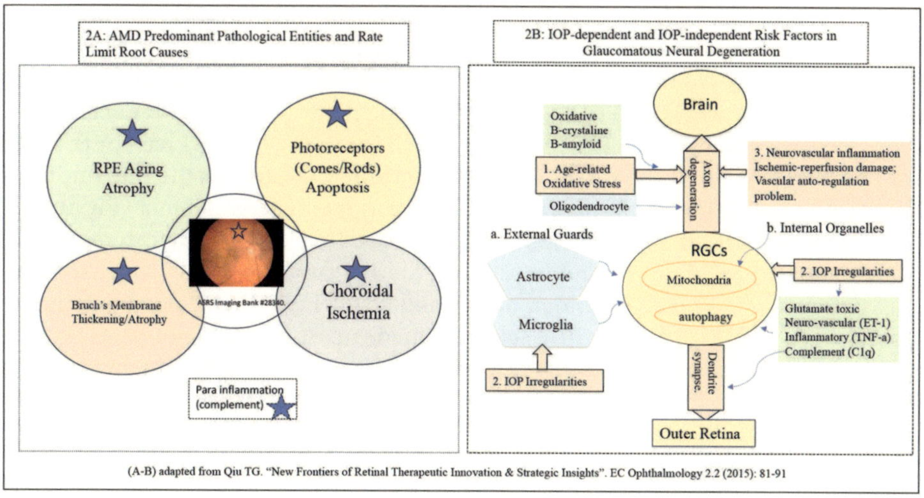

Figure 2.
Provides diagrams illustrating the rate limit disease root causes in AMD and glaucoma respectively. A) Illustrates the four key possible rate limit root causes associated with dry AMD: RPE aging oxidative damage, Bruch's membrane thickening, or atrophic thinning, choroidal ischemia and cone photoreceptor driven photoreceptor cell loss (unknown reasons). Recent clinical trials of C3 inhibitor (pegcetacoplan) and C5 inhibitor (Avacincaptad pegol) showed that removing subretinal inflammation did not stop but only slowed down GA growth rate at about 20% at 24 months, suggesting that complement inflammation or Para inflammation is not the rate limit root cause of GA secondary to AMD. B) Summarizes the IOP dependent and IOP independent risk factors contributing to the retinal ganglion cell death (apoptosis) in glaucoma including hypertensive glaucoma and normal tensive glaucoma (subset). All rights reserved @ 2015, 2023 Dr. Guanting Tina Qiu [7, 8].

less VEGF-dependent pathological entities with subretinal inflammatory or fibrotic scarring, surrounded by macular ischemia associated with the underneath choroidal microcapillary dropout or atrophy, which is similar to a GA lesion. In this sense, Wet AMD and GA represent a spectrum of AMD disease progression at a different time. The physio–pathological root causes associated with AMD can be categorized as RPE aging, Bruch's membrane thickening or atrophy, choroidal ischemia, photoreceptor loss by intricate metabolic abnormalities, and neuroinflammation or para-inflammation such as complement imbalance (**Figure 2A**) [7]. Recent development of the C3 inhibitor (e.g., Syfovre by Apellis Pharma) and C5 inhibitor (e.g., Izervay by Iveric Bio) has demonstrated that complement inhibition by Syfovre or Izervay can slow down GA progression by about 20% and reduce vison loss at some degrees [9]. This is an exciting and first step that we have a viable therapeutic drug to offer to GA patients other than vitamin supplement. Other pathway-based therapies such as removing N-retinylidene-N-retinylethanolamine (A2E, Gildeuretinol @Ph3 by Alkeus Pharma) and integrin modulation (Risuteganib@ Ph2b/3 by Allegro Pharma) are also being actively explored for treating early and intermediate AMD.

2.2 Rate limit root causes in AMD

Complement therapy has taught us that removing subretinal para inflammation is not sufficient to stop the disease progression in AMD. We also have learned that from real world evidence of Rescula eye drops in treating small subset refractory glaucoma. Rescula is a B-K channel activator [10], and it acts by tightening the gate to block inflammatory molecules from entering into the anterior chamber, which alleviates active metabolic or para inflammation at the trabecular meshwork ™; however, it cannot treat or remove the existing pathological processes that cause uncontrolled intraocular pressure (IOP), because Rescula does not have the right mechanism of action (MOA) to repair the existing damage to the TM. Recent discoveries by Dr. GQ Qiu (PCT application No.: 18/356,874. 2023) has for the first time shed light on the pressure sensor (dysfunction or failure) as the rate limit root cause of IOP diurnal irregularities or failure in patients with glaucoma (**Figure 2B**) [7, 8]. She also found that matrix metalloproteinase (MMP) therapy can rejuvenate TM by removing ECM debris and improving the TM functionality, ultimately leading to patients being on an extended drug holiday, during which period patients preserve vision [8, 11, 12]. Pressure sensor is made up of two integral parts of Schlemn's canal endothelium (sensing cells) and its underlying basement membrane (BM) in trabecular meshwork ™; their roles in TM outflow drainage share in common with RPE and Bruch's membrane as a blood retina barrier and a water pump in the retina health. Micro pulse laser retinal rejuvenation (2RT) in drusen resolution in early-stage AMD is a clinical validation that Bruch's membrane aging is a rate limit root cause [8]. Unlike the avascular TM outflow drainage system, retina has two vascular circulation systems and the complex neural circuitry; patients with GA or AMD undergo Muller glial driven subretinal remodeling processes, and the rate limit root causes of AMD could be much more complicated than Bruch's membrane aging problem alone (thickening, rigidity, atrophy). For example, choroidal ischemia within the macular area has received increasing attention as a rate limit to hRPE graft survival and genetic transfer as bottleneck challenges. Any effective treatment has to be able to remove the rate limit root causes in order to truly prevent and stop the disease from deterioration toward the end stage with irreversible vision loss [13].

3. Stargardt's macular degeneration (STGD)

3.1 Genetic epidemiology and clinical features

Stargardt's macular degeneration was first recognized in 1909 by Stargardts, who described 7 patients with recessive inherited macular dystrophy; later Franceschetti coined the term as fundus flavimaculatus (FFM) [14]. It is a single ABCA4-gene-mutant autosomal recessive form of juvenile macular degeneration that occurred 1 in 10,000 population, the most prevalent inherited macular degeneration, which is diagnosed during the first 1–2 decades, or the early 50s in late onset disease. It is estimated of 65,000 patients in the US/EU, less prevalent than retinitis pigmentosa. Clinically, it features as progressive center macular visual loss, central scotoma, and delayed dark adaptation. ABCA4 gene mutation causes RPE and photoreceptor cell loss (apoptosis) as a result of toxic A2E accumulation primarily at the RPE level. In ophthalmic clinical exams, STGD patients have distinguished macular atrophy and yellow-white flecks at the posterior pole on color fundus photography (**Figure 3**) [14, 15]. Fluorescein angiography (FA) sometimes shows "dark" choroid in the macular area, possibly related to significant A2E deposits at the RPE level that absorbs the blue fluorescence light and its underlying choroidal capillary loss or ischemia (non or poor perfusion). SD-OCT

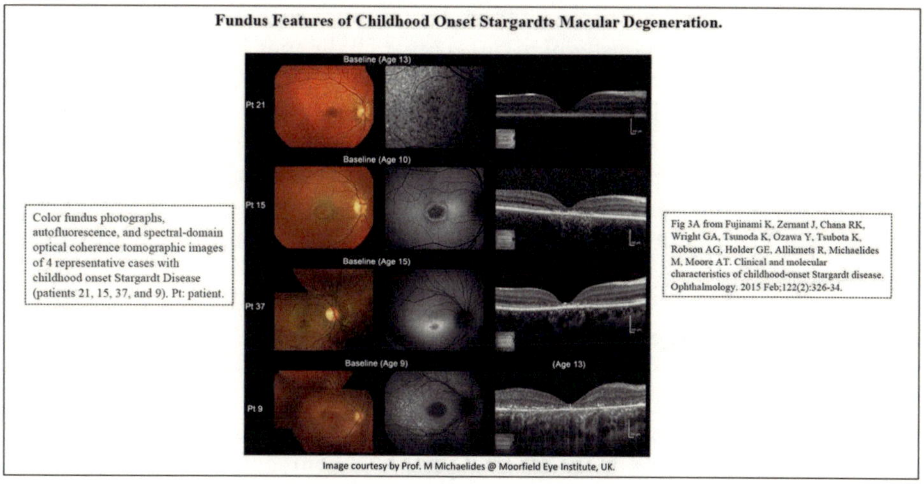

Figure 3.
Fundus features of childhood onset Stargardts macular degeneration in 4 representative cases (patients 21, 15, 37, and 9). Patient 21 has numerous flecks at the posterior pole without central atrophy (fundus grade: 2) and autofluorescence (AF) imaging demonstrates widespread multiple foci of high and low AF signal at the posterior pole with a heterogeneous background (AF type 2). SD-OCT identifies marked outer retinal loss at the central macula. Patient 15 has central atrophy without flecks (fundus grade: 3a) and AF imaging demonstrates a localized low AF signal at the fovea with a high signal edge surrounded by a homogeneous background (AF type: 1). SD-OCT detects marked outer retinal loss at the central macula. Patient 37 has central atrophy with macular flecks (fundus grade: 3b) and a localized low AF signal at the fovea surrounded by a homogeneous background with perifoveal foci of high signal (AF type: 1). SD-OCT shows outer retinal loss at the central macula. Patient 9 has central atrophy with peripheral flecks extending anterior to the vascular arcades (fundus grade: 3b) and a localized low AF signal at the macula surrounded by a heterogeneous background and widespread foci of high AF signal extending anterior to the vascular arcades (AF type: 2). SD-OCT reveals outer retinal disruption at the macula. Pt = patient. A) From Ref. [14]. Image courtesy by prof. M Michaelides (open access article under the CC BY license: http://creativecommons.org/licenses/by/3.0/).

shows progressive choroidal capillarity atrophy underneath the macular over time. By the age of 50 years old, a majority of patients become legally blind.

3.2 Initial attempts and lessons learned

Gene replacement is a preferable choice for treating STGD, and early treatment warrants better vision preservation. However, ABCR4 gene is a large gene with 6.8kd, which exceeds the maximal of adeno-associated virus (AAV) gene payload (5.0 kb). Between 2010 and 2017, Sanofi Aventis/Oxford Biomedical conducted the first lentiviral-ABCA4 gene replacement (StarGen/SAR422459) clinical trials (Ph1/2a), which did not achieve measurable visual functional improvement across low-, mid-, and high-dose cohorts in a total of 26 patients; hence, the company did not proceed to Ph2b/3 clinical trials [16–18]. The first retinal gene therapy success (voretigene neparvovec or Luxturna) was not by a chance; AAV2-RPE65 gene transfection into the RPE monolayer in LCA2 is relatively easier in comparison, and clinical endpoints (mobility score and retinal sensitivity test) are feasible and practical at a relatively lower bar to the end-stage terminally ill-sighted patients. On the other hand, ABCA4 gene codes for the photoreceptor outer segment disc protein (rim protein) [15]. In a diseased setting, subretinal Muller glial cell remodeling entangles the remaining photoreceptor soma and inner segment [19]. No photoreceptor outer segment remains, which poses great challenges for genetic transfection toward a wrapped photoreceptor (hibernating cones) in the form of cell clusters or islands, never mentioned of reconstructing the outersegment discs where the rim proteins reside. Using the remaining RPE (ectopic gene therapy) to produce the rim protein may not be sufficient to rescue the photoreceptors with inherited genetic abnormalities. In order to succeed, surgical delivery parameter design and endpoint measures require in-depth surgical and medical expertise along with meticulous study planning.

3.3 Challenges for a large gene delivery

AAV-based mini-gene (Iveric Bio), dual AAV (Biogen), RNA, and nanoparticle-based genetic delivery (Saliogen) are actively being explored for treating STGD1; however, these technologies so far have not yielded encouraging results. The gene transfer efficiency in animal models is fairly low (less than 50%), and there seems still a long way to go. For other large gene-mutated IRD, such as Retinitis pigmentosa-1 (RP1, 7 kb), RP25 (2.0 Mb), and MYO7A/usher1B (7.0 kb), the field faces a similar challenge. Gene editing potentially could be an alternative; however, the low editing efficiency of the current CRISPR technology remains a bottleneck hurdle [20] . Pharmacotherapy by removing A2E is also being studied for STGD1 in phase 2/3 clinical trials with a promise (Alkeus Pharma, Belite Bio) [21]. Once a patient passes a therapeutic window where little photoreceptor and RPE remain at the central macular region, cell replacement and optogenetic gene delivery may offer better alternatives. In 2012–2017, Advanced Cell Technology (now Astellas Pharma) tested their first

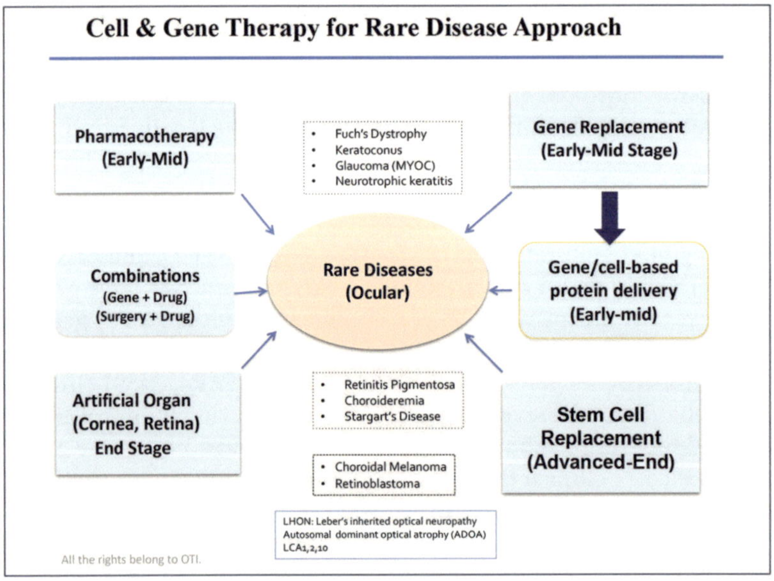

Figure 4.
Provides an overview of rare genetic disease approach, in principle, early intervention through gene replacement therapy in combination with pharmacological treatments are the key for preventing vision loss in inherited retinal disease or eye diseases. When disease advances to late stage or end stage where there are limited photoreceptor and RPE cells remained, artificial retina, cell transplant and optogenetic gene therapy offer alternative new hope. All rights reserved @ 2023 Dr. Guanting Tina Qiu.

hESC-hRPE line (MA09-hRPE) in 12 patients with end-stage STGD in Ph1/2 clinical trials, which provided the first glimpse of hESC-derived RPE cell behaviors and its interplay with the host in patients with end-stage macular degeneration [4, 22].

3.4 Holistic approach to complex problems

From early-stage disease intervention to late-stage cell replacement, we need to take a holistic approach in order to develop better strategies to treat a terminally ill inherited retinal disease such as STGD and RP, namely through combinations of pharmacotherapy with gene replacement or photoreceptor/hRPE transplant to address the underlying disease pathologies such as choroidal ischemia. **Figure 4** illustrates Cell & Gene Therapy Approach to Rare Genetic Disease in the eye care space. In principle, gene replacement needs to intervene early, whereas hRPE/photoreceptor transplant or Optogenetic treatment targets the advanced stage of AMD or STGD. Pharmacotherapy needs to gear toward disease staging and phenotypic pathological entities; for example, a STGD patient has extensive inflamed A2E depositions in the subretinal space, and a RP patient has extremely poor vascular circulation featuring ischemia inflammation (vascular sheath). A choroideremia patient suffers significant choroidal ischemia. These pathological entities pose significant inherited technical challenges for successful gene transfer and graft survival in transplant settings. Biogen failed CHM and XLRP gene therapy programs at pivotal phase 3 clinical trials in 2021, which could be attributed to such bottleneck hurdles, and clinical surgical delivery parameter design with improved tactics may or may not be able to circumvent.

4. Gene therapy for IRD and drug delivery bio factory

4.1 An evolving paradigm of retinal gene therapy

Since the first human genome project in 1990, Spark Therapeutics led by Prof. Jean Bennett and Dr. Katherine High has successfully developed the first retinal gene therapy, Luxturna (approved in late 2017), to treat LCA2 caused by RPE65 mutation, an early onset of RP with severe retinal photoreceptor and RPE degeneration. This success marks the beginning of gene therapy for retina and paves a clinical regulatory path forward; most importantly, it has validated AAV viral vector clinical safety and gene transfer efficiency in a diseased setting. Currently, there are hundreds of AAV-based gene therapies in clinical trials; dozens of AAV-based retinal gene therapies, including gene editing for IRD (CHM, LCA1, LCA10, STGD, achromatopsia, LCA5), are also in clinical trials, with XLRP being at the most advanced stage of phase 3 clinical development (Janssen Pharma/MeriaTGx, Syncona/AGTC). Using AAV-mediated protein delivery of therapeutic drugs, such as anti-VEGF, and complement factors are also being explored by Adverum, RegenxBio and Gyroscope/Novartis through subretinal, intravitreal, and suprachoroidal delivery routes in patients with wet AMD and GA, respectively. Optogenetic is another form of genetic medicine that uses genetic engineering to deliver photosensitive protein (e.g., channelrhodopsin) to the retinal ganglion cells or bipolar cells, for the purpose of replacing the photosensitive function of photoreceptors lost in the advanced disease of RP, AMD, or STGD [23]. GenSight Bio and Nanoscope have first reported encouraging results in early-stage clinical trials in patients with end-stage RP. **Figure 5** highlights an evolving paradigm of genetic medicine.

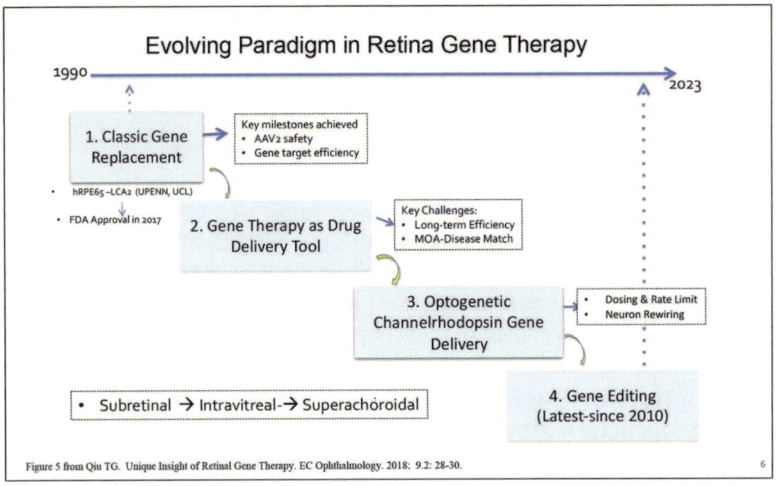

Figure 5.
Shows that retinal gene therapy has evolved from the classic gene replacement therapy (Luxtuna approved in 2017) to genetic based drug or protein delivery (bio factory) and optogenetic gene therapy to the latest gene editing technology. Gene delivery also has expanded from subretinal injection to office-based intravitreal injection and suprachoroidal gene delivery via microneedle (Clearside bio). So far, Luxtuna is the only FDA approved gene therapy product for retina. All rights reserved @ 2018 Dr. Guanting Tina Qiu,

4.2 Recent setbacks

In 2021, Biogen/Nightstar's two leading gene therapy programs: cotoretigene toliparvovec (BIIB112) for XLRP @ Ph2/3 and timrepigene emparvovec (BIIB111/AAV2-REP1) for choroideremia (CHM) @ Phase 3, did not meet clinical endpoints [24–26], which was quite unexpected and became the first awakening call to the field. In 2022, ProQR's Sepofarsen phase 3 RNA therapy for treating LCA10 with CEP290 p.Cys998X mutation also failed to meet the primary endpoint, despite that Ph2 clinical trials showed very promising results [27]. Editas Medicine recently also announced a pause of the world's first gene editing program using an *in vivo* CRISPR/Cas9 editing technology (EDIT-101 @ Ph ½) for treating LCA10 with CEP 290 mutation, because of gene editing efficiency issues. Theoretically, classic gene replacement for IRD should have high success in clinical translation, especially in phase 3 clinical trials if phase 2 study results are positive. In order to nail down the disease root cause, one must think outside the box with the right mindset and holistic approach; specifically, one has to understand the host pathological environment and its interplay between donor (genes) and targeted cells.

4.3 Understanding the host environment

First, one should view gene therapy as a cell tissue transplant; genetic medicine has to work through host tissue cells, not a singular play like anti-VEGF drugs removing excessive proteins in the retina and vitreous cavity, which does not require host cells to do additional work. Gene transfer involves high energy consumption of living cells with metabolic competence. Secondly, genetic delivery differs from protein/drug delivery; it requires high concentration viral particles per targeted cell (1e6:1 ratio) at a given time (millisecond). Inner limiting membrane (ILM) and/or external limiting membrane (ELM) become a rate limit barrier for most AAV viral vector penetrating through the sensory retina (at speed and quantity) toward the RPE layer from the intravitreal delivery route. Subretinal gene delivery is limited to a small size of bleb area being rescued, thus affecting the long-term durability [28]. Thirdly, retinal remodeling in IRD involves significant Muller glial scar formation (details see next section). Fourthly, choroidal ischemia in IRD presents significant challenges for gene transfer, especially to the photoreceptor cells that completely depend upon its underlying choroidal capillary network to supply oxygen and nutrients. Functional compensation through adaption is limited in IRD patients.

4.4 Suprachoroidal gene delivery via microneedle

It represents a new direction for future gene delivery, which has only been validated as a bio factory drug delivery of anti-VEGF or complement factor. In order to produce sufficient proteins, targeted genes are often ubiquitous to multiple cell types (RPE and vascular endothelium or Muller glial). For specific gene transfer toward RPE or photoreceptor, superachoroidal delivery route has not been tested for its clinical efficiency in IRD patients, though preclinical evidence points toward extensive gene transfection to the photoreceptor cells and RPE layers in healthy pig models. In principle, gene transfer is easier to the monolayer RPE than multi-layer photoreceptors, which often form cluster islands in a diseased condition. In retinal degenerative condition, when photoreceptors (rods) die, it triggers Muller glial proliferation and migration, extending its

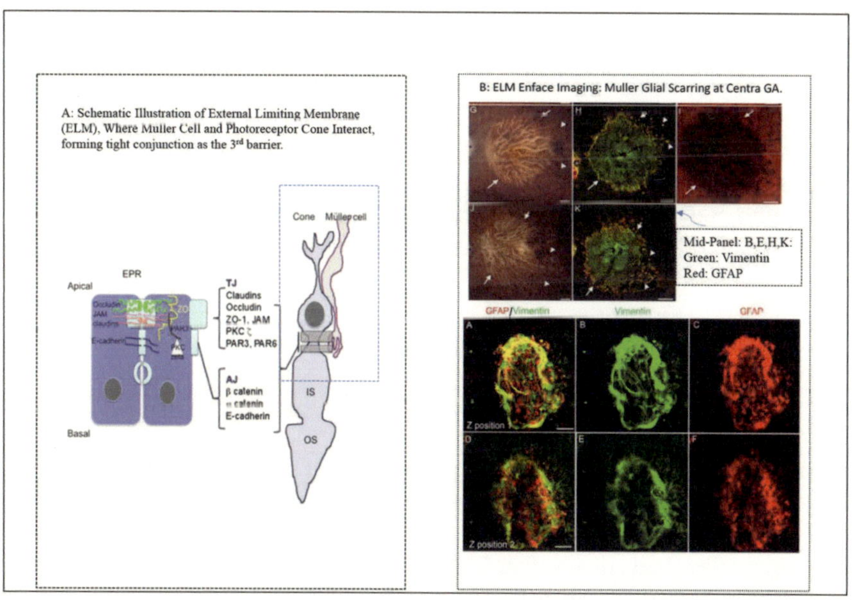

Figure 6.
(A-B): A) Shows a diagram of Muller glia and cone photoreceptor forming external limiting membrane (ELM) as the 3rd barrier of gene delivery toward the RPE and outer layer of the retina in human eye. B) Shows Muller glial scarring occupies and circles around the ELM platform, where remaining hibernating cone photoreceptor cells form islands or clusters, and being wrapped by the static Muller glial scars as the result of subretinal remodeling in patients suffering from aged related macular degeneration. A) From Ref. [29]. Copyright © 2010 Omri et al., publisher and licensee dove medical press ltd. (open access under a creative commons attribution-NonCommercial-NoDerivatives 4.0 international license). B) Is from Ref. [30]. Copyright @ 2017 the authors. Re-use of fig B is at the courtesy of ARVO journal under a creative commons attribution-NonCommercial-No derivatives 4.0 international license. (http://creativecommons.org/licenses/by/3.0/).

processes toward defected RPE layer to "repair or amend" blood-retinal barrier. During the course, Muller glial entangles with the remaining cones and disrupts ELM integrity, where the cone and Muller cell are in a parallel and hand-in-hand relation (**Figure 6**) [29–31]. Additionally, bipolar and amacrine often migrate toward the outer layer of the retina by taking residence where the rods were lost. In response to the injuries, microglial and macrophages are mobilized to clean up the dying or dead cell debris. One could imagine that the subretinal microenvironment is very harsh in GA or STGD patients. When we design clinical trials for a given gene therapy, the doing and surgical delivery parameters are some of the key considerations, surgeons begin to learn to navigate around these disease pathological entities in each individual eye, in order to achieve desirable clinical outcome.

4.5 Technical challenges for future development

While the field holds exciting promises, we must realize that gene therapy is still at a very early stage, even for basic AAV-mediated gene replacement for treating diseases, such as XLRP, CHM, and LCA1. Current technology has not been able to help patients to regain vision in a way that they can live independently. The only exception perhaps is LUMEVEQ, an AAV-mediated gene therapy for treating Leber's hereditary optic neuropathy (LHON ND4), a rare mitochondrial disease causing a sudden RGC cell loss in teens and young adults, and 98% of patients are bilateral with acute onset. The Ph2 and Ph3 clinical trials of LUMEVEQ have shown improvement in more than three lines, and patients have been able to back to school and engage in sports [32]. This case suggests that the host cell metabolic health determines the gene therapy outcome. Acute disease has better prognosis than chronic IRD. Genetic bio factory targeting AMD and DME will achieve better clinical outcomes than neural protection via gene transfer in chronic IRD with severe pathological conditions. In the future, we need more potent and safer viral vectors to enable office-based genetic medicine delivery, such as intravitreal or superachoroidal delivery via microneedles (Clearside Bio). Also, we need to develop novel genetic engineering technologies that will allow one genetic product to treat more than one gene mutations (gene agnostic approach).

5. Stem cell therapy for macular degeneration

5.1 Key problems

In transplant medicine, the quantity and quality of donor cells are of prerequisite condition. In retinal transplantation, the reconstruction of neural circuitry presents the most formidable challenge. Decades of scientific and clinical research efforts spending on fetal retinal sheet transplant have taught us many great lessons on this topic. For RPE suspension, selecting an appropriate cell seeding density (total dose needs to be based on the lesion size) is the key tactic to ensure a rapid graft survival without causing excessive metabolic burden to the remaining host RPE. Similar to cornea endothelium transplant (Aurion Bio) [33], hESC-RPE cell possesses its embryonic or intricate capacity to self-assembly, forming a monolayer RPE at the basement membrane following the subretinal transplantation in patients with GA; OpRegen transplant has demonstrated long-term survival (3–5 years) and visual functional improvement corresponding with the anatomic recovery, such as ELM reconstruction. The poor health of Bruch's membrane (BM), choroidal ischemia within the macular area, subretinal Muller glial scar, as well as local immune-inflammation are the four key prognostic factors in the host retina, which affect graft survival rate [4]. In a preclinical rat model of retinal degeneration, E17-derived rat retinal progenitor cell suspension transplant also showed its intricate embryonic competence to self-reorganize and form multilayer laminal sheet without the need for extracellular matrix scaffolding [34].

5.2 hESC-derived hRPE transplant

hESC or induced pluripotent stem cell or iPSC-derived hRPE cell lines will become the mainstay hRPE donor cell for treating macular degeneration. One of the key criteria of an ideal donor hRPE cell line is to obtain proficient biological competence from a short-term *in vitro* cell manipulation process; the cell biological competence should be equivalent to the native fetal hRPE cells. However, OpRegen hRPE transplant medicine is changing our views of what is possible and what additional capabilities may be required. In order to survive through a harsh subretinal environment in GA setting, the grafted young hRPE cells will need to remove subretinal inflammation, unwrap the metabolically hibernating cones from Muller glial entanglements, and refurbish atrophic Bruch's membranes. OpRegen hRPE cell line has demonstrated its superior therapeutic benefits in early-stage clinical trials in patients with GA (Ph1/2a), for example, blood-retinal repair and macular tissue restoration (PCT Publication No.: 2021/242788A1) [35].

The clinical regulatory path for hESC- or iPSC-derived hRPE or human photoreceptor progenitor cell line validation differs from conventional drug development. The first hESC-derived RPE line, MA09-hRPE has been studied in 38 human subjects

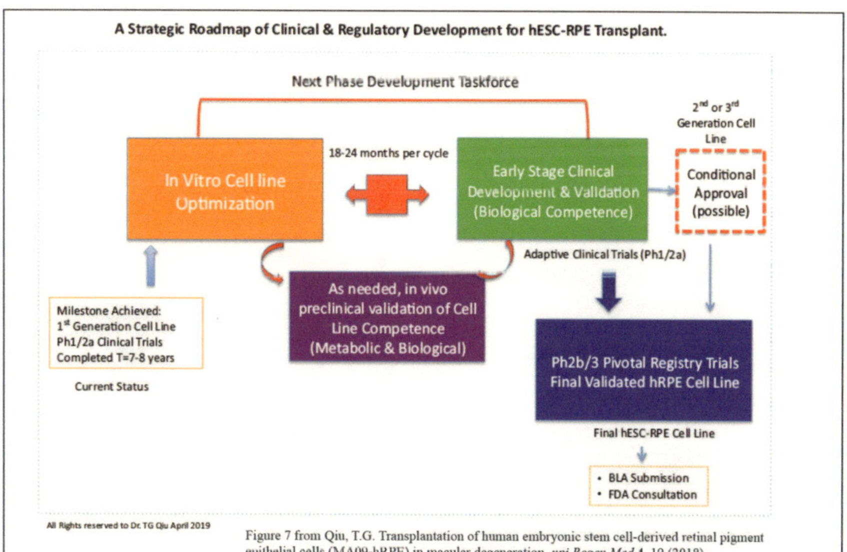

Figure 7.
Provides a strategic roadmap of clinical and regulatory development of hESC or iPSC derived RPE or photoreceptors as well as other lineage restricted cells for treating retinal degeneration or other human conditions, it may require back and forth between petri dish experimentation and early stage clinical studies in a small scale to validate the donor cell biological competences before moving toward pivotal clinical trials. All rights reserved @ 2019 author (Qiu GT).

for up to 10 years now; there is no report of tumorigenesis. OpRegen has been studied in 25 patients for up to 6 years; there is no tumorigenesis reported. The ethical issue of using human ESC has a clearance. The key technical hurdle lies ahead of the cell biological competence, which could take many years to fine tune for its clinical proficiency. **Figure 7** provides a brief summary of the hRPE cell line selection and validation process, between *in vitro* and Ph1/2 clinical trials in patients, through short cycle and small size clinical studies (Ph1/2). Most *in vitro* cultural-created hESC-hRPE lines lack biological competence; for example, MA09-hRPE only comprises 40–50% of genetic and protein profiles overlapping with native fetal human RPE cells. Astellas Institute of Regenerative Medicine is validating their 2nd generation hRPE line at the Ph1/2 stage (**Figure 8**) [4].

5.3 Photoreceptor transplantation and cell reprogramming

hESC- or iPSC-derived photoreceptor progenitor transplant is largely at the preclinical stage. State-of-the-art research conducted by Prof. Robin Ali at Kings College London in collaboration with Prof. James Bainbridge at UCL in England has shed light on the possibility of generating cone photoreceptors from pluripotent ESC cell lines through 3D retinal organoids *in vitro* cultural systems; the *in vivo* transplant experiment in mice degeneration model also demonstrated extensive material transfer between grafted cells (cones) and host retinal cells, suggesting possible neural protection benefit [36]. Generating commercial-scale donor cell sources remains the key challenge for successful clinical translation. These technical hurdles have driven scientists and clinicians to seek *in situ* regenerative approach via small molecule or genetic stimulation to the Muller glial at the ciliary margin zone or peripheral retina [37]. In 2009, Dr. Qiu first demonstrated that adult human

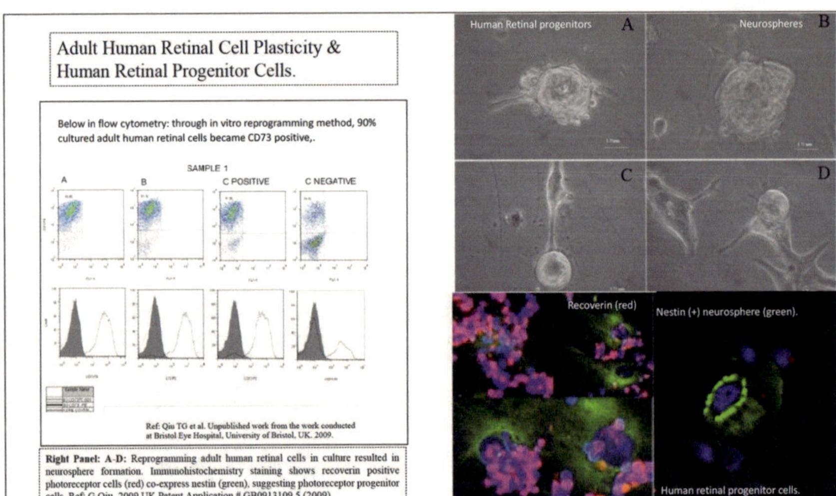

Figure 8.
(L-R): Left panel shows adult human retinal cells isolated from post-mortem human eyes are able to be reprogrammed in vitro cultural condition and regenerate clusters of neurospheres containing photoreceptor lineage specific progenitor cells, expressing nestin (green) and recoverin (red), showed in immunohistochemical assays. Right panel: Flow cytometry further confirmed that majorities of reprogrammed human retinal cells (90%) are possible photoreceptor lineage cells expressing CD73 biomarker, in correspondence with the results from immunohistochemical assays. This is the first time to challenge the century dogma of post mitotic human retinal cell plasticity. All rights @ 2009 author (Qiu GT).

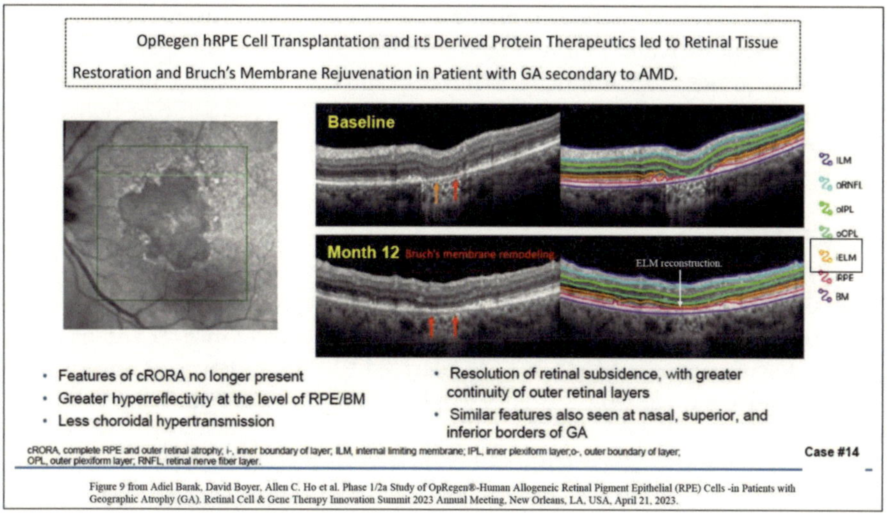

Figure 9.
(L-R). Shows an example of a female patient with GA/AMD receiving OpRegen hRPE transplant in her left eye, the grafted cells can self-assemble forming a monolayer RPE at GA lesion area and refurbish its underlying Bruch's membrane with increased elasticity, her BCVA gained more than 2 lines at 12 months post-transplant. Left panel is AF imaging showing a large well demarcated GA lesion. Right panel is SD-OCT imaging of a section line at the GA border showing the structure improvement and tissue restoration at 12 months post-transplant compared to the baseline. Specifically, reconstructing the integrity and continuity of the ELM is seen at 12-month, labeled in orange line on SD-OCT. the ELM integrity is corresponding to the functional BCVA gain. Image courtesy by lineage cell therapeutics, USA.

retinal cells can be reprogrammed, forming retinal neurospheres and expressing photoreceptor progenitor surface markers (recoverin + nestin co expression), which for the first time challenged the century-old dogma of adult human retinal plasticity (G Qiu, UK Patent Application No. GB0913109.5) [38–40]. Twelve years later, Lineage Cell Therapeutics first demonstrated photoreceptor cell regeneration following the subretinal transplantation of OpRegen hRPE cell (with high therapeutic potency) in patients with GA secondary to AMD; four patients were reported to have macular tissue restoration and 8–10 letters of BCVA gains. **Figure 9** provides an example of *in vivo* cell reprograming of retinal cells in a patient with GA following transplantation of OpRegen hRPE cell line with therapeutic benefits [41]. The question becomes why only a handful of patients have achieved such amazing results. Epigenetic variances and subretinal niche environment perhaps are the answers that deserve to be further investigated.

6. Conclusion

Retinal photoreceptor cell loss (apoptosis) is the principle and common pathological pathway that leads to irreversible vision loss in almost all the retinal diseases such as AMD, STGD, diabetic retinopathy, and IRD. These devasting age-related or genetically caused retinal diseases are increasingly becoming significant socioeconomic burdens. The conventional concept that post-mitotic human photoreceptor cells lose the embryonic competence to regenerate during adulthood has been the central dogma of developmental biology for decades, yet we have just begun to understand what is possible through the lens of *in vitro* and *in vivo* reprogramming of adult human retinal cells [11, 38]. Genetic medicine and pharmacotherapies should aim for an early intervention to prevent RPE and photoreceptor cell loss. Artificial intelligence, big data, and robotic surgeries are enabling us to develop and deliver better genetic medicine and cell therapies to treat individual patients with precision. The future holds great promise for patients with retinal degenerative diseases or neovascularization.

Acknowledgements

Special thanks to Lineage Cell Therapeutic and CEO, Brian Culley, who gave me the opportunity to work on OpRegen hRPE transplant project in 2021 and have made important discoveries to the field of hESC derived RPE therapeutics. I am also grateful to Prof. Andrew Dick, MD at Bristol Eye Hospital, University of Bristol, UK for hosting me in 2009 as Research Fellow of National Eye Research Center, UK during my sabbatical to the UK, along with his team's technical assistance on retinal stem cell research.

Conflict interest

None.

Author details

Tina Guanting Qiu
Ophthalmic Therapeutic Innovation, Massachusetts, Peabody, MA, USA

*Address all correspondence to: qiu-tina@ophthalmic-innovation.com

References

[1] Maguire AM, Russell S, Chung DC, et al. Durability of Voretigene Neparvovec for Biallelic RPE65-mediated inherited retinal disease: Phase 3 results at 3 and 4 years. Ophthalmology. 2021;**128**(10):1460-1468

[2] Hood L, Rowen L. The human genome project: Big science transforms biology and medicine. Genome Medicine. 2013;**5**:79

[3] Thomson JA, Itskovitz-Eldor J, Shapiro SS, et al. Embryonic stem cell lines derived from human blastocysts. Science. 1998;**282**(5391):1145-1147

[4] Qiu TG. Transplantation of human embryonic stem cell-derived retinal pigment epithelial cells (MA09-hRPE) in macular degeneration. npj Regenerative Medicine. 2019;**4**:19

[5] Fleckenstein M, Mitchell P, Freund KB, et al. The progression of geographic atrophy secondary to age-related macular degeneration. Ophthalmology. 2018;**125**(3):369-390

[6] Wolf AT, Harris A, Oddone F, et al. Disease progression pathways of wet AMD: Opportunities for new target discovery. Expert Opinion on Therapeutic Targets. 2022;**26**(1):5-12

[7] Qiu TG. New Frontiers of Retinal Therapeutic Innovation & Strategic Insights. EC Ophthalmology. 2015;**2**(2):81-91

[8] Qiu TG. Methods and compositions for treatments of glaucoma and related conditions. PCT Application No.: 18/356,874. Application date: July 21, 2023. Designee: OphthalmicTherapeutic Innovation LLC; 2023

[9] Shughoury A, Sevgi DD, Ciulla TA. The complement system: A novel therapeutic target for age-related macular degeneration. Expert Opinion on Pharmacotherapy. Sep-Dec 2023;**24**(17):1887-1899

[10] Qiu TG. Revisit Rescula and cystoid macular Edema and refractory glaucoma. Journal of Clinical and Experimental Ophthalmology. 2015;**6**:473

[11] Qiu TG. Trabodenoson on trabecular meshwork rejuvenation: A comprehensive review of clinical data. Expert Opinion on Investigational Drugs. 2021;**30**(3):227-236

[12] Bacharach J, Tatham A, Ferguson G, et al. ARTEMIS 2 study group. Phase 3, randomized, 20-month study of the efficacy and safety of Bimatoprost implant in patients with open-angle glaucoma and ocular hypertension (ARTEMIS 2). Drugs. 2021;**81**(17):2017-2033

[13] Qiu TG. Defining the problem in ophthalmic drug development and clinical translation. EC Ophthalmology. 2016;**3**:314-319

[14] Fujinami K, Zernant J, Chana RK, et al. Clinical and molecular characteristics of childhood-onset Stargardt disease. Ophthalmology. 2015;**122**(2):326-334

[15] Tsybovsky Y, Molday RS, Palczewski K. The ATP-binding cassette transporter ABCA4: Structural and functional properties and role in retinal disease. Advances in Experimental Medicine and Biology. 2010;**703**:105-125

[16] Kong J, Kim SR, Binley K, et al. Correction of the disease phenotype in the mouse model of Stargardt disease by

lentiviral gene therapy. Gene Therapy. 2008;**15**(19):1311-1320

[17] Binley K, Widdowson P, Loader J, et al. Transduction of photoreceptors with equine infectious anemia virus lentiviral vectors: Safety and biodistribution of StarGen for Stargardt disease. Investigative Ophthalmology & Visual Science. 2013;**54**:4061-4071

[18] Parker MA, Erker LR, Audo I, et al. Three-year safety results of SAR422459 (EIAV-ABCA4) gene therapy in patients with ABCA4-associated Stargardt disease: An open-label dose-escalation phase I/IIa clinical trial, cohorts 1-5. American Journal of Ophthalmology. 2022;**240**:285-301

[19] Marc RE, Jones BW, Watt CB, Strettoi E. Neural remodeling in retinal degeneration. Progress in Retinal and Eye Research. 2003;**22**(5):607-655

[20] McCullough KT, Boye SL, Fajardo D, et al. Somatic gene editing of *GUCY2D* by AAV-CRISPR/Cas9 alters retinal structure and function in mouse and macaque. Human Gene Therapy. 2019;**30**(5):571-589

[21] Charbel Issa P, Barnard AR, Herrmann P, et al. Rescue of the Stargardt phenotype in Abca4 knockout mice through inhibition of vitamin a dimerization. Proceedings of the National Academy of Sciences of the United States of America. 2015;**112**(27):8415-8420

[22] Mehat MS, Sundaram V, Ripamonti C, et al. Transplantation of human embryonic stem cell-derived retinal pigment epithelial cells in macular degeneration. Ophthalmology. 2019;**125**(11):1765-1775

[23] Sahel JA, Boulanger-Scemama E, Pagot C, et al. Partial recovery of visual function in a blind patient after optogenetic therapy. Nature Medicine. 2021;**27**:1223-1229

[24] Abbouda A, Avogaro F, Moosajee M, et al. Update on gene therapy clinical trials for Choroideremia and potential experimental therapies. Medicina (Kaunas, Lithuania). 2021;**57**(1):64

[25] MacLaren RE, Groppe M, Barnard AR, et al. Retinal gene therapy in patients with choroideremia: Initial findings from a phase 1/2 clinical trial. Lancet. 2014;**383**(9923):1129-1137

[26] MacLaren RE, Fischer MD, Gow JA, et al. Subretinal timrepigene emparvovec in adult men with choroideremia: A randomized phase 3 trial. Nature Medicine. 2023;**29**:2464-2472

[27] Russell SR, Drack AV, Cideciyan AV, et al. Intravitreal antisense oligonucleotide sepofarsen in Leber congenital amaurosis type 10: A phase 1b/2 trial. Nature Medicine. 2022;**28**(5):1014-1021

[28] Qiu TG. Unique insight of retina gene therapy. EC Ophthalmology. 2018;**9**(2):28-30

[29] Omri S, Omri B, Savoldelli M, Jonet L, Thillaye-Goldenberg B, Thuret G, et al. The outer limiting membrane (OLM) revisited: Clinical implications. Clinical Ophthalmology. 2010;**4**:183-195

[30] Edwards MM, McLeod DS, Bhutto IA, et al. Subretinal glial membranes in eyes with geographic atrophy. Investigative Ophthalmology & Visual Science. 2017;**58**(3):1352-1367

[31] Marshall J, Mellerio J. Disappearance of retino-epithelial scar tissue from ruby laser photocoagulations. Experimental Eye Research. 1971;**12**(2):173-174

[32] Newman NJ, Yu-Wai-Man P, Carelli V, et al. And LHON study group. Efficacy and safety of Intravitreal gene therapy for Leber hereditary optic neuropathy treated within 6 months of disease onset. Ophthalmology. 2021;**128**(5):649-660

[33] Numa K, Imai K, Ueno M, et al. Five-year follow-up of first 11 patients undergoing injection of cultured corneal endothelial cells for corneal endothelial failure. Ophthalmology. Apr 2021;**128**(4):504-514

[34] Qiu G, Seiler MJ, Mui C, et al. Photoreceptor differentiation and integration of retinal progenitor cells transplanted into transgenic rats. Experimental Eye Research. 2005;**80**(4):515-525

[35] Francois B, Hogge G, Rami S, Sha-Bat, A B, Jordi M, Eyal B, Qiu, TG. Methods and compositions for treating retinal diseases and conditions. PCT publication No.: 2021/242788A1. Designee: Lineage Cell Therapeutic, Inc. Patent publication date: 02 Dec 2021

[36] Ribeiro J, Procyk CA, West EL, et al. Restoration of visual function in advanced disease after transplantation of purified human pluripotent stem cell-derived cone photoreceptors. Cell Reports. 2021;**35**(3):109022

[37] Grisé KN, Coles BLK, Bautista NX, et al. Activation of adult mammalian retinal stem cells in vivo via antagonism of BMP and sFRP2. Stem Cell Research & Therapy. 2021;**12**:560

[38] Qiu TG. Retinal progenitor cells. UK Patent Application Number: GB0913109.5. 2009. Designee: University of Bristol, UK, patent application date: Aug 12 2009

[39] Koso H, Minami C, Tabata Y, et al. CD73, a novel cell surface antigen that characterizes retinal photoreceptor precursor cells. Investigative Ophthalmology & Visual Science. 2009;**50**(11):5411-5418

[40] Gagliardi G, Ben M'Barek K, Chaffiol A, et al. Characterization and transplantation of CD73-positive photoreceptors isolated from human iPSC-derived retinal organoids. Stem Cell Reports. 2018;**11**(3):665-680

[41] Barak A, Boyer D, Ho AC, et al. Phase 1/2a study of OpRegen®-human allogeneic retinal pigment epithelial (RPE). In: Cells -in Patients with Geographic Atrophy (GA). Retinal Cell & Gene Therapy Innovation Summit 2023 Annual Meeting. New Orleans, LA, USA: April 21, 2023

Section 2

Surgical Retina

Chapter 7

Epiretinal Membrane

Haroon Tayyab

Abstract

Epiretinal membrane (ERM) is formed at the vitreoretinal interface that leads to a myriad of visual disturbances includes decrease in visual acuity (VA), stereopsis, contrast sensitivity and metamorphopsia. Most common etiology of ERM is posterior vitreous detachment (PVD) and is usually labeled as idiopathic. Secondary ERMs arise from several causes including cataract surgery, retinal tears and detachment, diabetic retinopathy, uveitis etc. Multiple cell lines, cytokines, proteins, and genes play a role in the formation and progression of ERMs. In this chapter, we aim to summarize the current evidence related to etiology, pathophysiology, and management of ERM.

Keywords: epiretinal membrane, internal limiting membrane, optical coherence tomography, vitreo macular traction syndrome, lamellar macular hole

1. Introduction

Epiretinal membrane (ERM) is formed as a result of proliferative process involving myofibroblasts and extracellular matrix (ECM). There are many etiological pathways that eventually result in formation of ERM. Optical coherence tomography (OCT) is the most widely used investigative modality to diagnose, grade and plan intervention for ERMs but lacks the ability to classify according to histopathological variations that suggest it's multifactorial origin. In this chapter, we discuss the current evidence about the etiology, investigations and management of ERMs.

2. Epidemiology

The Blue Mountain Eye Study (BMES) and the Beaver Dam Eye Study (BDES) reported the initial prevalence of idiopathic ERMs (iERMs) as 7% and 11.8% respectively in large population-based analysis. This observation was based in colored retinal and macular photography showing cumulative 5-year incidence of 5.3% [1, 2]. iERMS were found to be bilateral in up to 31% with a 13.5% incidence of other eye involvement within 5 years [1, 3]. Later on, OCT was used in a 20-year follow-up of BDES that showed an overall prevalence of 34.1% which was significantly higher than that showed by retinal photography [4]. Therefore, now OCT is the most desirable investigation to detect the presence of ERM [5].

According to the published literature, there is significant ethnic variation in the prevalence of ERM. Care should be exercised when interpreting the results of ethnic variation due to possible confounders (reading methodology, imaging modalities, various differing OCT based imaging tools) and probable etiology (pigmentation may affect the ability to detect ERM on retinal photography) [6]. Various ethnic reported prevalence rates include 2.9% in Korean National Health and Nutrition Examination Study [7], 4.0% in Hisayama Study from Japan [8], 12.1% in Singapore Epidemiology of Eye Disease Study (SEED) [6], 7.6% in Singapore Indian Eye Study [9], 7.9% in Singapore Malay Eye Study [10], 2.2% in Beijing Eye Study from China [11], 11.8% in BDES from United States [2], 18.7% in Los Angeles Latino Eye Study [12] and 7% in BMES from Australia [1].

Another significant and consistent risk factor is age. BMES study showed increasing incidence from 1.9% (<60 years) to 7.2% (60–69 years) to 11.6% (70–79 years) and Melbourne Collaborative Cohort Study (MCCS) found further increasing incidence of 17% in population above 80 years [1, 13].

Gender does not play a major role as a risk fact although refractive errors have shown to play some inconsistent role where hyperopia [7] and myopia [5] have likelihood of increased ERM incidence.

3. Cellular architecture of ERM

3.1 Proteomic basis of ERM pathogenesis

Our knowledge of pathogenesis of iERMs and secondary ERM (sERM) have greatly improved in the last two decades due to advances in modern imaging coupled with new proteomic techniques and immunohistochemistry [14]. It has been shown in many literature reports that multiple genes and growth factors influence the formation of ERMs [15]. There is also a great range of cell types involved in the pathogenesis and formation of ERMs [16, 17].

3.2 Cellular basis of ERM pathogenesis

ERM is composed of an inner and an outer layer overlying the internal limiting membrane (ILM). The inner layer is composed of cellular sheets whereas the outer layer is a non-cellular protein constituting ECM and arranged in random orientation. With the progression in ERM, its contractile properties are further increased because of accumulation of further ECM and myofibroblasts [18]. The origin of myofibroblasts has been debated but now there is enough evidence from immunohistochemical studies that hyalocytes, retinal pigment epithelial (RPE) cells, fibroblasts and retinal glial cells, all contribute to formation of myofibroblasts [19–21].

There are three basic proposed mechanisms which explain the migration of ERM precursor cells to retinal surface. The earliest mechanism was proposed by Foos who theorized that precursor cells especially retinal glial cell travel to surface of retina after posterior vitreous detachment (PVD) leaving behind microdefects on retinal surface [22, 23]. This has been widely superseded by a more popular theory stating that hyalocytes left behind on retinal surface after PVD undergo metaplasia to form ERM [24]. However, ERMs do occur in the absence of PVD and there is possibility of precursor cells migrating to retinal surface through the retinal tissue and defects in ILM. Metaplasia of these cells then happens on the retinal surface [20]. Due to limitations in the process of ERM mechanism in all these theories, currently we do not have a consensus on this subject.

RPE cells are the most frequently found precursor cells of ERM occurring with a retinal detachment or retinal tears. These cells are not frequently found in iERMs [25]. Although the process of transretinal migration is still unclear, they can deposit on the surface of retina while migrating through retinal breaks in cases of rhegmatogenous retinal detachment. Once deposited on the retinal surface, they undergo transdifferentiation into myofibroblasts under stimulation of Transforming growth factor – beta (TGF-β) [26, 27].

The origin of fibroblasts as precursors of ERM is also not fully elucidated but they are found in ERMs associated with diabetic retinal disease [28]. Fibroblasts secrete ECM and can produce collagen fibers that can ultimately result in tractional retinal detachment [29]. Fibroblasts and myofibroblasts are responsible for the contractile properties of ERM and this happens with the expression of alpha smooth muscle actin protein. A-SMA is also responsible for production of collagen from fibroblasts and generation of contractile forces in ERM [30].

Müller cells can be activated to contribute in the formation of ERM by factors such as retinal ischemia, hyperglycemia, mechanical stress and by various growth factors and cytokines [31]. Traction on the macular surface can be a potential activator of Müller cells that can lead to reactive gliosis and differentiation into myofibroblasts [30].

Laminocytes and hyalocytes also contribute to the formation of iERMs. These are present in eye with PVD and in the cortical vitreous remnants [32]. TGF-β is produced and activated by both hyalocytes and Müllers cells that is involved in the formation of iERMs [33, 34].

Retinal microglia are now known to be found more frequently in the ERMs and PVR than once believed. They also have the capability to secrete TGF-B that aids in differentiation of epithelial cells to myofibroblasts [35]. Retinal astrocytes are flat cell body cells that are known to act as a scaffold for collagen production and fibroblast differentiation [21, 22]. These cell types are predominantly implicated in vitreomacular traction, lamellar macular holes, diabetic retinopathy associated ERMs and myopic traction maculopathies. Their role in formation of iERMs is not so consistent [36–38].

Macrophages have more role to play in secondary ERMs associated with vitreous hemorrhage [39]. They have an unclear role in iERMs formation, but they secrete TGF-β, insulin like growth factor – 1 (IGF-1), fibroblast growth factor (FGF) and platelet derived growth factor (PDGF) that are known to contribute in myofibroblastic transformation [40].

Hyalocytes are predominantly found in the vitreous base and posterior cortex [41]. At the posterior pole, they are positioned at 20–50 μm from ILM in a widely spaced single layer [24]. The presence of hyalocytes has been established in ERMs with their long fibers nested next to fibroblasts in cellular agglomerations [24, 42]. Studies have shown that hyalocytes display strong contractile properties in response to TGF-β2 stimulation that may have a role in enhancing the contractile properties of ERM [43]. It has been proposed that vitreoschisis can occur in the event of an anomalous PVD. The level of split in posterior vitreous (anterior or posterior to hyalocytes layer) determines the eventual role of hyalocytes in the contractile activity of ERMs [24]. Various studies have also proved the role of myofibroblastic differentiation from these cells in ERMs, vitreomacular traction syndrome (VMTS), lamellar macular hole (LM) and other proliferative vitreoretinopathies [44, 45].

Cell type	Role in pathogenesis of ERM
RPE	iERM and sERM (PVR, PDR)
Müller cells	iERM and sERM
Hyalocytes	iERM and sERM (PVR, PDR)
Glial cells	iERM and sERM (PVR, PDR)
Laminocytes	iERM
Fibroblasts	iERM and sERM (PDR)
Astrocytes	iERM
Endothelial cells	ERM formation
Macrophages	iERM and sERM (PVR)
Myofibroblasts	iERM and sERM (PVR, PDR)

iERM, idiopathic epiretinal membrane; sERM, secondary epiretinal membrane; PVR, proliferative vitreoretinopathy; PDR, proliferative diabetic retinopathy; RPE, retinal pigment epithelium.

Table 1.
Common cell types and their role in ERM formation.

Non cellular ECM forms the framework that promotes the proliferation and adhesion of epiretinal cells [46]. ECM is formed by the glial cells, RPE cells and myofibroblasts [47]. ECM is mainly composed of type I, II, III, IV and VI collagen [48]. Type I, II, and III are known to be newly formed collagen whereas type II and IV are native vitreous collagen present adjacent to ILM [49, 50]. Type VI collagen is known form the fine fibrillar network of ECM and interacts with type IV collagen of outer ILM boundaries of ECM to account for the biomechanical stability when removing surgically [16]. A summary of the cell types and their role in ERM formation are given in **Table 1**.

3.3 Genes involved in ERM pathogenesis

There has been keen interest to understand the role of genes in pathogenesis of ERM. A total of 52 genes are upregulated in PVR or sERM. Four genes in particular, PARP8, ZNF713, FN1 and MALAT1 are significantly upregulated in ERMs [51]. Out of these genes, MALAT1 is associated with progression of sERM such as PVR associated ERM. It also plays a role in activation of genes involved in metastasis and motility at the transcription level [52]. Other important genes involved in the pathogenesis of iERMs include RELA, tenscin C, glial fibrillary acidic protein and other cytokine encoding genes like TGF-β2, IL6 and VEGF-A [53]. PPM1D encodes wild type p53-induced phosphatase 1 (Wip1) that has been reported in PDR associated ERM formation. Another gene associated with encoding angiogenesis related factors in PDR associated ERM is SP1. It regulates expression of genes such as TGF-β, VEGF and many matrix genes [54].

3.4 Role of cytokines and growth factors in formation of ERMs

Cytokines and growth factors play their role in formation, growth and contraction of ERMs. Contraction and growth of ERMs is regulated by these molecules and their role is implicated in both iERMs and sERMs [55, 56].

3.4.1 The transforming growth factor-β family

The TGF-β family is involved in mediating the myofibroblast differentiation and inflammatory response. These are also involved in upregulation of ECM production. The retinal Müller cells and hyalocytes are involved in production and activation of TGF-β. This in return, leads to the process of Müller cell proliferation, transdifferentiation and migration [57, 58]. Both, TGF-β 1 and TGF-β2 are upregulated in ERMs and vitreous humor. Their expression seems to be secondary in cases of ERM although there is evidence, they may be involved in the initiation of iERM [17]. As studies have shown that there are differences in the levels of TGB-β1 and β2 in vitreous and that levels of the later are raised in vitreous in cases of iERMs, it is now believed that the role of TBF-β1 may be minimal in the pathogenesis of iERMs. This observed predominance of TGF-β2 in iERMs makes this a potential target for therapeutic agents targeted to control or limit/inhibit the formation of iERMs [14, 59].

3.4.2 Vascular endothelial growth factor (VEGF)

VEGF is known to contribute in development of iERMs. This is evidenced with high levels of VEGF in vitreous in patients of iERMs and retinal neovascularization leading to sERMs. Also, the VEGF-A gene is overexpressed in this clinical scenario [60, 61].

3.4.3 Nerve growth factor (NGF)

NGF is highly expressed and utilized in the formation of iERM through modulating intracellular signaling and there may play a part in the formation if iERMs [17].

3.4.4 Insulin like growth factor (IGF)

IGF has been shown to contribute to the growth, progression and contraction of ERM especially secondary to PDR [62, 63].

3.4.5 Platelet derived growth factor (PDGF)

RPE cells are known to stimulate the production of PDGF. As a result, PDGF enhances the interaction between RPE and glial cells after former have migrated to the retinal surface or vitreous [64]. This is most notably evidenced in ERM secondary to PVR [65, 66]. PDGF also stimulates other cells that lead to proliferation of ERM [66].

3.5 Proteins involved in pathogenesis of ERM

There are over 300 proteins that have been known to play a role in pathogenesis of iERMs and have been localized in aqueous fluid (AF) and vitreous fluid (VF) [32]. Out of these, 8 proteins are overexpressed in VF and 4 proteins are overexpressed in AF and rest of them are non-differentially expressed both in AF and VF. Of these, fibrinogen A is the most significant overexpressed protein in VF that plays a critical role in pathogenesis of iERMs [67].

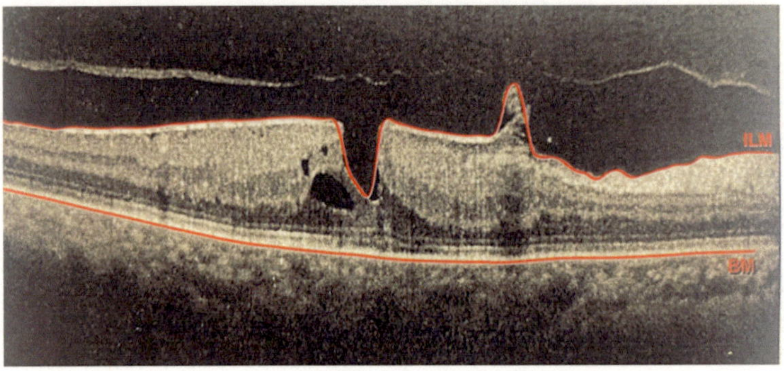

Figure 1.
Epiretinal membrane with no posterior vitreous detachment.

Idiopathic ERM
• No known pathology
• Posterior vitreous detachment
Secondary ERM
• Uveitis
• Retinal detachment
• Retinal tears
• Post cataract surgery
• Retinal laser
• Retinal cryotherapy
• Retinal surgery – vitrectomy
• Diabetic retinopathy
• Retinal vein occlusion
• Radiation retinopathy
• Sickle cell disease
• Retinal artery macroaneurysm
• Coats disease
• Retinal telangiectasia
• Trauma
• Pathological myopia
• Intraocular tumors
• Macular hole
• Vitreomacular traction syndrome
• Retinitis pigmentosa
• Age related macular degeneration

Table 2.
Etiology of idiopathic and secondary epiretinal membrane.

4. Etiology of iERMs and sERMs

Traditionally, ERMs are classified based on their causative factors and associated ocular conditions. A PVD is present in up to 95% of all iERMs and therefore suggest the role of PVD in iERM pathogenesis. 5% patients do not have PVD and still have iERM (**Figure 1**) [68, 69]. sERMs are found to coexist with other ocular conditions most common of which is recent cataract surgery, followed by diabetic retinopathy and retinal vein occlusion [70–72]. Common causes of iERMS and sERMs are listed in the **Table 2** above.

5. Signs and symptoms

Most common presenting complaints of patients with ERMs include decreased visual acuity (VA), hazy vision, anisokonia, micropsia, macropsia and reduced stereopsis. Binocular interference happens when the patient closes the involved eye to see better from the other eye in the absence of strabismus or diplopia. This symptom significantly reduces the quality of life [73, 74].

Clinical signs of ERM range from mild glistening of macular reflex to inner retinal distortion, disturbed vascular architecture, cystoid macular oedema (CMO), displaced fovea and full thickness or lamellar macular hole [75].

6. Clinical classification of ERMs

With the introduction of OCT, our understanding about the architecture, evaluation and prognosis of ERM has been revised. Original classification of ERM was from Gass who described ERM in terms of cellophane maculopathy (Grade 0), crinkled cellophane maculopathy (Grade 1), macular pucker (Grade 2) and pseudohole [76, 77].

7. Investigations

7.1 Optical coherence tomography

Various OCT based classifications of ERM have been proposed in the literature. Hwang et al. described ERMs based on their involvement of fovea and used multifocal electroretinogram (mfERG) to assess retinal function based on this classification [78]. Stevenson introduced an additional classification taking into account the presence or absence of PVD along with foveal involvement or sparing [79]. Konidaris et al. also proposed a complex classification of ERM while describing nine categories based on retinal architecture and PVD [80].

More recently, a simple classification proposed by Govetto et al. has gained attraction due to its simplicity and ease of application in clinical scenarios. It is a four-stage classification based on presence (**Figure 2**) or absence of foveal pit (**Figure 3**), ectopic inner foveal layers (**Figure 4**), and disorganization of retinal layers (**Figure 5**) [81]. Ectopic inner foveal layer is a continuous band extending form inner nuclear and plexiform layers across fovea [82]. Recent literature has validated the prognostic value

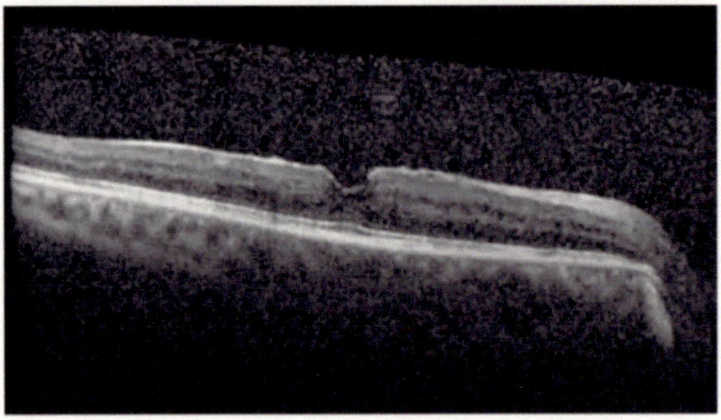

Figure 2.
Intact foveal pit with identifiable retinal layers. Reproduced with permission [81].

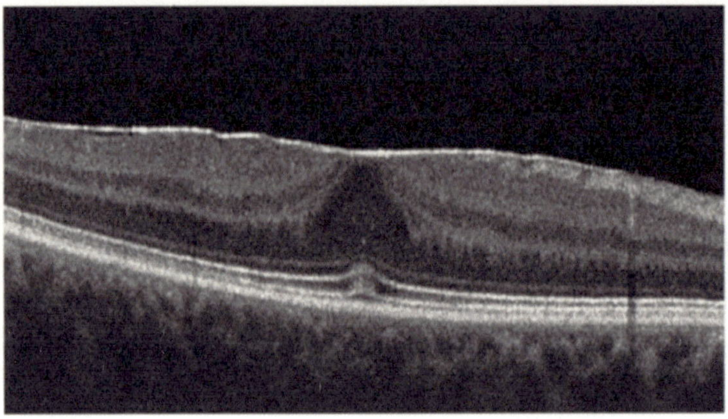

Figure 3.
Loss of foveal pit with identifiable retinal layers. Reproduced with permission [81].

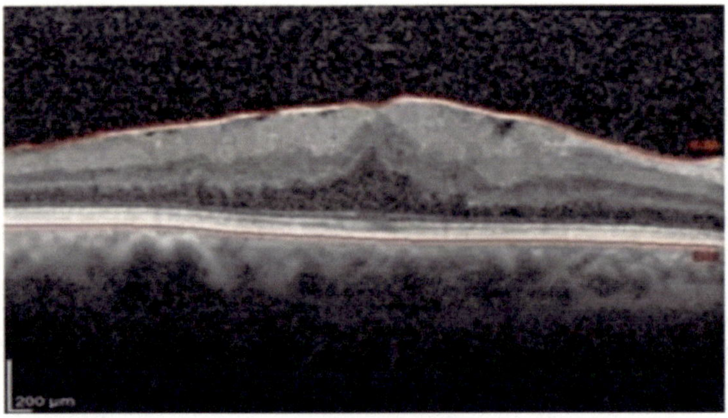

Figure 4.
Loss of foveal pit with identifiable ectopic inner retinal layers. Reproduced with permission [81].

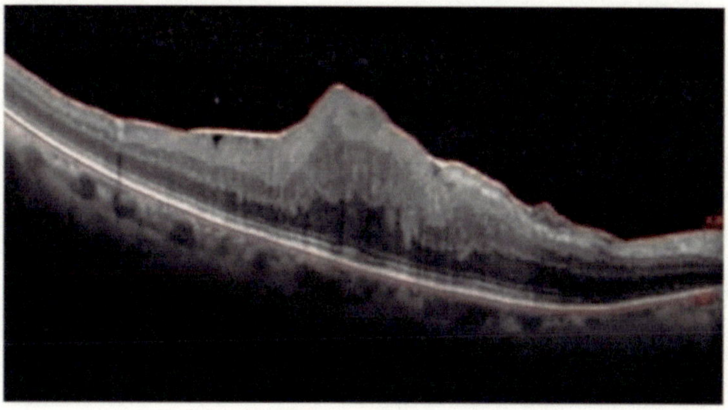

Figure 5.
Loss of foveal pit with disorganized inner retinal layers. Reproduced with permission [81].

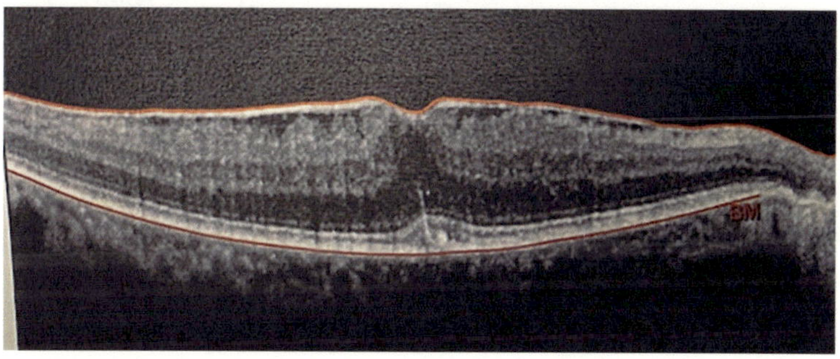

Figure 6.
Cotton ball sign visible at the center of fovea between ellipsoid zone and cone outer segment termination line.

of this staging with higher stage associated with poorer pre- and post-operative visual outcomes [83, 84].

Additional signs manifested and described in recent literature include cotton ball sign and center bouquet. The cotton ball sign is a round and reflective lesion at the center of fovea between ellipsoid zone (EZ) and cone outer segment termination (COST) line [85]. It has been suggested that cotton ball sign is a sign of chronic traction and may predict the severity of ERM. Based on the cotton ball sign, a central bouquet is an advancement of cotton ball sign and is described in 3 clinical variants according to their level of chronicity and severity of traction: cotton ball sign (**Figure 6**), acquired vitelliform lesion and central foveolar detachment (**Figure 7**) [86].

The eyes with cotton ball sign have better visual outcomes as compared to acquired vitelliform lesions and foveolar detachment [86].

OCT changes in ERMs are also being used as prognostic markers for visual outcomes and to the exact timing of intervention in ERM cases. OCT markers predicting better visual outcomes after surgery include absence of ectopic inner retinal foveal layer, inner retinal irregularity, CMO, acquired vitelliform lesion, normal EZ and COST [87–91]. There has been recent shift to the pathologies located in inner retinal layers in predicating the outcomes after intervention. This includes the presence or absence of ectopic inner foveal layer and surgeries performed before the formation of

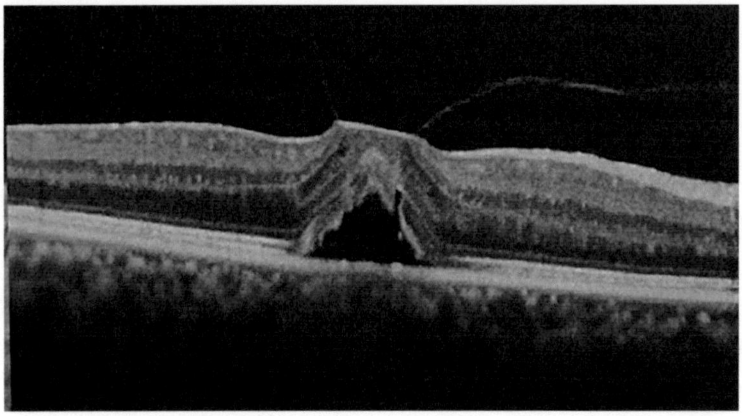

Figure 7.
Epiretinal membrane with vitreomacular traction syndrome and foveal elevation.

this layer carry better visual prognosis [92]. Another marker on OCT is the ratio of the length of inner plexiform layer to RPE in a 3 mm zone center on fovea. This marker is also significantly associated with predicting visual outcomes after surgical intervention [93]. Most of these studies have been done in cases of iERMs. It is difficult to deduce prognostic OCT markers in cases of sERMs. This is because the vision may be affected due to the primary disease process more than due to ERM and this acts as a confounder. Nevertheless, earlier intervention in cases of sERMs is favorable due to overall worse visual prognosis when compared to iERMs [94].

7.2 Angiography

Angiography can be helpful in accurately diagnosing the secondary causes of ERM and hence can be useful preoperatively [95]. Advanced ERMs can lead to alterations in foveal avascular zone because of displacement and stretching of superficial and deep capillary plexus as has been shown by OCT angiography (OCT-A). It has also been shown that there is reduced vascular density of superficial capillary plexus and increase in the density of deep vascular plexus after ERM surgery which may impact the post-operative visual function [96–98].

7.3 Microperimetry

It can be very useful to assess the subclinical abnormalities in visual function when other regular visual function tests are equivocal [99]. This has also clarified the role of additional ILM peeling in cases of ERMs that may at times lead to decreased retinal sensitivity and micro scotomas as shown by findings of microperimetry [100, 101].

7.4 Electroretinography (ERG)

Although ERG is not routinely used as an investigative tool for ERM management, several findings explain its novel role for research and investigative purpose. One such clinical finding is lower mfERG responses (P1) in cases of ERM with increased subfield retinal thickness [102]. Whereas some studies have shown decreased responses of dual peeling on microperimetry, mfERG has shown improved responses with this technique that shows improved retinal ganglion cell function [103–105]. mfERG also has predictive value as decreased pre-operative P1 values often signifies poorer post-operative results [106].

7.5 Artificial intelligence (AI)

There is a promising role of AI in detecting ERMs without human intervention as some studies have successfully identified ERMs based on OCT scans with high sensitivity (98.7%) and specificity (98%) [107, 108].

8. Management

8.1 Observation

It has been shown in natural history studies that ERMs progress very slowly. In the landmark BMES study, it was shown that only 10% of eyes with ERM progressed to pre retinal fibrosis over a follow up of 5 years [1]. Once we observe lamellar macular hole in presence of ERM, it is also a sign of long-term clinical stability and does not require intervention unless there is progressive decrease in VA [109].

8.2 Surgical management

There is no definitive medical management of ERMs and surgery is usually indicated when there is decline in visual functions. The optimal timing of surgery is still a question of debate but recently there has been preference to intervene before the formation of ectopic inner foveal layer. Often the surgery is reserved for cases where vision is <20/60 but modern-day surgery has decreased this threshold even further. Following surgery, there can be a prolonged period of up to 6–12 months over which the vision keeps on getting better. Studies have shown that up to 85% of patients achieve 2 or more lines of vision improvement and up to 55% of patients achieving vision >20/50 [110, 111]. Contrast sensitivity also improves significantly after ERM surgery even when vision does not improve, and this correlates well with Quality of Life measures and represents a better measure of surgical advantages [112, 113]. Stereopsis is another visual functional that improves after ERM surgery and it has been shown that stereopsis is worse in patients with ERM as compared with controls [114–116].

Often double peel is employed to ensure more complete removal of ERM and to ensure there are lesser chances of ERM recurrence [117, 118]. On the contrary, ILM peeling is associated with inner retinal dimpling, micro scotomas and has no impact on final VA. Therefore, some surgeons may reserve this for recurrent ERMs [119].

In modern day vitrectomy, the use of small gauge instruments has improved the surgical outcomes and post-operative rehabilitation after ERM surgery. Some studies have shown better outcome with 27-gauge vitrectomy plat form whereas others have shown equivocal results [120]. The surgery starts with core vitrectomy followed by check for PVD facilitated with triamcinolone acetonide. If PVD is not present, then induction of PVD is carried out. There has been recent interest in non vitrectemozing surgery with newer small gauge instruments. This technique potentially reduces the chances of post-operative cataract and retinal tears, but the general adaptation of this technique has been limited due to persistent presence of floaters due to vitreous debris

[121, 122]. ERM peel is facilitated by chromovitrectomy. The vital dyes used for ERM staining include trypan blue (TB) and for ILM, brilliant blue G (BBG) and indocyanine green (ICG) have been extensively used [123]. More recently, combinations of TB and BBG have been made available to facilitate dual membrane staining. The use of ICG has become less popular now because of purported macular toxicity [123]. This has been more pronounced in cases of macular hole and studies have shown no difference in macular toxicity in cases of ERM surgery [124, 125]. ICG has better binding with ILM as compared to ERM and a negative staining technique can also be used to peel ERM where ERM can be visualized as an area with no staining surrounded by clearly visible ILM [126, 127]. A number of studies reporting ICG toxicity have been published with varying incubation times, osmolarity, and concentrations. In general, RPE toxicity has been more commonly demonstrated with a solution that has an osmolarity of <270 mOsm, a concentration above 0.5%, and incubation time > 30 seconds. Additional factors that may be associated with RPE toxicity include application technique and duration of light exposure [128].

Usual application time of vital dyes to effectively stain the ERM and ILM range from 1 to 3 minutes. Once the staining of membranes is complete, there are a number of techniques to peel the ERM. Once way is to identify the edge of ERM and lift it with help of end grasping forceps. In cases where edge is not clearly visible, it can be created with bent picks or bent micro vitreo retinal (MVR) blades, flex loops or diamond dusted scrapers [129]. Peeling of ERM and ILM can also be facilitated with traditional pinch and peel technique using high magnification with contact or indirect posterior segment viewing systems. ILM peeling or end grasping forceps are used for peeling the membranes in a circular manner centered on the fovea and ranging up to the vascular arcades [130]. Peeling of secondary membranes employs similar techniques except that some additional maneuvers may be required to address the cause of sERMs. These may include laser or cryopexy for retinal tears or detachment, laser photocoagulation for PDR and retinal vein occlusions, anti VEGF treatment for neovessels arising from retina or choroid and intravitreal or preocular steroids of ERMs secondary to uveitis [131].

8.3 Surgical complications

As with any other vitrectomy surgery, ERM surgery is also associated with complications such as retinal detachment and tears, cataract formation, infection, and vitreous hemorrhage. With the advancements in OCT, certain particular complications of ERM surgery have surfaced which require additional discussion [132].

8.3.1 Swelling of arcuate nerve fiber layer (SANFL)

This is a temporary complication (lasts 3 months) which at times is followed by focal RNFL thinning in the temporal macula [133]. It is postulated that ILM peeling during ERM surgery causes swelling of arcuate nerve fiber layers especially in the papillomacular bundle (**Figure 8**). This may be caused by either damage to the Müller cell foot plates or direct retinal nerve fiber layer (RNFL) damage. It is noted as swelling of RNFL on OCT [134].

8.3.2 Nasal displacement of fovea

This condition arises after ERM peeling surgery when there is imbalance between the temporal and nasal mechanical forces due to release of traction caused

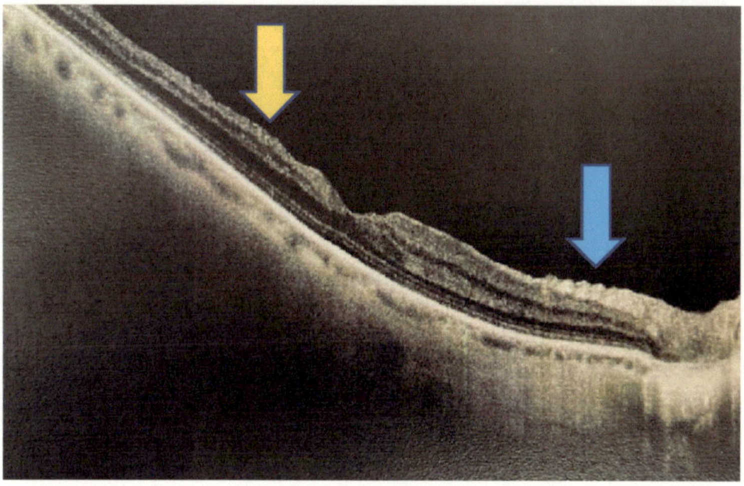

Figure 8.
Blue arrow shows swelling of arcuate nerve fiber layer and yellow arrow shows dissociated optic nerve fiber layer.

by ERM [135]. If there is a difference in the retinal thinning between temporal and nasal retina (temporal retinal thinning is more pronounced than nasal retina) after ERM surgery, then the chances of nasal displacement are higher [135].

8.3.3 Dissociated optic nerve fiber layer (DONFL)

Another name of DONFL is "inner retinal dimpling" proposed by Spaide who reclassified this condition in OCT scan (**Figure 8**). One hypothesis is that it represents changes secondary to regeneration of damaged Müller cells [136, 137].

8.3.4 Full thickness paracentral macular hole

There can be a full thickness paracentral macular hole that occurs at the point of start of ILM peel or where the ILM peel ends. These are asymptomatic and no intervention is usually needed [138].

8.4 Post operative functional results

There is usually a 2-line improvement after ERM surgery. In the absence of vision improvement, there is improvement in metamorphopsia [139]. Post-operative vision can keep on improving for next 3 years. This is because of continued resolution of macular edema and near normal organization of retinal layers [140].

9. Conclusion

The main risk factors the precedes the formation of iERMs is PVD and occurs in 2% of the population [1, 13, 68, 69]. One of the major associations of PVD is age [13]. With the advent of new diagnostic tools and molecular analysis methods, we now better understand the progressive and sequential processes that lead to formation of iERMs and sERMs [17]. Currently, we do not have the biochemical or diagnostic tools to predict the formation of ERMs but with improving knowledge about the cellular processes (proteins, cytokines, cellular lines), it is hoped that we may identify biochemical or genetic markers for the development and progression of ERMs. With advancements in the clinical classification of ERM severity, some simple and practical guidelines and grading systems have evolved in last decade that helps us understand the optimal timing for intervention and predicting functional outcomes after surgery [78–84]. We, currently do not have any prophylactic treatment of ERMs. With current small gauge instruments, our threshold to address ERMs has considerably decreased with safe outcomes and quick post-operative functional recovery [112, 113].

Conflict of interest

The author declares no conflict of interest.

Author details

Haroon Tayyab
Department of Ophthalmology and Visual Sciences, The Aga Khan University Hospital, Karachi, Pakistan

*Address all correspondence to: haroontayyab79@gmail.com

References

[1] Mitchell P, Smith W, Chey T, Wang JJ, Chang A. Prevalence and associations of epiretinal membranes. The Blue Mountains Eye Study, Australia. Ophthalmology. 1997;**104**(6):1033-1040

[2] Klein R, Klein BE, Wang Q, Moss SE. The epidemiology of epiretinal membranes. Transactions of the American Ophthalmological Society. 1994;**92**:403-425

[3] Fraser-Bell S, Guzowski M, Rochtchina E, Wang JJ, Mitchell P. Five-year cumulative incidence and progression of epiretinal membranes: The Blue Mountains Eye Study. Ophthalmology. 2003;**110**(1):34-40

[4] Meuer SM, Myers CE, Klein BE, et al. The epidemiology of vitreoretinal interface abnormalities as detected by spectral-domain optical coherence tomography: The beaver dam eye study. Ophthalmology. 2015;**122**(4):787-795

[5] Duan XR, Liang YB, Friedman DS, et al. Prevalence and associations of epiretinal membranes in a rural Chinese adult population: The Handan eye study. Investigative Ophthalmology & Visual Science. 2009;**50**(5):2018-2023

[6] Cheung N, Tan SP, Lee SY, et al. Prevalence and risk factors for epiretinal membrane: The Singapore epidemiology of eye disease study. The British Journal of Ophthalmology. 2017;**101**(3):371-376

[7] Kim JM, Lee H, Shin JP, et al. Epiretinal membrane: Prevalence and risk factors from the Korea National Health and Nutrition Examination Survey, 2008 through 2012. Korean Journal of Ophthalmology. 2017;**31**(6):514-523

[8] Miyazaki M, Nakamura H, Kubo M, et al. Prevalence and risk factors for epiretinal membranes in a Japanese population: The Hisayama study. Graefe's Archive for Clinical and Experimental Ophthalmology. 2003;**241**(8):642-646

[9] Koh V, Cheung CY, Wong WL, et al. Prevalence and risk factors of epiretinal membrane in Asian Indians. Investigative Ophthalmology & Visual Science. 2012;**53**(2):1018-1022

[10] Kawasaki R, Wang JJ, Mitchell P, et al. Racial difference in the prevalence of epiretinal membrane between Caucasians and Asians. The British Journal of Ophthalmology. 2008;**92**(10):1320-1324

[11] You Q, Xu L, Jonas JB. Prevalence and associations of epiretinal membranes in adult Chinese: The Beijing eye study. Eye (London, England). 2008;**22**(7):874-879

[12] Fraser-Bell S, Ying-Lai M, Klein R, Varma R, Los Angeles Latino Eye Study. Prevalence and associations of epiretinal membranes in latinos: The Los Angeles Latino Eye Study. Investigative Ophthalmology & Visual Science. 2004;**45**(6):1732-1736

[13] Aung KZ, Makeyeva G, Adams MK, et al. The prevalence and risk factors of epiretinal membranes: The Melbourne Collaborative Cohort Study. Retina. 2013;**33**(5):1026-1034

[14] Joshi M, Agrawal S, Christoforidis JB. Inflammatory mechanisms of idiopathic epiretinal membrane formation. Mediators of Inflammation. 2013;**2013**:192582

[15] Yoshida S, Ogura A, Ishikawa K, Yoshida A, Kohno R, Yamaji Y, et al.

Gene expression profile of fibrovascular membranes from patients with proliferative diabetic retinopathy. The British Journal of Ophthalmology. 2010;**94**(6):795-801

[16] Bu SC, Kuijer R, van der Worp RJ, Huiskamp EA, Renardel de Lavalette VW, Li XR, et al. Glial cells and collagens in epiretinal membranes associated with idiopathic macular holes. Retina. 2014;**34**(5):897-906

[17] Iannetti L, Accorinti M, Malagola R, Bozzoni-Pantaleoni F, Da Dalt S, Nicoletti F, et al. Role of the intravitreal growth factors in the pathogenesis of idiopathic epiretinal membrane. Investigative Ophthalmology & Visual Science. 2011;**52**(8):5786-5789

[18] Bu SC, Kuijer R, Li XR, Hooymans JM, Los LI. Idiopathic epiretinal membrane. Retina. 2014;**34**(12):2317-2335

[19] Vinores SA, Campochiaro PA, Conway BP. Ultrastructural and electron-immunocytochemical characterization of cells in epiretinal membranes. Investigative Ophthalmology & Visual Science. 1990;**31**(1):14-28

[20] Smiddy WE, Maguire AM, Green WR, et al. Idiopathic epiretinal membranes. Ultrastructural Characteristics and Clinicopathologic Correlation. Ophthalmology. 1989;**96**(6):811-820

[21] Hiscott PS, Grierson I, Trombetta CJ, Rahi AH, Marshall J, McLeod D. Retinal and epiretinal glia – An immunohisto-chemical study. The British Journal of Ophthalmology. 1984;**68**(10):698-707

[22] Foos RY. Vitreoretinal juncture – simple epiretinal membranes. Albrecht von Graefes Archiv für Klinische und Experimentelle Ophthalmologie. 1974;**189**(4):231-250

[23] Ngan ND, Cuong NV, Trung NL, Dat DT, Tuan HA, Dong PN, et al. Clinical characteristics and histopathology of idiopathic epiretinal membrane in Vietnam. Open Access Macedonian Journal of Medical Sciences. 2019;**7**(24):4324-4328

[24] Sebag J. The vitreoretinal interface and its role in the pathogenesis of vitreomaculopathies. Der Ophthalmologe. 2015;**112**(1):10-19

[25] Gandorfer A, Rohleder M, Kampik A. Epiretinal pathology of vitreomacular traction syndrome. The British Journal of Ophthalmology. 2002;**86**(8):902-909

[26] Reichenbach A, Bringmann A. Role of purines in Muller glia. Journal of Ocular Pharmacology and Therapeutics. 2016;**32**(8):518-533

[27] Kampik A, Kenyon KR, Michels RG, Green WR, de la Cruz ZC. Epiretinal and vitreous membranes. Comparative study of 56 cases. Archives of Ophthalmology. 1981;**99**(8):1445-1454

[28] Luo W, Hu L, Li W, Xu G, Xu L, Zhang C, et al. Epo inhibits the fibrosis and migration of Muller glial cells induced by TGF-beta and high glucose. Graefe's Archive for Clinical and Experimental Ophthalmology. 2016;**254**(5):881-890

[29] Feist RM Jr, King JL, Morris R, Witherspoon CD, Guidry C. Myofibroblast and extracellular matrix origins in proliferative vitreoretinopathy. Graefe's Archive for Clinical and Experimental Ophthalmology. 2014;**252**(2):347-357

[30] Bu SC, Kuijer R, van der Worp RJ, et al. Immunohistochemical evaluation

of idiopathic epiretinal membranes and in vitro studies on the effect of TGF-beta on Müller cells. Investigative Ophthalmology & Visual Science. 2015;**56**(11):6506-6514

[31] Bringmann A, Wiedemann P. Involvement of Muller glial cells in epiretinal membrane formation. Graefe's Archive for Clinical and Experimental Ophthalmology. 2009;**247**(7):865-883

[32] Yu J, Feng L, Wu Y, Wang H, Ba J, Zhu W, et al. Vitreous proteomic analysis of idiopathic epiretinal membranes. Molecular BioSystems. 2014;**10**(10):2558-2566

[33] Ikeda T, Homma Y, Nisida K, Hirase K, Sotozono C, Kinoshita S, et al. Expression of transforming growth factor-beta s and their receptors by human retinal glial cells. Current Eye Research. 1998;**17**(5):546-550

[34] Lazarus HS, Schoenfeld CL, Fekrat S, Cohen S, Carol A, Hageman GS, et al. Hyalocytes synthesize and secrete inhibitors of retinal pigment epithelial cell proliferation in vitro. Archives of Ophthalmology. 1996;**114**(6):731-736

[35] Jerdan JA, Pepose JS, Michels RG, et al. Proliferative vitreoretinopathy membranes. An immunohistochemical study. Ophthalmology. 1989;**96**(6):801-810

[36] Wang LC, Hung KH, Hsu CC, Chen SJ, Li WY, Lin TC. Assessment of retinal pigment epithelial cells in epiretinal membrane formation. Journal of the Chinese Medical Association. 2015;**78**(6):370-373

[37] Parolini B, Schumann RG, Cereda MG, Haritoglou C, Pertile G. Lamellar macular hole: A clinicopathologic correlation of surgically excised epiretinal membranes. Investigative Ophthalmology & Visual Science. 2011;**52**(12):9074-9083

[38] Yokota R, Hirakata A, Hayashi N, et al. Ultrastructural analyses of internal limiting membrane excised from highly myopic eyes with myopic traction maculopathy. Japanese Journal of Ophthalmology. 2018;**62**(1):84-91

[39] Bringmann A, Unterlauft JD, Barth T, Wiedemann R, Rehak M, Wiedemann P. Müller cells and astrocytes in tractional macular disorders. Progress in Retinal and Eye Research. 2022;**86**:100977

[40] Wiedemann P. Growth factors in retinal diseases: Proliferative vitreoretinopathy, proliferative diabetic retinopathy, and retinal degeneration. Survey of Ophthalmology. 1992;**36**(5):373-384

[41] Hamburg A. Some investigations on the cells of the vitreous body. Ophthalmologica. 1959;**138**:81-107

[42] Kohno RI, Hata Y, Kawahara S, et al. Possible contribution of hyalocytes to idiopathic epiretinal membrane formation and its contraction. The British Journal of Ophthalmology. 2009;**93**(8):1020-1026

[43] Hirayama K, Hata Y, Noda Y, et al. The involvement of the rho-kinase pathway and its regulation in cytokine-induced collagen gel contraction by hyalocytes. Investigative Ophthalmology & Visual Science. 2004;**45**(11):3896-3903

[44] Wertheimer C, Eibl-Lindner KH, Compera D, et al. A cell culture technique for human epiretinal membranes to describe cell behavior and membrane contraction in vitro. Graefe's Archive for Clinical and Experimental Ophthalmology. 2017;**255**(11):2147-2155

[45] Zhao F, Gandorfer A, Haritoglou C, et al. Epiretinal cell proliferation in macular pucker and vitreomacular traction syndrome: Analysis of flat-mounted internal limiting membrane specimens. Retina. 2013;**33**(1):77-88

[46] Regoli M, Tosi GM, Neri G, Altera A, Orazioli D, Bertelli E. The peculiar pattern of type IV collagen deposition in epiretinal membranes. The Journal of Histochemistry and Cytochemistry. 2020;**68**(2):149-162

[47] Snead DR, Cullen N, James S, et al. Hyperconvolution of the inner limiting membrane in vitreomaculopathies. Graefe's Archive for Clinical and Experimental Ophthalmology. 2004;**242**(10):853-862

[48] Telander DG, Yu AK, Forward KI, Morales SA, Morse LS, Park SS, et al. Epithelial membrane protein-2 in human proliferative vitreoretinopathy and epiretinal membranes. Investigative Ophthalmology & Visual Science. 2016;**57**(7):3112-3117

[49] Tsotridou E, Loukovitis E, Zapsalis K, Pentara I, Asteriadis S, Tranos P, et al. A review of last decade developments on epiretinal membrane pathogenesis. Medical Hypothesis, Discovery & Innovation in Ophthalmology. 2020;**9**(2):91-110

[50] Schumann RG, Gandorfer A, Kampik A, Haritoglou C. Clinicopathological correlations at the vitreoretinalinterface.DerOphthalmologe. 2015;**112**(1):20-28

[51] Asato R, Yoshida S, Ogura A, Nakama T, Ishikawa K, Nakao S, et al. Comparison of gene expression profile of epiretinal membranes obtained from eyes with proliferative vitreoretinopathy to that of secondary epiretinal membranes. PLoS One. 2013;**8**(1):e54191

[52] Tano K, Mizuno R, Okada T, Rakwal R, Shibato J, Masuo Y, et al. MALAT-1 enhances cell motility of lung adenocarcinoma cells by influencing the expression of motility-related genes. FEBS Letters. 2010;**584**(22):4575-4580

[53] Myojin S, Yoshimura T, Yoshida S, Takeda A, Murakami Y, Kawano Y, et al. Gene expression analysis of the irrigation solution samples collected during vitrectomy for idiopathic Epiretinal membrane. PLoS One. 2016;**11**(10):e0164355

[54] Yoshida-Hata N, Mitamura Y, Oshitari T, Namekata K, Harada C, Harada T, et al. Transcription factor, SP1, in epiretinal membranes of patients with proliferative diabetic retinopathy. Diabetes Research and Clinical Practice. 2010;**87**(3):e26-e28

[55] Elner SG, Elner VM, Jaffe GJ, Stuart A, Kunkel SL, Strieter RM. Cytokines in proliferative diabetic retinopathy and proliferative vitreoretinopathy. Current Eye Research. 1995;**14**(11):1045-1053

[56] El-Ghrably IA, Dua HS, Orr GM, Fischer D, Tighe PJ. Detection of cytokine mRNA production in infiltrating cells in proliferative vitreoretinopathy using reverse transcription polymerase chain reaction. The British Journal of Ophthalmology. 1999;**83**(11):1296-1299

[57] Bu SC, Kuijer R, van der Worp RJ, Postma G, Renardel de Lavalette VW, Li XR, et al. Immunohistochemical evaluation of idiopathic epiretinal membranes and In vitro studies on the effect of TGF-beta on Muller cells. Investigative Ophthalmology & Visual Science. 2015;**56**(11):6506-6514

[58] Hashimoto R, Jiang M, Shiba T, Hiruta N, Takahashi M, Higashi M, et al. Soluble form of LR11 is highly increased in the vitreous fluids of patients with idiopathic epiretinal membrane. Graefe's Archive for Clinical and Experimental Ophthalmology. 2017;**255**(5):885-891

[59] Zandi S, Tappeiner C, Pfister IB, Despont A, Rieben R, Garweg JG. Vitreal cytokine profile differences between eyes with Epiretinal membranes or macular holes. Investigative Ophthalmology & Visual Science. 2016;**57**(14):6320-6326

[60] Rollin R, Mediero A, Martinez-Montero JC, Roldan-Pallares M, Suarez-Leoz M, Vidal-Fernandez P, et al. Atrial natriuretic peptide in the vitreous humor and epiretinal membranes of patients with proliferative diabetic retinopathy. Molecular Vision. 2004;**10**:450-457

[61] Dong Z, Kase S, Ando R, Fukuhara J, Saito W, Kanda A, et al. Alphab-crystallin expression in epiretinal membrane of human proliferative diabetic retinopathy. Retina. 2012;**32**(6):1190-1196

[62] Kluge A, Zimmermann R, Weihrauch D, Mohri M, Sack S, Schaper J, et al. Coordinate expression of the insulin-like growth factor system after microembolisation in porcine heart. Cardiovascular Research. 1997;**33**(2):324-331

[63] Harada C, Mitamura Y, Harada T. The role of cytokines and trophic factors in epiretinal membranes: Involvement of signal transduction in glial cells. Progress in Retinal and Eye Research. 2006;**25**(2):149-164

[64] Vereb Z, Lumi X, Andjelic S, Globocnik-Petrovic M, Urbancic M, Hawlina M, et al. Functional and molecular characterization of ex vivo cultured epiretinal membrane cells from human proliferative diabetic retinopathy. BioMed Research International. 2013;**2013**:492376

[65] Campochiaro PA, Glaser BM. Platelet-derived growth factor is chemotactic for human retinal pigment epithelial cells. Archives of Ophthalmology. 1985;**103**(4):576-579

[66] Roldan-Pallares M, Rollin R, Martinez-Montero JC, Fernandez-Cruz A, Bravo-Llata C, Fernandez-Durango R. Immunoreactive endothelin-1 in the vitreous humor and epiretinal membranes of patients with proliferative diabetic retinopathy. Retina. 2007;**27**(2):222-235

[67] Pollreisz A, Funk M, Breitwieser FP, Parapatics K, Sacu S, Georgopoulos M, et al. Quantitative proteomics of aqueous and vitreous fluid from patients with idiopathic epiretinal membranes. Experimental Eye Research. 2013;**108**:48-58

[68] Hirokawa H, Jalkh AE, Takahashi M, Takahashi M, Trempe CL, Schepens CL. Role of the vitreous in idiopathic preretinal macular fibrosis. American Journal of Ophthalmology. 1986;**101**(2):166-169

[69] Wiznia RA. Posterior vitreous detachment and idiopathic preretinal macular gliosis. American Journal of Ophthalmology. 1986;**102**(2):196-198

[70] Tomita Y, Cagnone G, Fu Z, Cakir B, Kotoda Y, Asakage M, et al. Vitreous metabolomics profiling of proliferative diabetic retinopathy. Diabetologia. 2021;**64**(1):70-82

[71] Cicinelli MV, Chatziralli I, Touhami S, Smaoui A, Tombolini B, Nassisi M, et al. Epiretinal membrane peeling in eyes with retinal vein occlusion: Visual and morphologic

outcomes. Ophthalmology and Therapy. 2022;**11**(2):661-675

[72] Vallejo-Garcia JL, Romano M, Pagano L, Montericcio A, Borgia A, Morenghi E, et al. OCT changes of idiopathic epiretinal membrane after cataract surgery. International Journal of Retina and Vitreous. 2020;**6**:37

[73] Tanikawa A, Shimada Y, Horiguchi M. Comparison of visual acuity, metamorphopsia, and aniseikonia in patients with an idiopathic epiretinal membrane. Japanese Journal of Ophthalmology. 2018;**62**(3):280-285

[74] Hatt SR, Leske DA, Iezzi R, Holmes JM. Binocular interference vs diplopia in patients with epiretinal membrane. JAMA Ophthalmology. 2020;**138**(11):1121-1127

[75] Fang X, Chen Z, Weng Y, et al. Surgical outcome after removal of idiopathic macular epiretinal membrane in young patients. Eye (London, England). 2008;**22**(11):1430-1435

[76] Gass JDM. Stereoscopic Atlas of Macular Disease. St. Louis: Mosby; 1987. pp. 693-695

[77] Do DV, Cho M, Nguyen QD, et al. The impact of optical coherence tomography on surgical decision making in epiretinal membrane and vitreomacular traction. Transactions of the American Ophthalmological Society. 2006;**104**:161-166

[78] Hwang J-U, Sohn J, Moon BG, et al. Assessment of macular function for idiopathic epiretinal membranes classified by spectral-domain optical coherence tomography. Investigative Ophthalmology & Visual Science. 2012;**53**(7):3562-3569

[79] Stevenson W, Prospero Ponce CM, Agarwal DR, Gelman R, Christoforidis JB. Epiretinal membrane: Optical coherence tomography-based diagnosis and classification. Clinical Ophthalmology. 2016;**10**:527-534

[80] Konidaris V, Androudi S, Alexandridis A, Dastiridou A, Brazitikos P. Optical coherence tomography-guided classification of epiretinal membranes. International Ophthalmology. 2015;**35**(4):495-501

[81] Momin SNA, Choudhary RA, Siddiqui MAR, Hashmi S, Memon AS, Tayyab H. Post-operative visual outcomes based on morphological staging of idiopathic epiretinal membranes on OCT. International Journal of Ophthalmology. 2022;**15**(12):1966-1970

[82] Govetto A, Lalane RA 3rd, Sarraf D, Figueroa MS, Hubschman JP. Insights into epiretinal membranes: Presence of ectopic inner foveal layers and a new optical coherence tomography staging scheme. American Journal of Ophthalmology. 2017;**175**:99-113

[83] Doguizi S, Sekeroglu MA, Ozkoyuncu D, Omay AE, Yilmazbas P. Clinical significance of ectopic inner foveal layers in patients with idiopathic epiretinal membranes. Eye (London, England). 2018;**32**:1652-1660

[84] Alkabes M, Fogagnolo P, Vujosevic S, Rossetti L, Casini G, De Cilla S. Correlation between new OCT parameters and meta morphopsia in advanced stages of epiretinal membranes. Acta Ophthalmologica. 2020;**98**(8):780-786

[85] Tsunoda K, Watanabe K, Akiyama K, Usui T, Noda T. Highly reflective foveal region in optical coherence tomography in eyes with vitreomacular traction or epiretinal membrane. Ophthalmology. 2012;**119**(3):581-587

[86] Govetto A, Bhavsar KV, Virgili G, et al. Tractional abnormalities of the central foveal bouquet in epiretinal membranes: Clinical spectrum and pathophysiological perspectives. American Journal of Ophthalmology. 2017;**184**:167-180

[87] Gonzalez-Saldivar G, Berger A, Wong D, Juncal V, Chow DR. Ectopic inner foveal layer classification scheme predicts visual outcomes after epiretinal membrane surgery. Retina. 2020;**40**(4):710-717

[88] Fang IM, Hsu CC, Chen LL. Correlation between visual acuity changes and optical coherence tomography morphological findings in idiopathic epiretinal membranes. Graefe's Archive for Clinical and Experimental Ophthalmology. 2016;**254**(3):437-444

[89] Shimozono M, Oishi A, Hata M, et al. The significance of cone outer segment tips as a prognostic factor in epiretinal membrane surgery. American Journal of Ophthalmology. 2012;**153**(4):698-704

[90] Iuliano L, Fogliato G, Gorgoni F, Corbelli E, Bandello F, Codenotti M. Idiopathic epiretinal membrane surgery: Safety, efficacy and patient related outcomes. Clinical Ophthalmology. 2019;**13**:1253-1265

[91] Miguel AI, Legris A. Prognostic factors of epiretinal membranes: A systematic review. Journal Français d'Ophtalmologie. 2017;**40**(1):61-79

[92] Romano MR, Cennamo G, Amoroso F, et al. Intraretinal changes in the presence of epiretinal traction. Graefe's Archive for Clinical and Experimental Ophthalmology. 2017;**255**(1):31-38

[93] Cho KH, Park SJ, Cho JH, Woo SJ, Park KH. Inner-retinal irregularity index predicts postoperative visual prognosis in idiopathic epiretinal membrane. American Journal of Ophthalmology. 2016;**168**:139-149

[94] Yazici AT, Alagoz N, Celik HU, et al. Idiopathic and secondary epiretinal membranes: Do they differ in terms of morphology? An optical coherence tomography-based study. Retina. 2011;**31**(4):779-784

[95] Mastropasqua R, D'Aloisio R, Viggiano P, et al. Early retinal flow changes after vitreoretinal surgery in idiopathic epiretinal membrane using swept source optical coherence tomography angiography. Journal of Clinical Medicine. 2019;**8**(12):2067

[96] Mao J, Lao J, Liu C, et al. A study analyzing macular micro vasculature features after vitrectomy using OCT angiography in patients with idiopathic macular epiretinal membrane. BMC Ophthalmology. 2020;**20**(1):165

[97] Kim YJ, Kim S, Lee JY, Kim JG, Yoon YH. Macular capillary plexuses after epiretinal membrane surgery: An optical coherence tomography angiography study. The British Journal of Ophthalmology. 2018;**102**(8):1086-1091

[98] Osada U, Kunikata H, Yasuda M, Hashimoto K, Nishiguchi KM, Nakazawa T. Association of retinal vessel density with retinal sensitivity in surgery for idiopathic epiretinal membrane. Graefe's Archive for Clinical and Experimental Ophthalmology. 2020;**258**(9):1911-1920

[99] Cacciamani A, Cosimi P, Di Nicola M, Di Martino G, Ripandelli G, Scarinci F. Correlation between outer retinal thickening and retinal function impairment in patients with idiopathic epiretinal membranes. Retina. 2019;**39**(2):331-338

[100] Deltour JB, Grimbert P, Masse H, Lebreton O, Weber M. Detrimental effects of active internal limiting membrane peeling during epiretinal membrane surgery: Microperimetric analysis. Retina. 2017;**37**(3):544-552

[101] Tadayoni R, Svorenova I, Erginay A, Gaudric A, Massin P. Decreased retinal sensitivity after internal limiting membrane peeling for macular hole surgery. The British Journal of Ophthalmology. 2012;**96**(12):1513-1516

[102] Gao M, Wang Y, Liu W, et al. Assessment of macular function in patients with idiopathic epiretinal membrane by multifocal electroretinography: Correlation with visual acuity and optical coherence tomography. BMC Ophthalmology. 2017;**17**(1):221

[103] Si YJ, Kishi S, Aoyagi K. Assessment of macular function by multifocal electroretinogram before and after macular hole surgery. The British Journal of Ophthalmology. 1999;**83**(4):420-424

[104] Watanabe A, Gekka T, Arai K, Kohzaki K, Tsuneoka H. Early postoperative evaluation of retinal function by electroretinography after vitreous surgery for idiopathic epimacular membrane. Documenta Ophthalmologica. 2017;**134**(3):167-173

[105] Lim JW, Cho JH, Kim HK. Assessment of macular function by multifocal electroretinography following epiretinal membrane surgery with internal limiting membrane peeling. Clinical Ophthalmology. 2010;**4**:689-694

[106] Kim JH, Kim YM, Chung EJ, Lee SY, Koh HJ. Structural and functional predictors of visual outcome of epiretinal membrane surgery. American Journal of Ophthalmology. 2012;**153**(1):103-110

[107] Lo Y-C, Lin K-H, Bair H, et al. Epiretinal membrane detection at the ophthalmologist level using deep learning of optical coherence tomography. Scientific Reports. 2020;**10**(1):8424

[108] Sonobe T, Tabuchi H, Ohsugi H, et al. Comparison between support vector machine and deep learning, machine-learning technologies for detecting epiretinal membrane using 3D-OCT. International Ophthalmology. 2019;**39**(8):1871-1877

[109] Bottoni F, Deiro AP, Giani A, Orini C, Cigada M, Staurenghi G. The natural history of lamellar macular holes: A spectral domain optical coherence tomography study. Graefe's Archive for Clinical and Experimental Ophthalmology. 2013;**251**(2):467-475

[110] Wong JG, Sachdev N, Beaumont PE, Chang AA. Visual outcomes following vitrectomy and peeling of epiretinal membrane. Clinical & Experimental Ophthalmology. 2005;**33**(4):373-378

[111] Scheerlinck LM, van der Valk R, van Leeuwen R. Predictive factors for postoperative visual acuity in idiopathic epiretinal membrane: A systematic review. Acta Ophthalmologica. 2015;**93**(3):203-212

[112] Sugiura Y, Okamoto F, Okamoto Y, Hiraoka T, Oshika T. Contrast sensitivity and foveal microstructure following vitrectomy for epiretinal membrane. Investigative Ophthalmology & Visual Science. 2014;**55**(11):7594-7600

[113] Ghazi-Nouri SM, Tranos PG, Rubin GS, Adams ZC, Charteris DG. Visual function and quality of life following vitrectomy and epiretinal membrane peel surgery. The British Journal of Ophthalmology. 2006;**90**(5):559-562

[114] Okamoto F, Sugiura Y, Okamoto Y, Hiraoka T, Oshika T. Stereopsis and optical coherence tomography findings after epiretinal membrane surgery. Retina. 2015;**35**(7):1415-1421

[115] Kinoshita T, Imaizumi H, Miyamoto H, et al. Changes in meta morphopsia in daily life after successful epiretinal membrane surgery and correlation with M-CHARTS score. Clinical Ophthalmology. 2015;**9**:225-233

[116] Falkner-Radler CI, Glittenberg C, Hagen S, Benesch T, Binder S. Spectral-domain optical coherence tomography for monitoring epiretinal membrane surgery. Ophthalmology. 2010;**117**(4):798-805

[117] Jung JJ, Hoang QV, Ridley-Lane ML, Sebrow DB, et al. Long-term retrospective analysis of visual acuity and optical coherence topographic changes after single versus double peeling during vitrectomy for macular epiretinal membranes. Retina. 2016;**36**(11):2101-2109

[118] Schechet SA, DeVience E, Thompson JT. The effect of internal limiting membrane peeling on idiopathic epiretinal membrane surgery, with a review of the literature. Retina. 2017;**37**(5):873-880

[119] Azuma K, Ueta T, Eguchi S, Aihara M. Effects of internal limiting membrane peeling combined with removal of idiopathic epiretinal membrane: A systematic review of literature and meta-analysis. Retina. 2017;**37**(10):1813-1819

[120] Mitsui K, Kogo J, Takeda H, et al. Comparative study of 27-gauge vs 25-gauge vitrectomy for epiretinal membrane. Eye. 2016;**30**(4):538-544

[121] Reibaldi M, Longo A, Avitabile T, et al. Transconjunctival non-vitrecomizing vitreous surgery versus 25-gauge vitrectomy in patients with epiretinal membrane: A prospective randomized study. Retina. 2015;**35**(5):873-879

[122] Saito Y, Lewis JM, Park I, et al. Nonvitrectomizing vitreous surgery: A strategy to prevent postoperative nuclear sclerosis. Ophthalmology. 1999;**106**(8):1541-1545

[123] Hernández F, Alpizar-Alvarez N, Wu L. Chromovitrectomy: An update. J. Ophthalmic Vis. Res. 2014;**9**(2):251-259

[124] Hillenkamp J, Saikia P, Gora F, et al. Macular function and morphology after peeling of idiopathic epiretinal membrane with and without the assistance of indocyanine green. The British Journal of Ophthalmology. 2005;**89**(4):437-443

[125] Kocstinger A, Bovey EH. Visual acuity after vitrectomy and epiretinal membrane peeling with or without premacular indocyanine green injection. European Journal of Ophthalmology. 2005;**15**(6):795-799

[126] Foster RE, Petersen MR, Da Mata AP, Burk SE, Rosa RH Jr, Riemann CD. Negative indocyanine green staining of epiretinal membranes. Retina. 2002;**22**(1):106-108

[127] Sakamoto H, Yamanaka I, Kubota T, Ishibashi T. Indocyanine green-assisted peeling of the epiretinal membrane in proliferative vitreoretinopathy. Graefe's Archive for Clinical and Experimental Ophthalmology. 2003;**241**(3):204-207

[128] Rodrigues EB, Costa EF, Penha FM, et al. The use of vital dyes in ocular surgery. Survey of Ophthalmology. 2009;**54**(5):576-617

[129] Bopp S. Is there room for improvement in pucker surgery? In: Kirchhof B, Wong D, editors. Vitreo-Retinal Surgery. Berlin, Heidelberg: Springer Berlin Heidelberg; 2005. pp. 37-65

[130] Charles S. Techniques and tools for dissection of epiretinal membranes. Graefe's Archive for Clinical and Experimental Ophthalmology. 2003;**241**(5):347-352

[131] Chen W, Shen X, Zhang P, et al. Clinical characteristics, long-term surgical outcomes, and prognostic factors of epiretinal membrane in young patients. Retina. 2019;**39**(8):1478-1487

[132] Fabian ID, Moisseiev J. Sutureless vitrectomy: Evolution and current practices. The British Journal of Ophthalmology. 2011;**95**(3):318-324

[133] Pichi F, Lembo A, Morara M, et al. Early and late inner retinal changes after inner limiting membrane peeling. International Ophthalmology. 2014;**34**(2):437-446

[134] Scupola A, Grimaldi G, Abed E, et al. Arcuate nerve fiber layer changes after internal limiting membrane peeling in idiopathic epiretinal membrane. Retina. 2018;**38**(9):1777-1785

[135] Loiudice P, Pellegrini M, Montesel A, et al. Negative correlation between retinal displacement and ganglion cell layer thickness changes in eyes with epiretinal membrane. European Journal of Ophthalmology. 2019;**30**(6):1424-1431

[136] Tadayoni R, Paques M, Massin P, Mouki-Benani S, Mikol J, Gaudric A. Dissociated optic nerve fiber layer appearance of the fundus after idiopathic epiretinal membrane removal. Ophthalmology. 2001;**108**(12):2279-2283

[137] Spaide RF. "Dissociated optic nerve fiber layer appearance" after internal limiting membrane removal is inner retinal dimpling. Retina. 2012;**32**(9):1719-1726

[138] Sandali O, El Sanharawi M, Basli E, et al. Paracentral retinal holes occurring after macular surgery: Incidence, clinical features, and evolution. Graefe's Archive for Clinical and Experimental Ophthalmology. 2012;**250**(8):1137-1142

[139] Matoba R, Morizane Y. Surgical treatment of epiretinal membrane. Acta Medica Okayama. 2021;**75**(4):403-413

[140] Donati S, Caprani SM, Semeraro F, et al. Morphological and functional retinal assessment in epiretinal membrane surgery. Seminars in Ophthalmology. 2017;**32**(6):751-758

Chapter 8

Persistent Macular Hole Management Options

Andrea Tamine Hoyos Dumar and Juan Carlos Lugo Prada

Abstract

The widely accepted gold standard technique for the treatment of Macular holes is pars plana vitrectomy combined with internal limiting membrane peeling, resulting in closure rates of 80–100%. Results are influenced by the base diameter, inner opening size, and chronicity, with outcomes less favorable for larger holes and those persisting for over a year. In recent years, surgical attention has shifted toward addressing the closure of refractory or very large holes. Literature has published significant data showing satisfactory anatomical and promising visual outcomes. These techniques can be categorized based on the presumed mechanisms of closure induction. Retinal expansion, autologous retinal transplant, ILM flaps, lens capsules, or amniotic membranes within the MH, each yielding varying closure rates. Modulation of intraretinal gliosis through growth and neurotrophic factors using autologous blood-derived plugs or scaffolds to facilitate Muller cell migration and proliferation have also been documented. Plasma rich in growth factors (PRGF) exhibits anti-inflammatory, anti-fibrotic, and regenerative functions lead to high MH closure rates, garnering attention from retinal surgeons globally. The growing volume of publications suggests benefits from Plasma Rich in Growth Factors over other plasma derivatives. While there is no definitive method for treating macular holes, these newer techniques offer a promising future.

Keywords: macular hole, surgical management, plasma rich in growth factors, tissue transplantation, scaffolds

1. Introduction

A full-thickness macular hole (FTMH) is characterized by a structural defect in the fovea where all neural retinal layers from the ILM to the retinal pigment epithelium (RPE) are interrupted [1]. This condition is diagnosed through clinical assessment and imaging modalities like optical coherence tomography (OCT), which provide additional information, characteristics, and prognostic indicators.

The central opening in the fovea can result from various mechanical factors, including tractional forces within a foveal cystoid space, breakdown and elevation of central photoreceptors, and tangential traction on the inner retinal layers. Some FTMHs might also exhibit a true retinal operculum. The hole's edges tend to be rounded and may contain intraretinal pseudocysts. Additionally, due to the accumulation of intraretinal fluid, the edge might appear slightly elevated compared to the RPE plane. Full-thickness macular hole often exhibit an hourglass shape, which can vary based on the orientation of the OCT scan. The vitreous may or may not be attached to the edge of the MH [2].

Macular hole pose challenges for vitreoretinal surgeons. Idiopathic FTMH are relatively common, with a prevalence of about 0.3–5% in the general population over 60 years of age. This prevalence increases with age and is more common in females [3, 4]. The widely accepted gold standard treatment technique is PPV combined with ILM peeling, resulting in closure rates ranging from 80 to 100%. The outcomes are influenced by factors such as base diameter, inner opening size, and chronicity. Poorer outcomes are observed in cases of holes larger than 400 microns and those present for over a year (with a closure rate around 77%) [5–7].

In recent years, attention has shifted to surgical techniques targeting refractory, recurrent, persistent, or very large holes with limited closure potential using conventional approaches. New techniques have emerged in the literature, demonstrating satisfactory and promising anatomical and visual outcomes.

2. Pathogenesis

This passage offers an overview of the evolving comprehension of MH pathogenesis, with a specific focus on the vitreous's role and the mechanisms that underlie hole formation and progression.

Initial theories postulated that MH might stem from a degenerative process, potentially linked to vascular insufficiency. Moreover, certain theories centered on the vitreous's role in MH development, suggesting that tangential traction, potentially resulting from Müller cell proliferation and contraction within the vitreoretinal interface, played a substantial part [8, 9].

2.1 Involvement of the vitreous

The significance of the vitreous in MH pathogenesis is underscored. This notion is substantiated by the observation that eyes with complete posterior vitreous detachment (PVD) exhibit fewer occurrences of MH. Furthermore, MHs are less prone to enlargement when PVD is evident at the time of diagnosis [9, 10].

2.2 Gass's theory

A pivotal aspect of Gass's theory is that MHs arise from the centrifugal displacement of photoreceptors, rather than a mere loss of these cells. This concept elucidates the restoration of visual acuity to nearly normal levels following MH surgery [8–12].

2.3 Histopathological discoveries

Histopathological evaluations of operculae (tissue overlaying MHs) surgically removed have demonstrated their frequent inclusion of glial elements, albeit not necessarily implying a loss of foveal cones. However, more recent findings suggest

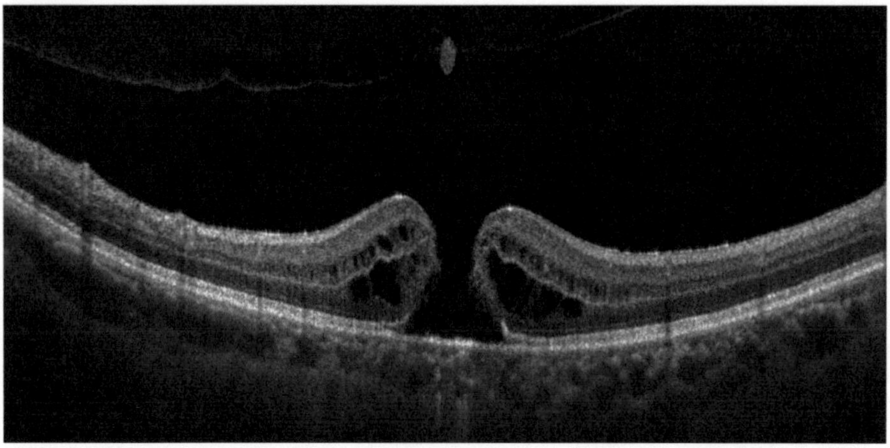

Figure 1.
A 65-year-old male patient with a FTMH with vitreous detachment and an operculum.

that, in certain MH cases, substantial amounts of foveal tissue, including cones, can become torn from the foveal region (**Figure 1**) [5, 9].

2.4 Lateral displacement of photoreceptors

Some studies, including one utilizing binocular kinetic perimetry, have directly substantiated the lateral displacement of photoreceptors during MH development, explaining the typical distortion reported by MH patients [9, 12].

2.5 Revised theory with optical coherence tomography

With the arrival of OCT, Gass's theory has undergone revision. Recent studies utilizing OCT and ultrasound have unveiled that impending macular holes often encompass perifoveal vitreous detachment with localized vitreous attachment to the foveal umbo. A division emerges between the Müller cell cone (central glial element) and foveal photoreceptors due to posterior-anterior vitreomacular traction, fostering the development of a cystic lesion [2, 5, 12].

2.6 Transition to FTMH

The progression from an impending MH to a FTMH typically commences with a disruption in the roof of the cystic lesion. Centrifugal traction, the origin of which remains enigmatic, triggers the expansion of the disruption into the photoreceptor layer, resulting in a full-thickness defect. The hole may subsequently increase in size and assume a more rounded shape over time [12].

After conducting a comprehensive review of the literature and taking clinical experience into account, we posit that MH development is a complex interplay of various factors. The interplay of posterior-anterior vitreous traction, combined with tangential traction of the inner layers, notably the ILM, contributes to this process. This perspective elucidates why solely performing PPV on small holes, or in the case of moderately sized holes, peeling the ILM, leads to lesion closure (**Figure 2**).

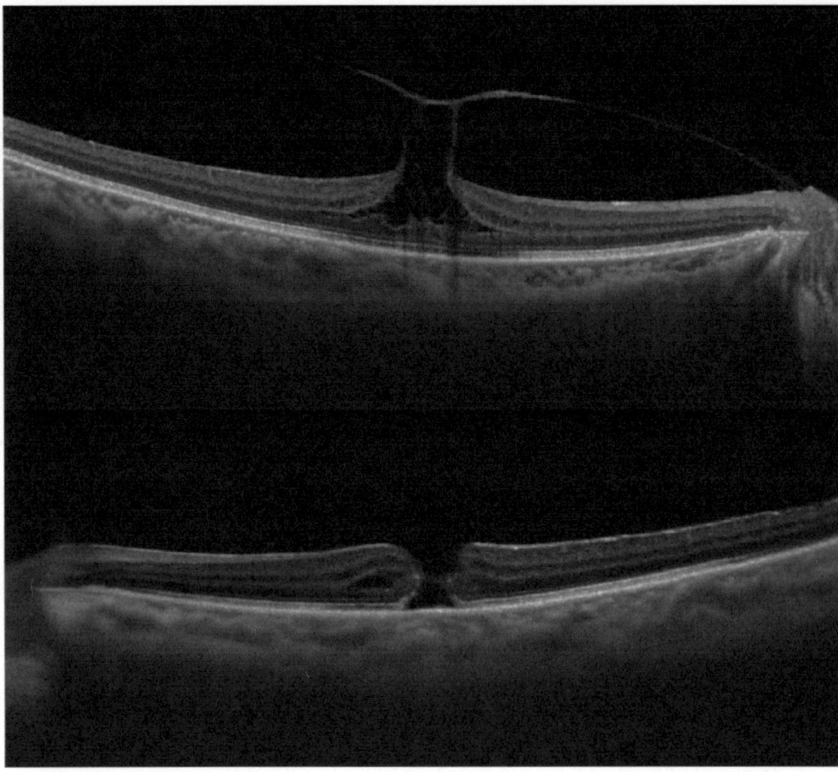

Figure 2.
A 64-year-old female patient with vitro macular traction syndrome in the right eye (upper image) and a FMTH en left eye (inferior image).

3. Natural history

The natural history of MH comprises several distinct stages. The prognosis and likelihood of spontaneous closure or progression hinge on the MH's size and the presence of PVD [12].

3.1 Impending macular holes (stage 1)

Impending MH may lead to different outcomes. They can either resolve spontaneously, remain unchanged, or progress to FTMH. The presence of complete PVD seems to have a positive prognosis for stage 1 MH. Initial visual acuity of 20/40 or better in some cases indicates a better outcome [12].

3.2 Spontaneous resolution

In one study, about 48% of stage 1 MHs regressed, 29% remained the same, and 23% evolved into a FTMH within a year. Regressions often correlated with a posterior vitreous separation, either at baseline or during follow-up [12].

3.3 Stage 2 macular holes

Stage 2 MH also demonstrate varying outcomes. They may remain stable, close spontaneously (though full closure might not result in a normal foveal appearance), or expand over time. In a study, a significant percentage (74%) of stage 2 MH advanced to stage 3 within a year. Some spontaneously closed stage 2 MH did not regain normal foveal morphology but displayed flattened hole edges. However, reports exist of spontaneous closure with a minority of cases reverting to normal foveal contour [12].

3.4 Stage 3 and stage 4 macular holes

Spontaneous closure is rare in these advanced MH stages. Such closure, characterized by the flattening of hole edges (not necessarily returning to normal foveal morphology), was observed in a small portion of cases. Generally, stage 3 and stage 4 macular holes remain steady or enlarge with time [12].

3.5 Rhegmatogenous retinal detachment (RRD)

MH typically do not precipitate RRD. However, highly myopic eyes with a posterior staphyloma are at a rare risk of developing retinal detachment [12].

4. Classification

4.1 International Vitreomacular traction study (IVTS)

Traditionally, FTMHs were categorized using the Gass classification, which divided them into the aforementioned four stages based on clinical examination. However, advancements in OCT technology have yielded a more precise understanding of FTMH pathogenesis and progression [1, 2].

Optical Coherence Tomography-Based FTMH Classification System (Based on Size, Presence or Absence of Vitreomacular Traction, and Cause):

- Hole Size: An OCT-based system permits exact anatomical measurements of FTMHs. The minimum hole width, also referred to as aperture size, holds crucial significance. Small FTMHs boast an aperture size under 250 microns, while medium FTMHs span from 250 to 400 microns. Large FTMHs exceed 400 micrometers in diameter. These size classifications are pivotal, as they influence treatment strategies [2, 13].

- Vitreomacular Traction (VMT) Presence or Absence: FTMHs can be grouped based on the presence or absence of vitreous attachment. For the consideration of pharmacologic vitreolysis, only macular holes concurrently exhibiting VMT should be selected [2, 14].

- Primary Versus Secondary FTMH: Full-thickness macular hole can be further categorized into primary and secondary forms. Primary FTMHs, previously termed idiopathic, stem from vitreous traction on the fovea, often linked to anomalous PVD and VMT. Secondary FTMHs result directly from underlying pathologies, devoid of pre-existing or concurrent VMT. These secondary FTMHs may arise from factors such as trauma, high myopia, macular schisis, macular telangiectasia type 2, wet macular degeneration treated with anti-vascular endothelial growth factor therapy, macroaneurysm, or surgical trauma [2, 14].

It's important to note that FTMHs can co-occur with macular edema related to various retinal diseases, including diabetic macular edema, age-related macular degeneration, retinal vascular occlusions, and uveitis. The classification as primary or secondary FTMH hinges on VMT presence or absence. This OCT-based classification system offers a more comprehensive and precise approach to understand and manage FTMHs based on their size, underlying vitreous condition, and causative factors [1].

5. Optical coherence tomography prognosis biomarkers

Structural OCT imaging is pivotal in the diagnosis and management of FTMHs. This imaging technique has long been essential for accurately diagnosing FTMHs, distinguishing them from other vitreomacular pathologies, and predicting visual outcomes following successful surgery [15].

OCT is essential in measuring various aspects of FTMHs, including their size, base diameter, height, and the macular hole index (height/maximum basal diameter). The minimum linear dimension, representing the horizontal span between the closest retinal components, is a critical factor in assessing anatomical success post-surgery and forms the basis of an international OCT-based classification system for FTMH [16].

Smaller hole diameters tend to lead to better postoperative visual acuity. Recent investigations have explored additional OCT structural features as predictors of functional recovery after surgery [16].

Structural OCT also allows the identification of three hyper-reflective bands within the external retinal layers: the external limiting membrane (ELM), the ellipsoid zone (EZ), and the interdigitation zone (IZ). Restoration of these bands is often associated with improved visual acuity after FTMH surgery, with the preoperative length of defects serving as a strong predictor of visual acuity outcomes [16].

Furthermore, FTMHs may be associated with intraretinal cystoid cavities around their edges, which expand and separate retinal layers during hole formation. The presence of these cysts has shown mixed correlations with postoperative outcomes, varying by study [16].

Supra-RPE granular deposits have been investigated as potential biomarkers of negative prognosis. These deposits, often found in cases with lower postoperative visual acuity, may indicate photoreceptor disruption [16].

Finally, the presence of epiretinal proliferation, distinct from traditional epiretinal membranes, has been observed in some macular holes. Holes with epiretinal proliferation tend to have worse clinical and surgical outcomes compared to those without it [16].

In summary, OCT imaging is a critical tool in understanding and managing FTMHs, offering insights into their dimensions, structural features, and prognostic implications for visual outcomes after surgery.

6. Macular hole associated with other vitreoretinal interface pathologies

6.1 Macular hole and epiretinal membrane (ERM)

An ERM results from the growth of fibrous-like tissue on the inner surface of the retina. ERMs are often idiopathic but can also be linked to pre-existing conditions or caused by medical procedures. Several studies explore the connection and underlying mechanisms between ERM and FTMH [17].

6.2 Macular hole and epiretinal proliferation (EP)

EP is now considered a distinct clinical entity from conventional ERM, histological analysis supports Müller cell involvement in EP development but it is required a more specific immunohistochemical studies for other etiologies; EP has an impact on vision and surgical treatment. It is reported that almost 90% of EP cases remain stable without surgery, intervention is required for exacerbated cases or those associated with FTMH. Postoperative outcomes remain controversial but in surgery it is important to perform a gentle handling of EP to avoid further rise of FTMH [18].

The connection between ERM or EP and the success of surgical closure for FTMH has stirred controversy. Traditionally, it was believed that removing an ERM during macular hole surgery had no significant impact on postoperative results. However, recent studies, though limited in patient numbers and lacking rigorous statistical analysis, have brought this belief into question. The presence of an ERM during surgery can inadvertently introduce tangential tension on the MH, making procedures like the inverted ILM flap challenging. Additionally, ERM-induced chronic mechanical stress may trigger inflammation and neurodegeneration, hindering sufficient gliosis for closure. Regarding EP, it is mainly composed of noncontractile gliotic tissue from Müller cells, and its relationship with FTMH is still relatively unexplored due to recent improvements in OCT resolution. Although some studies suggest EP as a preoperative risk factor for adverse surgical outcomes, they involve a small patient sample and lack adjustment for baseline factors, such as age, sex, and ERM presence. Therefore, whether ERM or EP affects FTMH surgical outcomes remains controversial and necessitates further investigation [19].

We consider that vitreomacular interface pathologies can play a role in the evolution and progression of MHs. In the case of ERM, by generating additional tangential traction and thickening of the neuroepithelium, they can, in some cases, lead to FTMH and therefore require surgery for removal. Cases of EP may lead to FTMH, but in a very different and poorly understood manner. However, in the majority of published studies, removal of the EP is not recommended due to the potential iatrogenic progression to FTMH. Therefore, it has been considered that EPs contain internal components of the neuroepithelium, and removing them could lead to tissue disruption and worsen the anatomic and visual prognosis.

7. Risk factors of the fellow eye

These risk factors underscore the importance of evaluating both MH stage and posterior vitreous status in fellow eyes when contemplating treatment options for patients with newly diagnosed MHs. Vigilant monitoring and timely intervention may be imperative, especially in high-risk factor cases, to avert macular hole development in the other eye [12, 20].

- Presence of Stage 1 macular hole: A stage 1 macular hole in the opposite eye bears a high risk of progressing to a FTMH within a year. This highlights the significant risk that fellow eyes with early-stage macular holes face in terms of MH development [1, 12].

- Posterior vitreous status: The posterior vitreous status in the fellow eye is another pivotal factor. In cases where the posterior vitreous is detached in the fellow eye (complete posterior vitreous detachment), the risk of it evolving into a FTMH is minimal, estimated at less than 2%. Essentially, a PVD appears to safeguard against MH development in the fellow eye [10, 12].

- Risk in fellow eyes with normal macula and attached posterior vitreous: In fellow eyes featuring a normal macula (no evidence of macular hole) and an attached posterior vitreous, the risk of developing a full-thickness macular hole within 5 years was approximately 15.6%, as indicated by one prospective study. A similar risk value emerged from a retrospective study. This suggests that even in fellow eyes lacking early-stage MH, a noteworthy risk of macular hole development persists [12, 21].

8. Surgical techniques

8.1 Primary FTMH

The standard approach for repairing primary FTMHs involves PPV with ILM peeling and gas tamponade. This method boasts a high success rate of 80–100%. The inverted ILM flap technique is gaining popularity, especially for large or myopic FTMHs [22].

8.2 ILM peeling

ILM peeling is associated with a lower risk of reopening and better outcomes in FTMH surgery [22].

- Conventional ILM peeling: This technique entails PPV, PVD, and ILM removal. It addresses posterior-anterior tractional forces and eliminates tangential tractions on the foveal region. ILM peeling triggers mechanical trauma to the retina, stimulating Müller cells' gliosis, migration, and potentially proliferation. This procedure also eliminates potential vitreous remnants, reducing postoperative epiretinal membrane occurrence and hole reopening. Gas tamponade is employed to seal the hole, creating retinal isolation that promotes subretinal fluid absorption and Müller cell gliosis and migration [22–24].

- Inverted ILM flap: In this method, the ILM is peeled circumferentially but left attached to the hole's borders. The central remnants are manipulated to cover the hole, adopting an "inverted" configuration where the vitreous side of the ILM faces the retinal pigment epithelium (RPE). This approach proves particularly effective for large and myopic macular holes, boasting higher closure rates and

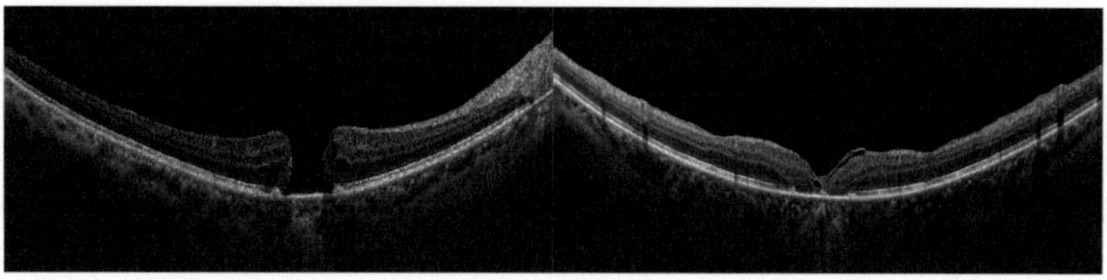

Figure 3.
A 65-year-old female patient with a full-thickness macular hole (FTMH) in the right eye. The left image displays the FTMH with isoreflective pseudocysts at the edges. The right image depicts the postoperative outcome with macular hole closure and evidence of an inverted internal limiting membrane (ILM) flap filling the central area.

improved postoperative visual acuity compared to conventional ILM peeling. The inverted ILM flap may serve as a scaffold for Müller cell migration and proliferation, facilitating hole closure. Immunohistochemical analyses suggest the flap's presence stimulates Müller cells' gliosis and migration. ILM components also enhance Müller cell proliferative and migratory activities in vitro (**Figure 3**) [25, 26].

8.3 Refractory and recurrent cases

Some FTMHs remain open after primary surgery (refractory), or they reopen after initial closure (recurrent), necessitating secondary surgery. Secondary closure proves successful in over 75% of patients, not often leading to substantial visual improvement [27].

Unsuccessful FTMH closure after primary surgery is linked to factors such as large size (> 500 μm), chronicity, high myopia, insufficient ILM peeling, Inadequate postoperative positioning, among others. Recurrent FTMHs share risk factors including cataract surgery, high axial length, and postoperative complications [13, 26].

Multiple surgical techniques are available for repairing refractory or recurrent FTMHs, but consensus on the optimal approach remains elusive due to limited literature on newer methods. These techniques can be grouped according to the presumed mechanisms driving closure [9].

8.4 Revisional vitrectomy (rePPV) with ILM peeling enlargement

This procedure involves enlarging the primary ILM peeling, if necessary, and intraocular tamponade using gases, silicone oils, or heavy silicone oils. The rationale is to weaken tangential tractions, boost retinal elasticity, activate Müller cells, and plug the hole for subretinal fluid reabsorption. The tamponade material choice depends on factors including patient posturing capabilities [9].

These techniques aim to achieve MH closure through distinct mechanisms, including Müller cell gliosis, migration, proliferation, tractional force elimination, and fostering a healing environment. The choice of technique may hinge on factors like macular hole size, type, and desired visual outcomes [5, 9].

8.5 Subretinal fluid injection

This technique causes macular detachment by injecting balanced salt solution (BSS) into the subretinal space. It's believed to promote closure by disrupting abnormal adhesions between neuroretina and RPE, enhancing hole edge elasticity. Subretinal fluid injection may benefit refractory MHs with robust neuroretina-RPE adhesions, such as chronic, large, or traumatic holes [28].

Tissue transplantation: Autologous or heterologous tissue transplantation:

- Lens capsular flap (LCF) or posterior lens capsule (PLC) transplantation: Studies indicate positive immunoreactivity of macroglia and microglia cells in transplanted PLC. This implies a potential similarity between MH closure mechanisms in the inverted ILM flap technique and PLC transplantation. Graft size and orientation are crucial, ensuring the graft is slightly larger than the MH diameter, with the smoother outer surface facing the hole. Differences exist between anterior and posterior capsules, with the anterior capsule adhering firmly with perfluorocarbon liquid (PFCL) tamponade. The posterior capsule may require silicone oil tamponade to prevent flap dislocation. The technique demonstrated partial MH closure through flap incorporation into retinal tissue, leading to visual acuity improvement [29, 30].

- Autologous retinal trasplantation (ART): Proposed for refractory myopic MHs, ART involves a graft twice the MH size, using thicker retina for stability, and positioning under the hole edges. Autologous Neurosensory Retinal Flap showed visual acuity improvement and graft integration, but its value for chronic MHs with poor baseline vision is debated. Postoperative recovery of outer retinal structure, particularly the ellipsoid zone (EZ) and the external limiting membrane (ELM), is vital for improved vision. However, retinal free flap signal transmission remains unclear due to retinal circulation disruption [31, 32].

We consider it could be an alternative in cases of retinal detachment associated with MH.

- Human amniotic membrane (hAM) graft: Is a layer of tissue from the innermost part of the human placenta. It is known for its rich content of growth factors and possesses various beneficial properties, including anti-inflammatory, anti-fibrotic, anti-microbial, and anti-angiogenic effects. Are used in ocular surface reconstruction, and their potential to integrate into host tissue makes them a candidate for macular hole repair. The use of hAM grafts in MH surgery is based on their potential to act as a scaffold for tissue repair and to promote healing. The hAM's basement membrane contains components similar to those found in the internal limiting membrane (ILM), such as collagens IV, laminins, and fibronectin, which may support the adhesion and migration of retinal cells [33, 34].

The surgical procedure involves a standard PPV, similar to other MH repair techniques. After the necessary steps of PPV and confirmation of ILM peeling status, a piece of hAM is harvested from the placenta and prepared. The graft can be placed over the MH in different ways, such as epiretinally (flattened to cover the hole), intraretinally (inserted into the hole), or subretinally (inserted under the hole's edges). The graft is usually manipulated and positioned under perfluorocarbon liquid (PFCL) to aid in its placement. Depending on the specific case and surgeon's preference, tamponade agents like gases, silicone oil (SO), or PFCL can be used. Postoperative positioning, including face-down positioning, is determined based on the choice of tamponade agent [33, 34].

The closure rate of refractory macular holes treated with hAM grafts varies, with reported rates ranging from 66.7 to 100%. However, while successful macular hole closure can be achieved, the functional success, defined as a significant improvement in visual acuity, appears to be less common. The results suggest that while hAM grafts may effectively seal the hole, they may not always lead to substantial visual improvement. The final visual acuity can be influenced by factors such as baseline visual acuity, hole closure, and the reconstitution of the ellipsoid zone (EZ) and ELM on OCT. In summary, hAM grafts represent a potential option for the surgical repair of complex macular holes, especially those that were previously considered untreatable, such as large, recurrent, or highly myopic macular holes. While hAM grafts can effectively close macular holes, the extent of visual improvement may vary, and the graft's integration into host tissue remains a subject of research. The choice to use hAM grafts depends on the specific characteristics of the macular hole and the surgeon's experience and judgment [33, 34].

Autologous blood-derived plugs or scaffolds

- Autologous Platelet-Rich Plasma (aPRP): The use of autologous aPRP aims to modulate intraretinal gliosis through growth and neurotrophic factors, stimulating Müller cell activation and closure. This technique involves using a portion of plasma with a higher concentration of platelets than peripheral blood. It is obtained by centrifuging the patient's blood sample under sterile conditions to prevent contamination. The rationale for using aPRP is based on experimental evidence of the influence of platelets and their growth factors on Müller cells and RPE cells. aPRP stimulate the proliferation and migration of retinal glial cells, Müller cells, and RPE cells in vitro, aiding in macular hole closure. However, it may contain a high concentration of leukocytes that can lead to the release of free radicals and proinflammatory substances that alter or prevent tissue regeneration. Whole blood has the same disadvantage [9, 35, 36].

- Plasma Rich in Growth Factors (PRGF): Is a subtype of aPRP, characterized by a moderate concentration of platelets, in the absence of leukocytes. It involves platelet activation before using it. This absence of leukocytes is based on the fact that they synthesize matrix metalloproteinases (MMPs), free radicals and proinflammatory cytokines, which do not contribute and even impair the altered tissue regeneration [37–40]. Additionally, the clotted PRGF may mechanically contribute to MH closure by sealing the hole and acting as a scaffold for cell migration and proliferation.

The following procedure was standardized at Instituto de Terapias Avanzadas (ITA, Barranquilla, Colombia); the patient's whole blood is collected in 4.5 ml vacutainer tubes containing sodium citrate as an anticoagulant. The samples were processed immediately after collection. Each tube underwent centrifugation for 5 minutes at 300 g. Three components are extracted: fraction 1 (F1), which has a similar platelet concentration as peripheral blood; fraction 2 (F2), with 2 or 3 times the platelet concentration of peripheral blood; and the lowest fraction containing erythrocytes. In this case we took fraction 1 and fraction 2 and place them into a tube. The falcon tube went under centrifugation for a second time for 18 minutes at 700 g. Two milliliters of F2 are taken to prepare the leukocyte-free PRGF. To form the three-dimensional structure, the sample is activated with $C12H22CaO14$ and incubated at 40°C until the membrane coagulates. This process yields three structures: fibrin, scaffold, and eye drops. The prepared material is transported to the operating room under strict aseptic and sterile conditions. The above has been carried out based on the first case report published in Latin America by the retina group of FOSCAL, Colombia [36].

In this approach, a rePPV is performed to address the MH. The previously peeled area of the internal limiting membrane is visualized, and additional peeling may be performed if necessary. After fluid-air exchange, the PRGF membrane is placed over the MH. Gas or silicone oil can be used as a tamponade, and the patient is instructed to assume a specific postoperative position, often involving a period of supine positioning followed by face-down positioning.

In the scarce published studies using this technique, a closure rate of 87.5–100% is reported for refractory macular holes, with significant improvement in visual function. We bring up a representative patient with primary macular hole in both eyes associated with epiretinal membrane and proliferation. This latter factor is a marker of poor prognosis due to the neurodegenerative association in MH formation. This type of pathology associated with MH is usually linked to a low closure rate and poor visual improvement with conventional surgery, and even manipulation of epiretinal proliferation remains a topic of debate due to atrophic changes and post-surgical visual losses. In this case, we performed conventional surgery in one eye and PRGF without EP or ILM peeling in the contralateral eye. We found anatomical closure and visual improvement in both eyes. However, the tomographic characteristics of the outer layers of the neuroepithelium showed greater approximation and regeneration in the PRFG case compared to the eye managed with conventional surgery. Nevertheless, it's important to note that the size of the macular hole managed with ILM peeling was larger (**Figures 4** and 5).

8.6 Other surgical techniques

Outpatient fluid/gas exchange: Intravitreal injection of gas to improve hole closure. Closure rates vary, and complications can include transient raised intraocular pressure (IOP) and retinal detachment [41].

Relaxing retinotomies: Creating retinal incisions around the FTMH to reduce traction. Closure rates vary, and there can be concerns about postoperative scotomas [42, 43].

Retinal massage: Gentle manipulation of the FTMH edges to facilitate closure. Closure rates vary, and visual improvement is often observed [44].

Microdrain: Using a backflush to aid in the drainage of subretinal fluid. Closure rates vary [45].

Macular buckling: This technique is utilized for macular pathologies, including FTMHs associated with macular detachment. It involves employing various macular explants to provide support to the retina and create a flatter configuration of the posterior ocular wall. These techniques are aimed at enhancing the closure of FTMHs, particularly in myopic patients and when traditional surgical approaches like PPV

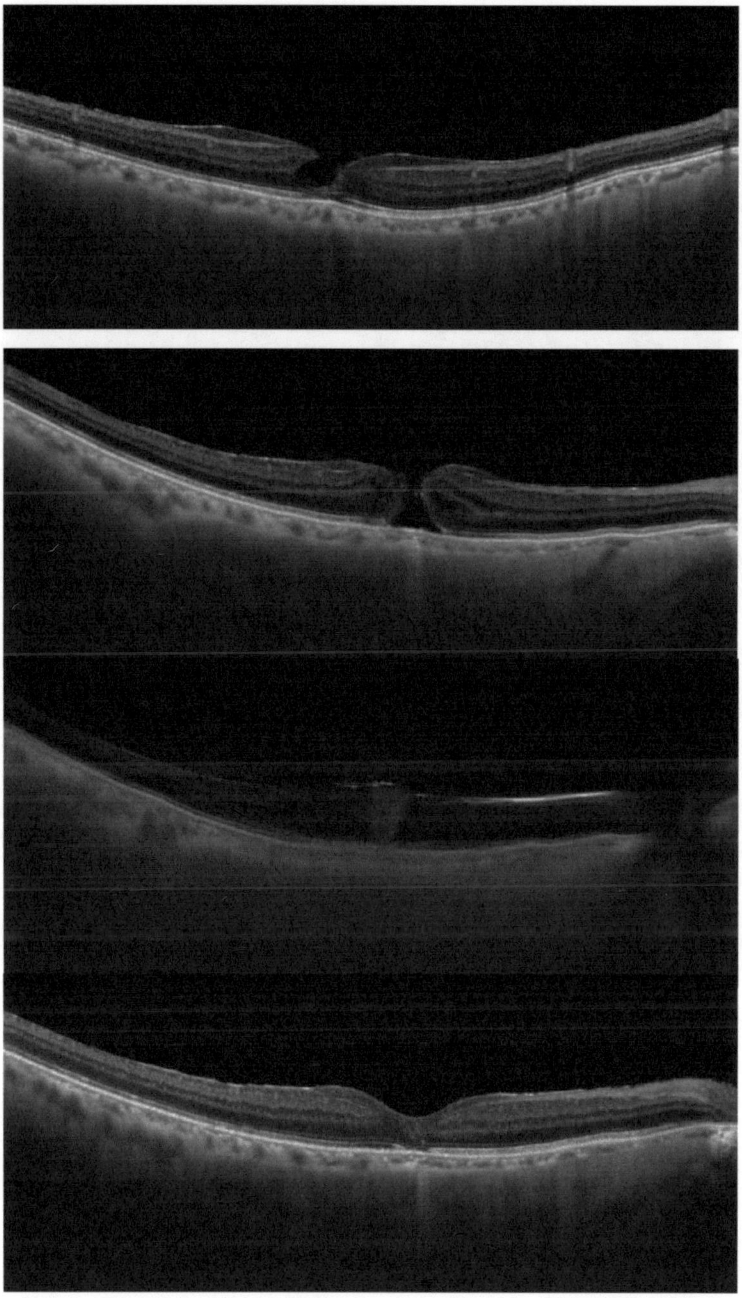

Figure 4.
The right eye of a 74-year-old female patient. OCT B-scans, demonstrates the disease progression. It starts with a lamellar hole-associated epiretinal proliferation and ERM. Then progresses into a FTMH with epiretinal proliferation (EP). The next image is from the first day postoperative after pars plana vitrectomy (PPV) without membrane or EP peeling, using the PRGF membrane. The final image depicts the evolution one month after surgery, showing partial restoration of external layers at the foveal level.

with ILM peeling and gas tamponade have not yielded success. The selection of the technique depends on the specific attributes of the FTMH and the patient's condition [9].

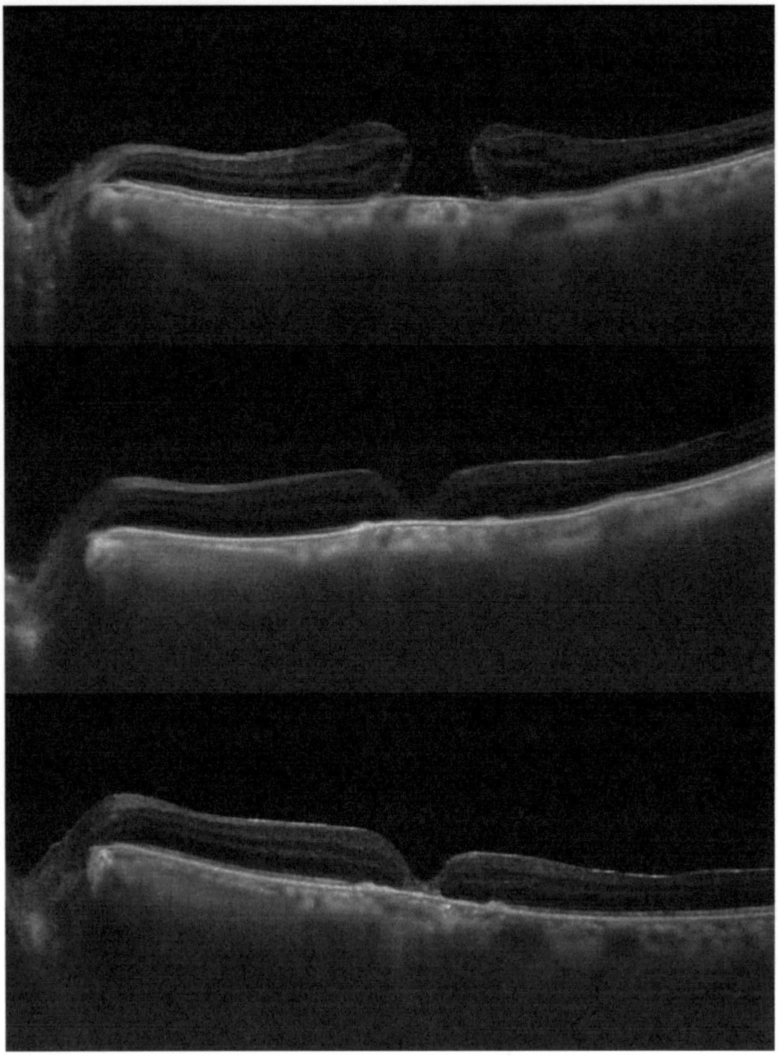

Figure 5.
Left eye of the previous 74-year-old female patient, upper image with FTMH and EP, then postoperative day 1 of PPV with ILM inverted flap, then 1 month postoperative.

8.7 Choice of tamponade

Gases are generally preferred over silicon oil (SO) or heavy silicone oil (HSO) as tamponades, as they do not require additional removal procedures and are not associated with typical SO/HSO-related complications like intraocular emulsification, hypertension and inflammation [46].

8.8 Use of face down position after surgery

Despite the high success rate of the recent techniques, there remains ongoing debate about the best surgical approach. Also Different intraocular tamponade agents such as sulfur hexafluoride (SF6) perfluoroethane (C2F6), perfluoropropane (C3F8), silicone oil, or air have also been employed [15].

For many years, there has been a debate surrounding the ideal duration of postoperative face-down positioning following MH surgery. Although it was once deemed essential, recent optical coherence tomography (OCT) studies have hinted at the possibility of macular holes closing as early as one day after the procedure. This has prompted questions about the necessity of prolonged face-down posturing, which many patients, including older individuals, those with obesity, individuals living alone, or those with limited mobility, find challenging. Additionally, extended posturing may pose an increased risk of thromboembolism [15].

Interestingly, approximately 80% of surgeons still recommend face-down posturing, typically for a period ranging from 5 to 10 days. The rationale behind this practice is that it assists in MH closure by ensuring the buoyant force of the intraocular gas bubble, which is most potent at its apex, maintains contact with the macula. This gas bubble serves to keep the edges of the macular hole dry, prevents vitreous intrusion, and acts as a scaffold for the growth of glial cells. It is worth noting that surface tension around the bubble's interface with the retina remains consistent. Therefore, as long as there is an adequate volume of intraocular gas (approximately two-thirds to three-quarters of the vitreous cavity) and the patient avoids a supine position, the macular hole remains covered [15].

Historical studies indicated better surgical outcomes with prolonged face-down posturing, such as a closure rate of 94.4% for patients posturing face-down for 14 days (90% of the time) followed by 14 days (50% of the time) compared to a 65.6% closure rate for patients posturing face-down for 7 days (90% of the time). However, recent research has demonstrated favorable MH closure rates even with shorter posturing periods, especially when combined with internal limiting membrane (ILM) peeling. In cases with ILM peeling, closure rates reached 92.9% compared to 79.3% without [15].

Recent findings also suggest that the rate of MH closure with face-down posturing for less than 24 hours is comparable to posturing for 5 to 10 days. Nevertheless, there's currently insufficient evidence to definitively determine whether face-down posturing significantly influences MH closure rates after surgery. Additional research is required to establish the precise role of face-down posturing in MH surgery [15].

8.9 Less invasive vs. more invasive procedures

Less invasive revisional surgical procedures (e.g., rePPV with ILM free flap, PRGF or aPRP) appear to be at least as effective as more invasive techniques (e.g., hAM graft and autologous retinal transplantation). The choice of procedure may depend on the complexity of the FTMH, with more invasive techniques reserved for complex cases.

We believe that the choice of surgical technique to use is based on various factors, including the type of MH (primary or refractory), its size, association with vitreoretinal interface pathologies, and the retinal status (attached or detached). Taking these considerations into account, in the case of small primary macular holes, it might be appropriate to consider conventional PPV, with or without ILM peeling. For larger primary macular holes, ILM peeling with or without inverted flap technique, or even the use of PRGF, could be contemplated. For macular holes associated with retinal detachment, we could consider the use of PRGF, hAM, or ART. In the case of myopic macular holes with macular detachment, macular indentation could be complemented with PRGF, hAM, or PRP. Regarding refractory macular holes, we hold the opinion that both anatomical and visual outcomes could be improved by using blood derivatives such as PRP and PRGF. However, it's important to highlight that these suggestions are based on our own experience and we recognize the need for further studies and publications in this field.

9. Conclusions

There is a lack of randomized controlled trials and large prospective studies comparing different surgical techniques for refractory FTMHs. The existing studies have limitations, including heterogeneity in methods, samples, and surgical approaches, as well as small sample sizes.

More research is needed to better understand the mechanisms of FTMH closure, especially when using autologous or heterologous tissue transplantation. Investigating the healing mechanisms could help optimize both anatomical and functional outcomes.

Some experimental and preliminary clinical studies have introduced potential adjuvants for treating refractory and recurrent FTMHs, such as nerve growth factor, mesenchymal stem cells, and mesenchymal stem cell-derived exosomes. These emerging therapies may hold promise for the future.

When dealing with unsuccessful closure or reopening of FTMHs, there is a trend toward surgical approaches that involve adjuvants capable of inducing and modulating intraretinal gliosis and/or membranes that can also act as a mechanical scaffold.

Acknowledgements

Thanks to Dr. Juan David Arias, Dr. Valentina Perez Vergara, Clinica Carriazo, Clinica Yepes Porto, Instituto de Terapias Avanzadas.

Conflict of interest

The authors declare no conflict of interest.

Appendices and nomenclature

MH	macular holes
ILM	internal limiting membrane
ELM	external limiting membrane
PRGF	plasma rich in growth factors
FTMH	full-thickness macular hole
OCT	optical coherence tomography
PVD	posterior vitreous detachment
RRD	rhegmatogenous retinal detachment
IVTS	international vitreomacular traction study
VMT	vitreomacular traction
ERM	epiretinal membrane

EP	epiretinal proliferation
RPE	retinal pigment epithelium
LCF	lens capsular flap
PLC	posterior Lens Capsule
PFCL	perfluorocarbon liquid
hAM	human amniotic membrane
EZ	ellipsoid zone
aPRP	autologous platelet-rich plasma
MMPs	matrix metalloproteinases
rePPV	revisional vitrectomy
IOP	intraocular pressure
SO	silicon oil
HSO	heavy silicone oil

Author details

Andrea Tamine Hoyos Dumar* and Juan Carlos Lugo Prada
Carriazo Clinic, Barranquilla, Colombia

*Address all correspondence to: andrea.tamine.h@gmail.com

References

[1] Premi E, Donati S, Azzi L, Porta G, Metrangolo C, Fontanel L, et al. Macular holes: Main clinical presentations, diagnosis, and therapies. Journal of Ophthalmology. 2022;**2022**:2270861. DOI: 10.1155/2022/2270861. PMID: 35450323; PMCID: PMC9017549

[2] Duker JS, Kaiser PK, Binder S, De Smet MD, Gaudric A, Reichel E, et al. The international Vitreomacular traction study group classification of Vitreomacular adhesion, traction, and macular hole. Ophthalmology. 2013;**120**:2611-2619. DOI: 10.1016/j.ophtha.2013.07.042

[3] Reid GA, McDonagh N, Wright DM, Yek JTO, Essex RW, Lois N. First failed macular hole surgery or reopening of a previously closed hole: Do we gain by re-operating?—A systematic review and meta-analysis. Retina. 2020;**40**(1):1-15. DOI: 10.1097/IAE.0000000000002564. PMID: 31335482; PMCID: PMC6924931

[4] Hwang S, Kang SW, Kim SJ, Choi J, Son KY, Lim DH, et al. Risk factors for the development of idiopathic macular hole: A nationwide population-based cohort study. Scientific Reports. 2022;**12**(1):21778. DOI: 10.1038/s41598-022-25791-1. PMID: 36526695; PMCID: PMC9758209

[5] Caporossi T, Carlà MM, Gambini G, De Vico U, Baldascino A, Rizzo S. Spotlight on the internal limiting membrane technique for macular holes: Current perspectives. Clinical Ophthalmology. 2022;**16**:1069-1084. DOI: 10.2147/OPTH.S284620

[6] Li K, Zhou Y, Yang W, Jiang Q, Xu X. Modified internal limiting membrane flap technique for large chronic macular hole two case reports. Medicine (United States). 2022;**101**:E28412. DOI: 10.1097/MD.0000000000028412

[7] Khodabande A, Mahmoudi A, Faghihi H, Bazvand F, Ebrahimi E, Riazi-Esfahani H. Outcomes of idiopathic full-thickness macular hole surgery: Comparing two different ILM peeling sizes. Journal of Ophthalmology. 2020;**2020**:1619450. DOI: 10.1155/2020/1619450. PMID: 32908679; PMCID: PMC7450298

[8] Bringmann A, Unterlauft JD, Barth T, Wiedemann R, Rehak M, Wiedemann P. Müller cells and astrocytes in tractional macular disorders. Progress in Retinal and Eye Research. 2022;**86**:100977. DOI: 10.1016/j.preteyeres.2021.100977. Epub 2021 Jun 5. PMID: 34102317

[9] Romano MR, Rossi T, Borgia A, Catania F, Sorrentino T, Ferrara M. Management of Refractory and Recurrent Macular Holes: A comprehensive review. Survey of Ophthalmology. 2022;**67**:908-931

[10] Bikbova G, Oshitari T, Baba T, Yamamoto S, Mori K. Pathogenesis and management of macular hole: Review of current advances. Journal of Ophthalmology. 2019;**2019**:3467381. DOI: 10.1155/2019/3467381. PMID: 31191994; PMCID: PMC6525843

[11] Smiddy WE, Flynn HW. Pathogenesis of macular holes and therapeutic implications. American Journal of Ophthalmology. 2004;**137**:525-537. DOI: 10.1016/j.ajo.2003.12.011

[12] La Cour M, Friis J. Macular holes: Classification, epidemiology, natural history and treatment. Acta Ophthalmologica Scandinavica. 2002;**80**:579-587

[13] Rezende FA, Ferreira BG, Rampakakis E, Steel DH, Koss MJ, Nawrocka ZA, et al. Surgical

classification for large macular hole: Based on different surgical techniques results: The CLOSE study group. International Journal of Retina and Vitreous. 2023;**9**(1):4. DOI: 10.1186/s40942-022-00439-4. PMID: 36717928; PMCID: PMC9885593

[14] García-Layana A, García-Arumí J, Ruiz-Moreno JM, Arias-Barquet L, Cabrera-López F, Figueroa MS. A review of current management of vitreomacular traction and macular hole. Journal of Ophthalmology. 2015;**2015**:809640. DOI: 10.1155/2015/809640. Epub 2015 Mar 3. PMID: 25821592; PMCID: PMC4363823

[15] Tatham A, Banerjee S. Face-down posturing after macular hole surgery: A meta-analysis. British Journal of Ophthalmology. 2010;**94**:626-631. DOI: 10.1136/bjo.2009.163741

[16] Nicolosi C, Vicini G, Bacherini D, Giattini D, Lombardi N, Esposito C, Rizzo S, Giansanti F. Non-invasive retinal imaging modalities for the identification of prognostic factors in vitreoretinal surgery for full-thickness macular holes. Diagnostics (Basel). 2023; **13**(4):589. DOI: 10.3390/diagnostics13040589. PMID: 36832078; PMCID: PMC9955111

[17] Gonzalez-Cortes JH, Bilgic A, De Los Santos Polanco J, Treviño-Herrera AB, Sudhalkar A, Gonzalez-Cantu JE, et al. Spontaneous closure of an idiopathic macular hole after epiretinal membrane development. American Journal of Ophthalmology Case Reports. 2023;**29**. DOI: 10.1016/j.ajoc.2022.101767

[18] Yang YS, Lee JS, Son G, Sohn J. Epiretinal proliferation associated with lamellar hole or macular hole: Origin and surgical prognosis. Korean Journal of Ophthalmology. 2019;**33**:142. DOI: 10.3341/kjo.2018.0070

[19] Yang JM, Choi SU, Kim YJ, Kim R, Yon DK, Lee SW, et al. Association between epiretinal membrane, epiretinal proliferation, and prognosis of full-thickness macular hole closure. Retina. 2022;**42**(1):46-54. DOI: 10.1097/IAE.0000000000003262. PMID: 34267114

[20] Staropoli PC, Moolani HV, Elhusseiny AM, Flynn HW, Smiddy WE. Rates of fellow eye macular hole development during long term follow-up. Clinical Ophthalmology. 2023;**17**: 47-52. DOI: 10.2147/OPTH.S394933

[21] Ezra E, Wells JA, Gray RH, Kinsella FM, Orr GM, Grego J, et al. Incidence of idiopathic full-thickness macular holes in fellow eyes. A 5-year prospective natural history study. Ophthalmology. 1998;**105** (2):353-359. DOI: 10.1016/s0161-6420(98)93562-x. PMID: 9479299

[22] Ruban A, Petrovski BÉ, Petrovski G, Lytvynchuk LM. Internal limiting membrane peeling and gas tamponade for full-thickness macular holes of different etiology – Is it still relevant? Clinical Ophthalmology. 2022;**16**: 3391-3404. DOI: 10.2147/OPTH.S373675

[23] Abdul-Kadir MA, Lim LT. Update on surgical management of complex macular holes: A review. International Journal of Retina and Vitreous. 2021;**7** (1):75. DOI: 10.1186/s40942-021-00350-4. PMID: 34930488; PMCID: PMC8686572

[24] Rahimy E, McCannel CA. Impact of internal limiting membrane peeling on macular hole reopening: A systematic review and meta-analysis. Retina. 2016; **36**(4):679-687. DOI: 10.1097/IAE.0000000000000782. PMID: 26441264

[25] Kastl G, Heidenkummer P. ILM flap repositioning for persistent macular

hole. Case Reports in Ophthalmology. 2022;**13**:499-503. DOI: 10.1159/000525303

[26] Cao JL, Kaiser PK. Surgical Management of Recurrent and Persistent Macular Holes: A practical approach. Ophthalmology and Therapy. 2021;**10**: 1137-1153. DOI: 10.1007/s40123-021-00388-5

[27] Lorenzi U, Mehech J, Caporossi T, Romano MR, De Fazio R, Parrat E, et al. A retrospective, multicenter study on the Management of Macular Holes without residual internal limiting membrane: The refractory macular hole (ReMaHo) study. Graefe's Archive for Clinical and Experimental Ophthalmology. 2022;**260**: 3837-3845. DOI: 10.1007/s00417-022-05739-x

[28] Khan TH, Rizvi SF, Mahmood SA, Feroz L. Treatment of chronic large and persistent macular hole by a new technique in a tertiary care hospital. Pakistan Journal of Medical Sciences. 2021;**37**(4):979-982. DOI: 10.12669/pjms.37.4.3618. PMID: 34290769; PMCID: PMC8281167

[29] Yepez JB, Murati FA, De Yepez J, Petitto M, Arevalo JF. Aanterior lens capsule in the management of chronic full-thickness macular hole. Retinal Cases and Brief Reports. 2018;**12**(4): 286-290. DOI: 10.1097/ICB.0000000000000513. PMID: 28033231

[30] Cisiecki S, Bonińska K, Bednarski M. Autologous lens capsule flap transplantation for persistent macular holes. Journal of Ophthalmology. 2021;**2021**: 8148792. DOI: 10.1155/2021/8148792. PMID: 33728059; PMCID: PMC7937468

[31] Yamada K, Maeno T, Kusaka S, Arroyo JG, Yamada M. Recalcitrant macular hole closure by autologous retinal transplant using the peripheral retina. Clinical Ophthalmology. 2020;**14**: 2301-2306. DOI: 10.2147/OPTH.S236592

[32] Rojas-Juárez S, Cisneros-Cortés J, Ramirez-Estudillo A, Velez-Montoya R. Autologous full-thickness retinal transplant for refractory large macular holes. International Journal of Retina and Vitreous. 2020;**6**(1):60. DOI: 10.1186/s40942-020-00266-5. PMID: 33292851; PMCID: PMC7685585

[33] Lipková B, Rosocha J, Maurská A. Report on amniotic membrane for surgery of persistent macular hole. Cesk Slov Oftalmol. 2022 Spring;**78**(3):130-137. English. DOI: 10.31348/2022/15. PMID: 35760584

[34] Ferreira MA, Maia A, Machado AJ, Ferreira REA, Hagemann LF, Júnior PHER, et al. Human amniotic membrane for the treatment of large and refractory macular holes: A retrospective, multicentric, interventional study. International Journal of Retina and Vitreous. 2021;**7**(1):38. DOI: 10.1186/s40942-021-00308-6. PMID: 33964971; PMCID: PMC8105940

[35] Shpak AA, Shkvorchenko DO, Krupina EA. Surgical treatment of macular holes with and without the use of autologous platelet-rich plasma. International Ophthalmology. 2021;**41**: 1043-1052. DOI: 10.1007/s10792-020-01662-4

[36] Arias JD, Hoyos AT, Alcántara B, Sanchez-Avila RM, Arango FJ, Galvis V. Plasma rich in growth factors for persistent macular hole: A pilot study. Retinal Cases and Brief Reports. 2022;**16**(2):155-160. DOI: 10.1097/ICB.0000000000000957. PMID: 31895724

[37] McCarrel TM, Minas T, Fortier LA. Optimization of leukocyte concentration in platelet-rich plasma for the treatment

of tendinopathy. Journal of Bone and Joint Surgery. 2012;**94**:e143(1). DOI: 10.2106/JBJS.L.00019

[38] Schnabel LV, Mohammed HO, Miller BJ, McDermott WG, Jacobson MS, Santangelo KS, et al. Platelet rich plasma (PRP) enhances anabolic gene expression patterns in flexor Digitorum Superficialis tendons. Journal of Orthopaedic Research. 2007;**25**:230-240. DOI: 10.1002/jor.20278

[39] Scott A, Khan KM, Roberts CR, Cook JL, Duronio V. What do we mean by the term "inflammation"? A contemporary basic science update for sports medicine. British Journal of Sports Medicine. 2004;**38**:372-380

[40] Sundman EA, Cole BJ, Fortier LA. Growth factor and catabolic cytokine concentrations are influenced by the cellular composition of platelet-rich plasma. American Journal of Sports Medicine. 2011;**39**:2135-2140. DOI: 10.1177/0363546511417792

[41] Imai M, Gotoh T, Iijima H. Additional intravitreal gas injection in the early postoperative period for an unclosed macular hole treated with internal limiting membrane peeling. Retina. 2005;**25**(2):158-161. DOI: 10.1097/00006982-200502000-00007. PMID: 15689805

[42] Charles S, Randolph JC, Neekhra A, Salisbury CD, Littlejohn N, Calzada JI. Arcuate Retinotomy for the repair of large macular holes. Ophthalmic Surgery Lasers and Imaging. 2013;**44**:69-72. DOI: 10.3928/23258160-20121221-15

[43] Zas M, Lasave AF, Alfano A, Saravia M. Surgical technique for approaching chronic or persistent macular holes: Two case reports. American Journal of Ophthalmology Case Reports. 2020;**18**: 100692. DOI: 10.1016/j.ajoc.2020. 100692. PMID: 32322749; PMCID: PMC7160520

[44] Wang H, Ji M, Di R, Qi Y, Pei C, Gao S, et al. Parafoveal retinal massage combined with autologous blood cover in the Management of Giant, persistent or recurrent macular holes. International Journal of Ophthalmology. 2020;**13**: 1773-1779. DOI: 10.18240/ijo.2020.11.14

[45] Maguire MJ, Steel DH, Yorston D, Hind J, El-Faouri M, Jalil A, et al. Outcome of revision procedures for failed primary macular hole surgery. Retina. 2021;**41**(7):1389-1395. DOI: 10.1097/IAE.0000000000003072. PMID: 33315821

[46] Nicolai M, Lassandro N, Franceschi A, Rosati A, De Turris S, Pelliccioni P, et al. Intraocular pressure rise linked to silicone oil in retinal surgery: A review. Vision (Switzerland). 2020;**4**:1-18

Chapter 9

Choroidal Perfusion after Macular Surgery in Myopic Traction Maculopathy

Miguel A. Quiroz-Reyes and Erick A. Quiroz-Gonzalez

Abstract

Myopic traction maculopathy (MTM) is a vision-threatening condition associated with high myopia, posing public health concerns due to the global rise in the prevalence of myopia. MTM encompasses various pathological changes, including foveoschisis, macular hole formation, and retinal detachment, which can lead to irreversible vision loss if not detected or managed early. Understanding choroidal perfusion, particularly in highly myopic eyes, is crucial because the choroid undergoes changes such as thinning and reduced perfusion, which may influence the onset and severity of myopic maculopathy. This chapter explores the importance of choroidal perfusion in MTM and its role in guiding surgical interventions. This chapter investigates two key hypotheses: the impact of various surgical approaches on the postoperative choroidal vascularity index (CVI) and the correlation between the CVI and postoperative visual outcomes following current surgical techniques. This chapter discusses the advantages and limitations of CVI, future research directions, and potential therapeutic implications.

Keywords: central macular thickness, choriocapillaris flow area, choroidal vascularity index, foveoretinal detachment, foveoschisis, macular hole, macular hole-related retinal detachment, myopic traction maculopathy, pathologic myopia, vitreomacular traction

1. Introduction

Myopic traction maculopathy (MTM), a vision-threatening condition due to high myopia (HM) considered an eye with an anteroposterior axial length of ≥26.5 mm or more, has received considerable attention for its timely diagnosis and management, as it leads to multiple retinal pathologies if untreated on time [1]. Pathologic myopia (PM), which is defined as the progressive deterioration of chorioretinal tissue owing to scleral elongation and posterior staphyloma (PS) development, is characterized by the existence of myopic lesions in the back of the eye consistent with chorioretinal atrophy, choroidal neovascularization (CNV), and slow vitreomacular traction (VMT) linked to the progressive emergence of different MTM manifestations in approximately 30% of high myopia cases with the common occurrence of PS [2].

The global prevalence of myopia has been steadily increasing globally, making MTM an emerging public health issue [3]. The World Health Organization estimates that by 2050, approximately 50% of the world's population will be affected by myopia, with nearly 10% of patients suffering from HM [4]. HM is a significant contributor to legal blindness in industrialized nations, and its prevalence has steadily increased in recent decades. Projections suggest that by 2050, it could affect nearly one billion individuals. Studies analyzing regional and temporal trends have observed a sharp increase in myopia cases worldwide, particularly in East and Southeast Asia, affecting approximately 80–90% of the population, with up to 20% suffering from HM [5]. In the United States, nearly 2% of the general population aged between 12 and 54 years is estimated to be affected by HM, underscoring the need to focus on preventive measures and treatment strategies [6]. These approaches aim to prevent vision loss and blindness caused by PM. Notably, in Japan, PM is identified as the fifth leading cause of blindness, while in China (among people over 40 years of age), it ranks as the second leading cause [7]. As the prevalence of myopia increases, so does the incidence of associated complications, such as MTM, making it essential to understand the disease mechanisms and optimize treatment strategies.

MTM is explained in numerous forms by different researchers, ranging from retinal thickening resembling macular schisis (MS) to foveoschisis (FS), foveoretinal detachment (FRD), and shallow macular detachment (MD) [8]. The first mention of "retinomacular schisis" was by Phillips in 1958 [9], who described posterior retinal detachment (RD) without a macular hole (MH) in patients with myopic staphyloma, suggesting traction as the cause. In 1999, Takano and Kishi used optical coherence tomography (OCT) for anatomical characteristics, which they refer to as "foveal retinomacular schisis" [10]. Panozzo et al. introduced the term "myopic traction maculopathy," which affects 9–34% of HM patients with PS [11]. Shimada et al. [12] described the stages of macular FS that lead to FRD through an outer lamellar macular hole (O-LMH). Ruiz-Medrano et al. [13] provided a comprehensive classification of myopic maculopathy, including MTM as a tractional aspect [13]. Parolini et al. proposed a novel MTM staging system (MSS) that defines it as a progressive disease starting with inner MS (I-MS) and culminating in MD, reflecting the dynamic nature of the condition [14].

The current understanding is that MTM with all these pathological changes may result in a spectrum of different and very complex clinical manifestations with distinct OCT structural phenotypes, including isolated macular thickening without schisis (**Figure 1a**), extrafoveal MS (**Figure 1b**), myopic MS (**Figure 1c**), MS with inner lamellar macular hole (I-LMH) (**Figure 1d**), localized or extensive FRD (**Figure 1e**), inner LMH (**Figure 1f**), inner LMH with epiretinal membrane (ERM) (**Figure 1g**), full-thickness macular hole (FTMH) (**Figure 1h**), and posterior pole or more extensive MH-related rhegmatogenous RD (MHRD) (**Figure 1i**) [15], all of which can severely impair visual function [11, 14, 16]. As MTM progresses, it can lead to irreversible vision loss, emphasizing the importance of early detection and intervention.

MTM pathogenesis is multifactorial and involves tangential retinal traction and combined anteroposterior traction induced by VMT, vitreomacular adhesions, vitreous cortex remnants, PS, and epiretinal membrane (ERM) proliferation [17, 18]. The internal limiting membrane (ILM), retinal vascular microfolds, and paravascular vitreal adhesions may also contribute to its pathogenesis [19–21]. In highly myopic eyes, the choroid undergoes changes, including thinning and reduced perfusion,

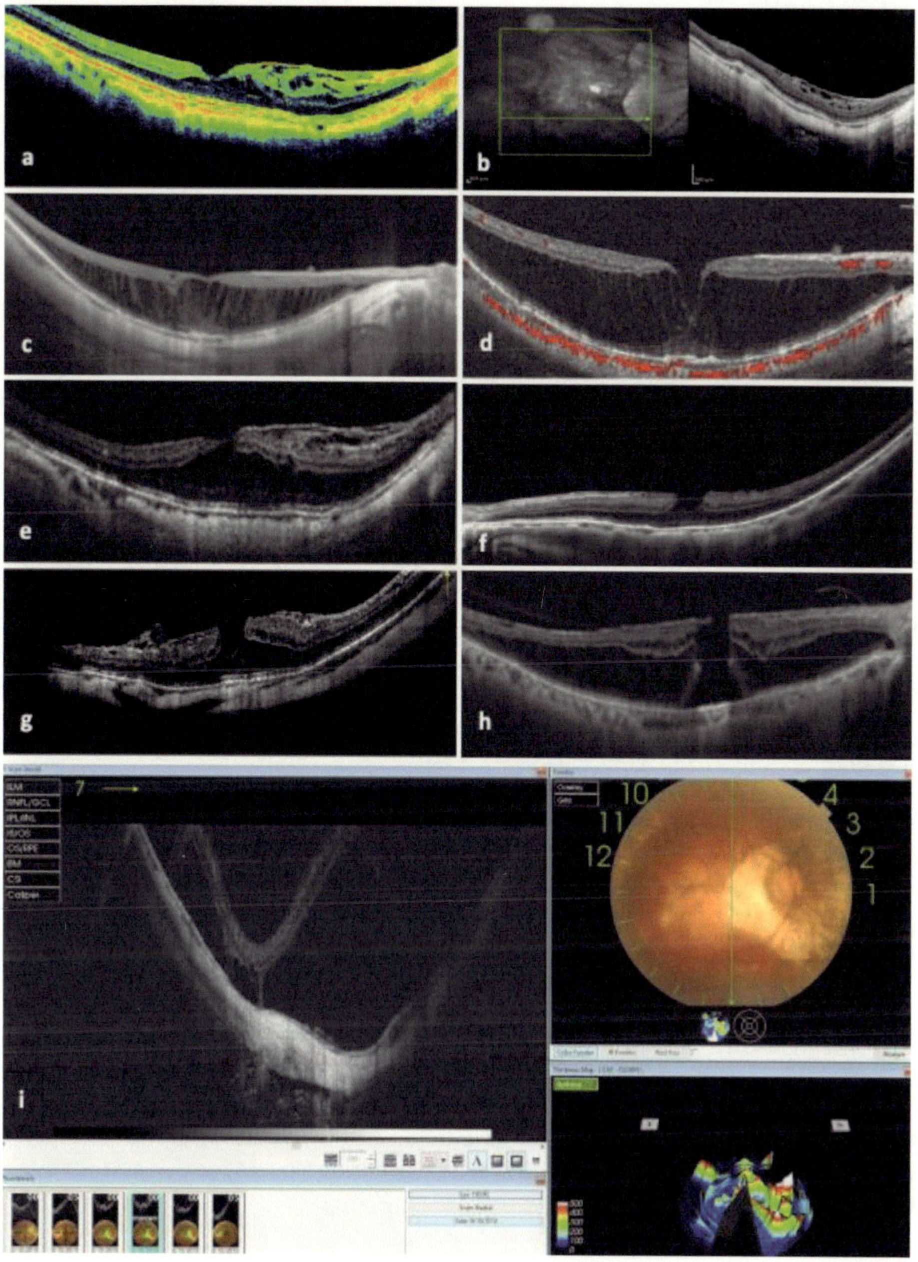

Figure 1.
Different stages of myopic traction maculopathy (a) Schisis-like thickening of the macula nasally to the fovea. (b) Extrafoveal schisis-like thickening of the macula with epiretinal membrane proliferation (ERM). (c) Elevated macular foveoschisis (FS) with tractional elongation of Henle's nerve fiber layer. (d) Macular FS and severe tractional elongation of Henle's nerve fiber layer with an inner lamellar macular hole (I-LMH). (e) Magnified image of macular foveoretinal detachment with ERM and schisis-like thickening on the nasal side; there is subretinal retinal fluid. (f) Highly myopic eye with I-LMH. (g) Complex FRD and I-LMH with inner and outer schisis-like thickening of the macula and some hyaloidal remnants on the nasal side. (h) High-definition horizontal line 12 mm image of a very elevated macular FS with a full-thickness macular hole (FTMH) and severe traction of Henle's nerve fiber layer. (i) Spectralis B-scan examination consistent with retinal detachment and confirmed presence of FTMH (not shown); deep and irregular scleral staphyloma is depicted.

which have been linked to the onset and severity of myopic maculopathy [22]. Thus, assessing choroidal circulation in patients with MTM can offer valuable insights into disease progression and treatment response, thereby aiding the development of targeted therapeutic approaches.

Currently, the optimal stage for patients with MTM to benefit the most from surgical intervention remains uncertain. Some researchers have proposed that surgery should be considered in all cases of MTM where there is a risk of sight-threatening complications or when such complications are already evident [23, 24]. However, some experts recommend a wait-and-see approach for patients in the early stages, advising at least six months of observation [25], as there is a chance of spontaneous remission [26]. Surgery is necessary in cases of reduced visual acuity, symptomatic FS and FRD, full-thickness macular holes (FTMHs), or RS with a schisis pattern resembling a champagne flute [17, 27]. To address RS, the primary goal is to release traction forces from the front of the retina and to counteract the posterior elongation force caused by the staphyloma. Surgical treatment options for this condition include pars plana vitrectomy (PPV) with or without internal limiting membrane (ILM) peeling or macular buckling (MB) [28, 29]. However, the selection of surgical methods could influence postoperative outcomes such as the integrity of the choroidal circulation. Understanding the consequences of various surgical approaches on choroidal perfusion is essential for optimizing visual outcomes in patients with MTM.

Moreover, while best-corrected visual acuity (BCVA) is a commonly used measure to evaluate visual function, it may not fully encompass the intricacies of visual performance influenced by changes in choroidal perfusion. Recent studies have indicated that choroidal perfusion might be evaluated using the choroidal vascularity index (CVI), which has been linked to various visual outcomes beyond BCVA, including contrast sensitivity, central macular thickness (CMT), and microperimetry [1, 30]. Therefore, investigating the correlation between the CVI and visual outcomes can offer a more comprehensive assessment of visual function in patients with postoperative MTM, leading to improved management and enhanced patient care.

This chapter aimed to examine the importance of choroidal perfusion in MTM and its role in guiding surgical intervention. We will explore two key hypotheses: first, the impact of various surgical approaches on postoperative CVI and second, the correlation between CVI and visual outcomes beyond BCVA following surgical interventions. Through a comprehensive analysis of peer-reviewed literature and the exploration of these hypotheses, we aimed to enhance the comprehension of MTM management and ultimately improve patient outcomes for this serious eye condition.

2. Pathophysiology of myopic traction maculopathy

MTM development has been attributed to two distinct groups of forces exerting influence on the retina: preretinal and subretinal factors [31]. Preretinal factors include forces that generate centrifugal and tangential traction on the retina, such as incomplete posterior vitreous detachment (PVD), VMT, and ERM. However, subretinal factors involve forces that induce centrifugal traction on the retina, such as the deformation of the scleral eyewall. If either group of forces surpasses the retina's limited elasticity, which is constrained by small retinal vessels, a thickened or stiffened ILM, or vitreous remnants, it can potentially cause damage to the retina [20, 27, 32, 33]. Understanding the pathophysiology of MTM is crucial for developing effective management strategies to preserve vision in affected individuals. The pathophysiology of MTM is multifactorial and involves several interrelated mechanisms.

2.1 Posterior vitreous detachment

PVD is linked to serious ocular conditions, such as retinal tears, rhegmatogenous RD, vitreous hemorrhage, MHs, and VMT syndrome, as reported in multiple studies [34–40]. Retinal complications associated with PVD are more commonly observed in individuals with HM than in those without HM [12, 17, 27, 40–44]. As a result, it is presumed that PVD advancement differs between highly myopic and nonhighly myopic eyes. The vitreous humor in highly myopic eyes tends to liquefy, leading to PVD [45]. The occurrence of partial or complete PVD was identified as a contributing factor to the increased development of traction, particularly in myopic eyes compared with emmetropic eyes [46, 47]. Moreover, highly myopic eyes were found to exhibit the formation of a specific gap termed the posterior precortical vitreous pocket (PPVP) between the vitreous cortex, which is in contact with the ILM, and the vitreous itself, which could mimic the effects of PVD [47]. PVD is rare in eyes with MTM, but the reason for this has not been determined [48–50]. Prior investigations employing different techniques to study the posterior vitreous revealed that PVD occurs at an earlier age in individuals with HM than in those without HM (nonhighly myopic patients) [46, 47, 51, 52]. Until the advent of swept-source optical coherence tomography (SS-OCT), precise visualization of the posterior vitreous was not feasible [53–55].

A study conducted by Itakura et al. [47] utilized SS-OCT and demonstrated that both partial and complete PVD occur earlier in highly myopic patients than in nonhighly myopic patients. However, their investigation did not include a detailed classification of the subtle progression of partial PVD, although they had a three-stage classification system for partial PVD that covered paramacular, perifoveal, and peripapillary PVD [56]. Additionally, Takahashi et al. [57], employing ultrawide field SS-OCT, reported various abnormal PVD patterns specific to the PM. More recently, among highly myopic patients aged ≥60 years, PVD tended to occur at a younger age in women than in men [58]. Therefore, to gain a better understanding of the situation, it is crucial to compare the status of PVD between patients with and without high myopia using cohorts matched for age and sex. Furthermore, a more intricate classification of partial PVD stages is necessary.

2.2 Bruch's membrane and choroidal changes

HM is strongly associated with various retinal and macular complications, including FS, FRD, and MHs, which are partly caused by vitreous traction. MTM has been demonstrated to occur in approximately 9.0–34.4% of highly myopic eyes with PS [10, 16]. Approximately 10% of highly myopic eyes have macular Bruch's membrane (BM) defects, which could be closely linked to other chorioretinopathies [59]. The BM is a 2–4 μm-thick acellular sheet positioned between the choroid and RPE [60]. The BM serves as a barrier between the retinal pigment epithelium (RPE) and choriocapillaris. In addition to spatially separating the retinal and choroidal compartments, BM potentially plays a biomechanical role in supporting the shape and form of the eyeball. For eyes with myopia, there is a hypothesis suggesting that axial elongation could be influenced by BM production in the retro-equatorial region [61]. Regarding chorioretinopathy, scientists have discovered that macular BM abnormalities could serve as a distinctive feature in cases of patchy atrophy or myopic CNV, leading to foveal atrophy [62, 63]. Additionally, the presence of a dome-shaped macula (DSM) appears to be significantly associated with macular BM defects [64]. The root cause of these BM abnormalities appears to be related to increased tension within the membrane; however, the precise underlying mechanism remains unclear. Similarly, the myopization process and development of fundus lesions in highly myopic eyes pose a challenge to elucidate [65].

The vascular choroid supplies nutrients and a high concentration of oxygen to the outer layers of the retina [66]. This vascular network is crucial for maintaining homeostasis and normal functioning of the outer layers of the retina, including the RPE. Changes in the choroid structure may indicate the presence of an underlying disease. To effectively assess the condition of the choroid in both healthy and diseased retinas, clinicians often rely on choroidal thickness measurements in their research [67]. However, it is important to note that choroidal thickness alone has limitations as it cannot fully characterize the vascular flow between the stromal and luminal vascular regions."

2.3 Foveoschisis

During MTM progression, the earliest change in the retina is known as retinoschisis (RS). When it involves the macula, it is termed MS; when it involves only the fovea, it is called FS [68] (**Figure 2**). These changes occur in approximately 8–34% of individuals diagnosed with PM [10, 16, 69]. This condition was first described by Calbert Phillips in 1959 when he observed localized posterior RD occurring over a PS without a detectable MH. He speculated that conditions such as FS may explain this RD [70].

The term "myopic foveoschisis" was introduced by Takano and Kishi in 1999. They described it as the splitting of the macular inner retinal layers, resulting in a thinner outer layer and thicker inner layer [10]. In 2003, Baba et al. found a correlation between FS and PS, suggesting that FS may be due to scleral protrusion, which surpasses the stretching capacity of the retina [16]. Benhamou et al. characterized FS as a thickening of the outer retinal layer, with perpendicular columns of tissue bridging the outer and inner layers known as tractional elongation of Henle's layer

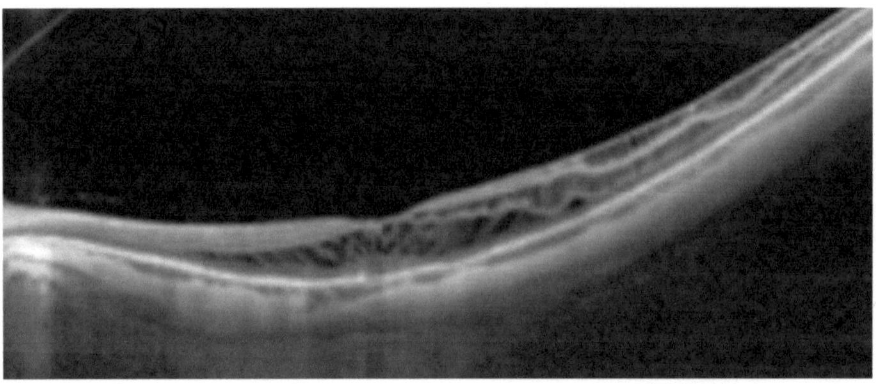

Figure 2.
Macular foveoschisis with extensive tractional elongation of Henle's nerve fiber layer, foveal thinning, inner and outer schisis-like retinal thickening, and epiretinal membrane (ERM) on the temporal side.

[18]. This progressive separation of the retinal layers appears as long, straight, and highly reflective lines at the fovea and throughout the RS area when observed using OCT [71]. FS is often accompanied by other OCT features, such as ERMs, detachment of the ILM, retinal microfolds, defects in the ellipsoid zone (EZ) line, paravascular micro holes, inner or outer LMHs, FTMHs, and chorioretinopathy [72]. According to Wu et al. [69] OCT images of myopic FS or early-stage MTM reveal splitting of the neurosensory retina into two distinct layers. One layer is a thin outer retinal layer positioned on the RPE, and the other is a thicker inner retinal layer [69].

Various classifications have been proposed for FS. Shimada et al. suggested five categories of outer FS based on its location and extension: no apparent FS (S0), extrafoveal FS (S1), foveal FS (S2), foveal FS without involvement of the entire macula (S3), and FS with complete macular involvement (S4) [27]. In contrast, Fujimoto et al. and Ceklic et al. classified FS based on the location of the splitting of the retina into inner, outer, or both inner and outer FS [71, 73]. The exact cause of myopic FS remains uncertain; however, several factors have been proposed to contribute to its development, including posterior vitreous traction, reduced ILM flexibility, inflexibility of retinal vessels, presence of an ERM in conjunction with elongation of the axial length (AXL), and retinal stretching due to staphyloma [18, 21, 69, 74].

2.4 Foveoretinal detachment

FS can progress to FRD over time (**Figure 3**), but its progression is generally slow. In some instances, FS may remain stable or even improve if traction on the retina is spontaneously relieved [75]. According to Gaucher et al., myopic FS can trigger the formation of ERMs, FRD, MH, LMH, and MHRD, which are usually responsible for the dramatic deterioration of the patient's BCVA [17]. A study conducted by Shimada et al. monitored 207 highly myopic eyes for a minimum period of 24 months. They observed a decrease or complete resolution of FS in 3.9% of the eyes, while 11.6% of the eyes exhibited progression from FS to FRD or more advanced stages of MTM. Notably, eyes with more extensive FS tend to experience a higher likelihood of progression than those with less extensive FS [27].

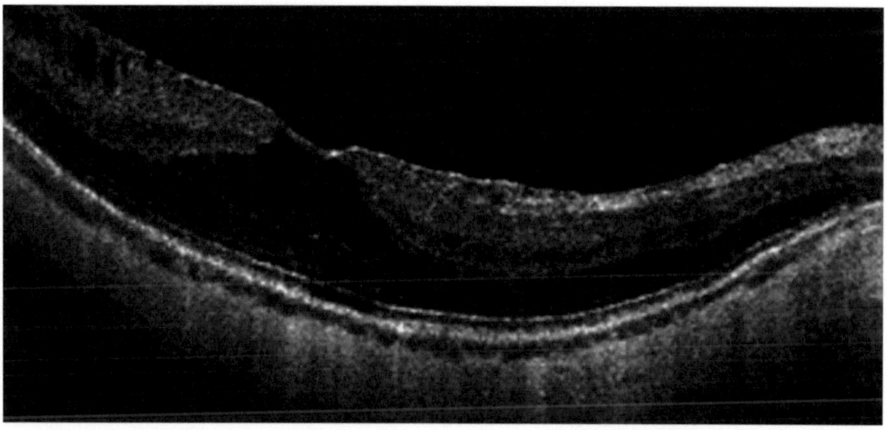

Figure 3.
Magnified macular image of moderately elevated foveoretinal detachment (FRD) with thinning of the foveal roof and outer schisis-like macular thickening and evidence of epiretinal macular proliferation.

Another study conducted by the same authors [12] categorized the stages of progression from FS to RD by using OCT.

- Stage 1: Characterized by irregularity in external retinal layer thickness with localized retinal elevation.
- Stage 2: The development of an outer lamellar macular hole (O-LMH) occurs either in the foveal or extrafoveal region and is associated with a small RD.
- Stage 3: The O-LMH increases vertically and horizontally, separating the column-like structures within the RS layer, with concurrent enlargement of the RD.
- Stage 4: RD further enlarges, and the RS resolves.

These findings shed light on the possible evolution of FS to more severe conditions such as FRD, O-LMH, I-LMH, FTMH, and MHRD, highlighting the importance of close monitoring in eyes with high myopia.

2.5 Lamellar macular hole

LMH is characterized by irregularities in the foveal contour, where there is a defect in the inner retina with or without splitting within the retinal layers [76]. In some instances, there may be disruptions in the outer retinal layers, including the external limiting membrane (ELM) and EZ [77–82]. LMHs can be further classified into two types: inner LMHs (I-LMHs), characterized by the splitting of the inner foveal layers (**Figure 4**), and outer LMHs (O-LMHs), characterized by the splitting of photoreceptors [14] (**Figure 5**). However, the mechanisms underlying LMH formation are subject to ongoing debate in the scientific community. The emergence of OCT has enabled the identification of structural changes associated with LMH, such as ERMs and VMT [81, 83, 84]. Govetto et al. observed two distinct morphologies of LMHs and proposed that they may arise through either a tractional process or degenerative evolution [85]. More recently, Hubschman et al. redefined LMH-related lesions as "LMH," "ERM with foveoschisis," and "macular pseudohole," supporting the hypotheses of both tractional and degenerative evolutionary pathways [86].

In nonmyopic eyes, LMH is associated with two types of ERM: conventional ERM, commonly found in macular pucker, appearing as a highly reflective line overlying the

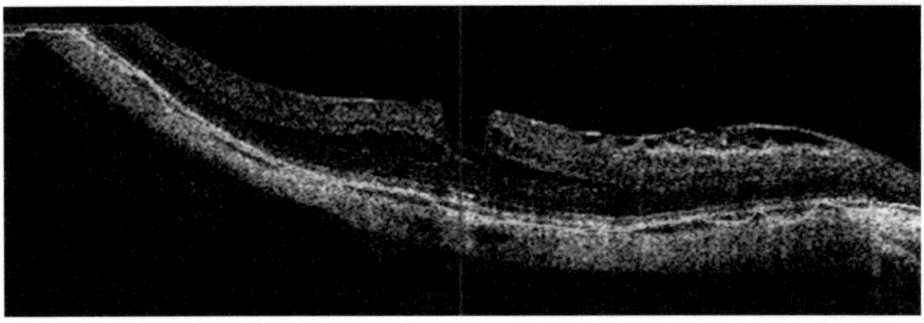

Figure 4.
Inner lamellar macular hole (I-LMH) with nasal epiretinal macular proliferation; automated red and blue segmentation lines in this horizontal B-scan partial-thickness macular hole indicate tissue irregularities.

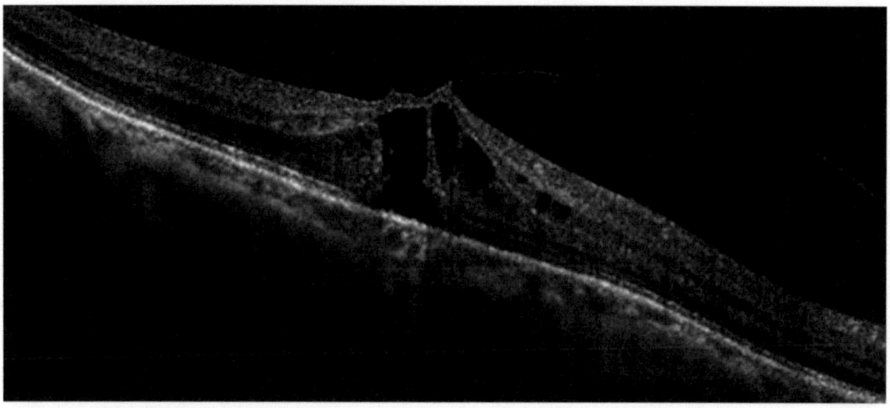

Figure 5.
Complex localized foveoretinal detachment (FRD) with evidence of outer lamellar macular hole (O-LMH), there is evidence of outer schisis-like macular thickening and vitreomacular traction.

retinal nerve fiber layer (RNFL) with tractional properties, and atypical ERM, which is a thicker membrane delineated by a highly reflective line filled with moderately reflective material that lacks tractional properties [80]. In eyes with HM, the clinical progression of LMHs is characterized by increased complexity and instability due to the presence of intricate forces, including the adherent posterior hyaloid, ERM, rigid ILM, PS, and the occurrence of macular RS [87–90].

The stability of myopic LMH is a subject of ongoing debate. Dell'Omo et al. conducted a retrospective observational case series of 44 myopic eyes with LMH and found that they were often linked with ERMs and LMH-associated epiretinal proliferation (LMHEP). Over time, they observed both morphological and functional stability in these patients [89]. In contrast, Frisina et al. performed a retrospective observational longitudinal study of 40 myopic eyes affected by LMH and pseudoholes. They discovered that myopic LMHs, particularly those associated with atypical ERMs, represent a more severe condition than those associated with conventional ERMs. Moreover, they observed that myopic LMHs may not be stable and may progress to FTMH [91]. In conclusion, understanding LMH variations and progression is crucial for better outcomes and requires advancements in imaging technology.

2.6 Macular hole and macular hole retinal detachment

Myopic FTMH is an advanced stage of MTM that is associated with significant visual impairment [92] (**Figure 6**). Ikuno et al. [93] observed 44 eyes with myopic FS and noted that its natural progression typically advanced from RS to MH and then to MHRD (**Figure 7**). The status of the fovea was identified as a prognostic indicator for the success of surgical interventions, such as vitrectomy and ILM peeling, with better surgical outcomes observed in the RS group and poorer outcomes in the MH group [93]. According to Jo et al. [94], myopic MH can be classified into two types: the "flat type" and the "schisis type." The "flat type" closely resembles idiopathic macular holes (IMHs) and typically does not progress to MHRD. On the other hand, the "schisis type" is characterized by a tall and straight-sided configuration with a sharp angle at the top, forming an acute-angled edge that is shorter than the base diameter. The "schisis type" is associated with a higher risk of developing MHRD.

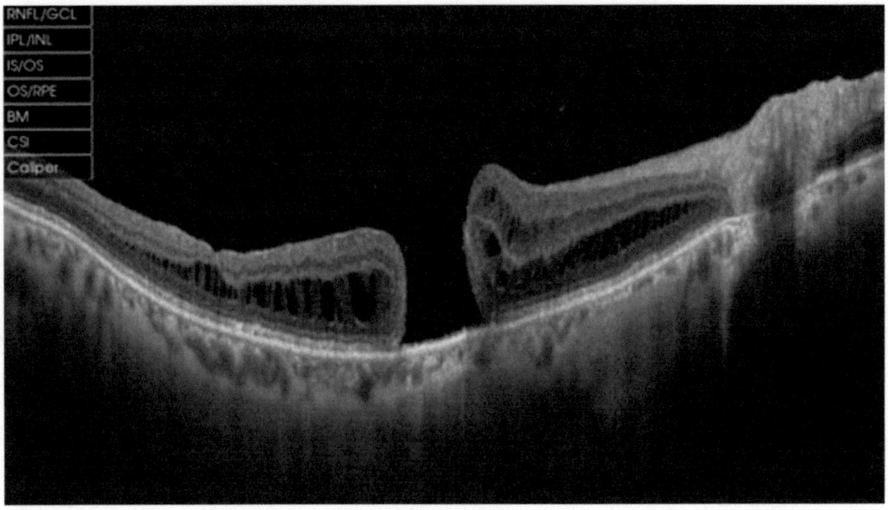

Figure 6.
Irregular full-thickness macular hole (FTMH) with moderate schisis-like thickening of the macula due to tractional elongation of Henle's nerve fiber layer and epiretinal traction on the nasal border of the hole.

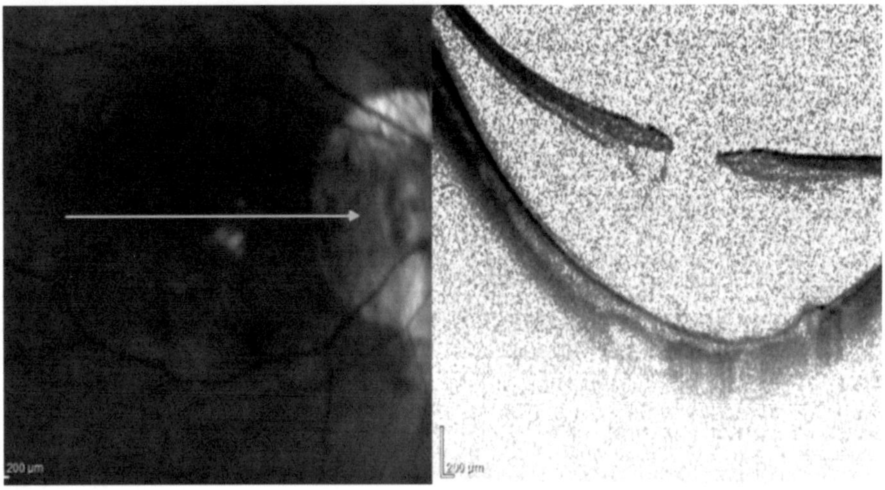

Figure 7.
Full-thickness irregular macular hole and retinal detachment associated with a shallow posterior staphyloma.

2.7 Different stages of MTM and clinical manifestations

Previously, MTM grading was not commonly practiced and primarily relied on clinical examination using slit-lamp biomicroscopy or fundus photographs. Some classification systems based on fundus photography, such as the International Photographic Classification Grading System, exist [95]. However, with the widespread adoption of OCT machines in clinical settings, the diagnosis of MTM has become increasingly accurate.

Parolini et al. introduced the Myopic Traction Maculopathy Staging System (MSS), which classifies MTM into two evolutionary patterns based on OCT images. They also determined the average time of progression of MTM, confirmed a decline in visual acuity with advancing stage, and observed a correlation between MTM staging and age. They investigated the pathogenesis of MTM by describing various centrifugal forces acting on the retina and fovea, counteracting the centripetal forces exerted by Müller cells, the external limiting membrane (ELM), and the ILM that maintain retinal integrity. Based on these theories, Parolini et al. outlined two evolutionary patterns in MTM: retinal and foveal patterns. Retinal patterns evolve from inner MS (I-MS) or inner and outer MS (IO-MS) in stage 1 to predominantly outer MS (O-MS) in stage 2 and then progress to MS with macular detachment (MS-MD) in stage 3 and eventually to MD in stage 4. Conversely, the foveal patterns evolved from a normal foveal profile in stage a to I-LMH in stage b and finally to FTMH in stage c. The presence of O-LMHs and any epiretinal abnormalities are additional findings associated with each pattern and are denoted in the MSS as "O" and "+", respectively. Moreover, Parolini et al. observed a gradual reduction in the mean MTM evolution as it progressed from stages 1 to 2 (20 months), stages 2 to 3 (12 months), and stages 3 to 4 (3 months), with BCVA decreasing as the stages advanced. Additionally, they found a correlation between MTM stage and patient age [14].

In 2019, Ruiz-Medrano et al. proposed the ATN classification system that combines clinical examinations and OCT findings to categorize MTM. This system classifies MTM based on macular appearance (atrophic, A), presence of traction observed on OCT (tractional, T), and the presence or history of neovascularization (neovascularization, N) [13, 96]. The ATN classification accounts for tractional and neovascularization-related changes and has demonstrated high consistency and agreement among different observers [97]. Precise pathological staging of MTM plays a crucial role in making well-informed decisions regarding the optimal timing of surgical intervention for both the affected and fellow eyes [98].

3. Surgical approaches in myopic traction maculopathy

The historical development of the ab externo approach to MTM dates back to 1930, before the formal definition of MTM. The initial concept involved reinforcing the posterior sclera to prevent the progressive elongation of the myopic eye. Various materials, such as fascia lata [12], donor sclera [99], and lyodura (derived from processed cadaver dura mater) [100], have been used for this purpose. A modified posterior scleral reinforcement (PSR) technique was proposed by Snyder and Thompson and further refined by several researchers [100–104]. Additionally, the MB technique, introduced by Schepens et al., is considered the primary surgical approach for treating MTM [105].

3.1 Macular/scleral buckling

MB in combination with scleral imbrication has proven to be an effective treatment that significantly enhances the surgical success rate of MH-associated macular degeneration. MB is essential for alleviating both anteroposterior traction resulting from PS and tangential traction exerted by the vitreous cortex [106, 107]. The rationale behind MB was to counteract pathological posterior bulging and stretching of the sclera, particularly in eyes with pronounced PS, which is a significant risk factor for MTM development [108, 109]. The evolution of macular buckling is shown in **Figure 8**. For a considerable period of time, the ab externo approach was overshadowed by the ab interno approach. However, in the 2000s, the MB technique made

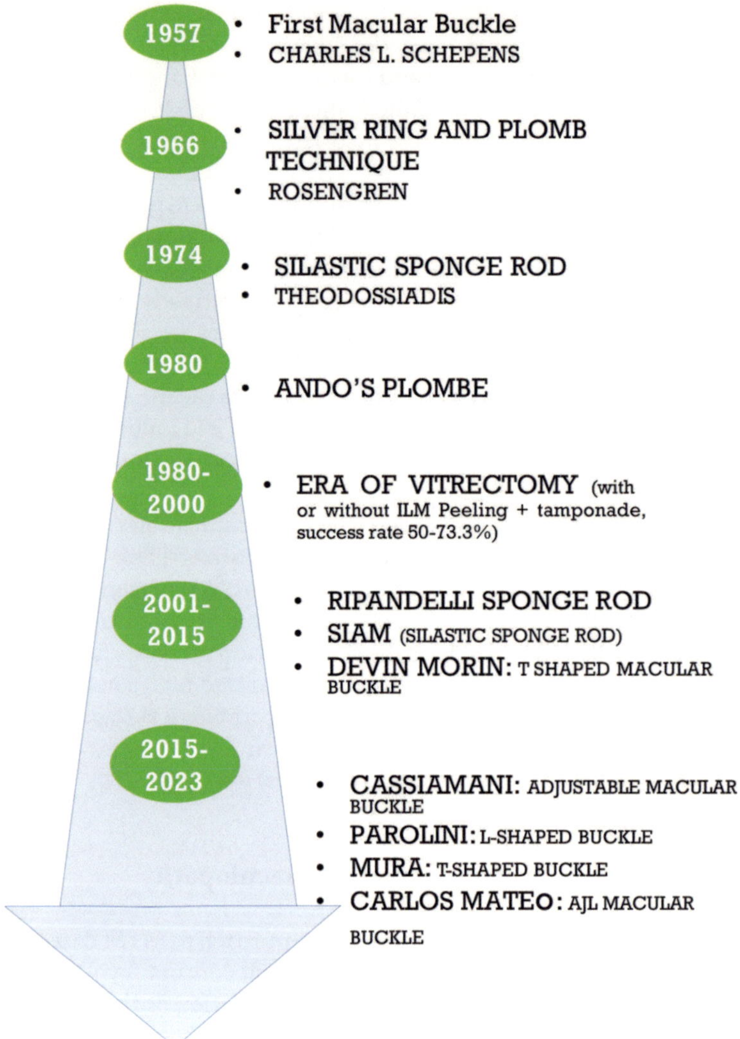

Figure 8.
The evolution of macular buckling with historical depiction.

a comeback with the use of sponges or solid silicone exoplants, resulting in a high rate of reattachment [107, 110]. The MB technique was reported in 2009 by Ward to effectively control axial myopia by shortening the AXL in HM, exhibiting better visual outcomes than PPV [111], and was regarded as the gold standard for treating MTM when compared to the ab interno approach, as per Alkabes and Mateo's 16-year review of MB for MTM [112].

3.2 Pars plana vitrectomy

PPV is currently considered the gold standard treatment for MTM, resulting in maintenance and improvement of vision in most cases [16, 113]. The most commonly employed surgical approach for MTM involves PPV with complete ILM removal, a procedure known as ILM peeling (ILMP) [33, 114]. The introduction of surgical techniques such as ILMP and laser treatment around the edges of the MH yielded promising anatomical results with success rates of up to 90% but limited functional recovery [115–118]. However, MH occurs in approximately 5–28.6% of eyes that have undergone PPV with ILMP for the treatment of MTM, resulting in unfavorable visual outcomes even after a repeated surgical procedure [28, 87, 93, 119–130]. Recently, a novel approach called fovea-sparing internal limiting membrane peeling (FSIP), described by Shimada et al. [120], has emerged in the scientific community (**Figure 9**). This technique aims to prevent postoperative MH formation after surgery by preserving the foveal Müller cell cone [121]. Shimada et al. [120] compared the FSIP and complete ILMP groups. The study showed a relatively higher occurrence of MH formation in the complete ILMP group; however, this difference was not statistically significant. Additionally, there was no substantial improvement in postoperative BCVA in the FSIP group compared to that in the complete ILMP group. However, subsequent studies with larger sample sizes reported contrasting results. These studies revealed a significant difference in postoperative BCVA [121] and CMT [131] between the two groups. Furthermore, various outcome measures were explored to compare the complete ILMP and FSIP groups. PPV combined with ILM has been effective in relieving major traction in some cases [33, 114]. However, postoperative FTMH can develop in up to 28.6% of cases [121]. To overcome these complications, FSIP has gained attention [120, 121, 131–134], and this approach is not entirely free from FTMH formation, particularly because of the vulnerability of the thin fovea to mechanical forces during surgery [131]. To address larger or persistent FTMH, an alternative method known as the inverted internal limiting membrane flap (ILMF or modified ILMF) has been utilized [134, 135]. According to Lin and Yang, both the

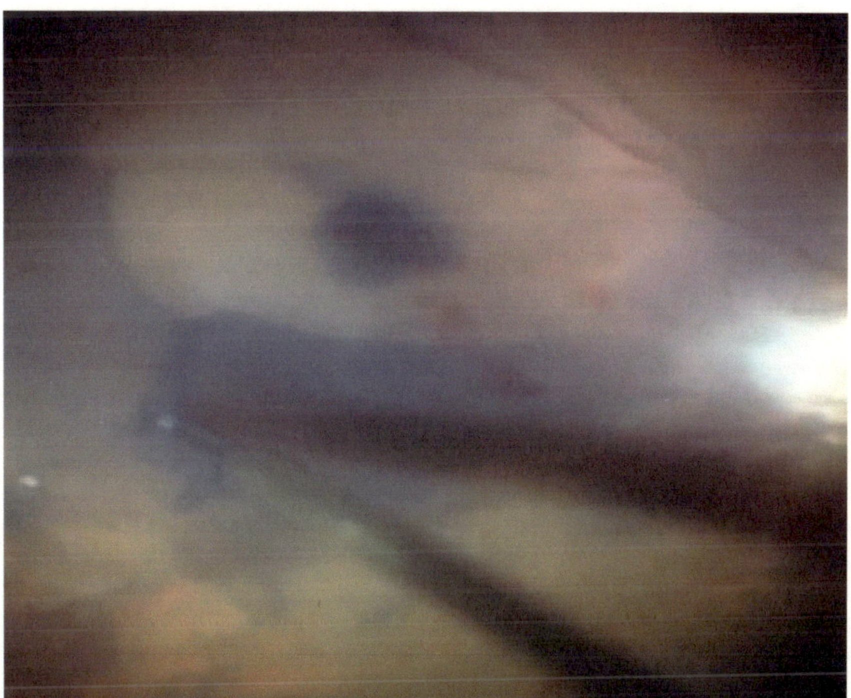

Figure 9.
Intraoperative image of the fovea-sparing internal limiting membrane peeling approach.

FSIP technique and the combined FSIP and ILMP technique demonstrated the ability to enhance both BCVA and central macular thickness (CMT). Nevertheless, none of the 35 eyes in the modified ILMF group developed postoperative MH after surgery. In contrast, in the FSIP control group, two eyes experienced immediate MH development after surgery, and one eye had a delayed occurrence of MH [136].

Furthermore, different intravitreal tamponades, such as gas and silicone oil (SO), were combined with PPV. Although SO showed a higher anatomical success rate than gas, several authors have reported unsatisfactory functional outcomes [137, 138]. PPV was subsequently adopted for the treatment of RS, MS, and RD without MH. However, PPV has limitations, such as the limited power of tamponades due to the configuration of the PS, the potential weakening of an already fragile retina through ILM peeling, and difficulties in visualizing atrophic changes in the myopic choroid. Consequently, the success rate of PPV in MTM remains variable across different studies, leading to ongoing debates regarding its use in such cases [23, 139–142].

3.3 Combined vitrectomy and macular buckling

The combination of MB and vitrectomy allows simultaneous treatment of tangential and anteroposterior tractions of the MTM [29]. MTM management has evolved over the years, and combined vitrectomy and MB surgery have emerged as promising treatment approaches [143]. Vitrectomy was performed to address anteroposterior traction caused by the vitreous. To counteract tangential force, the surgeon peels the ILM, achieves complete PVD from the optic nerve and macula, and removes the ERM if present [93, 119, 127, 144]. In cases where there are recent or unsuccessful macular tractional changes despite vitrectomy, attention should be given to the third component of the tractional force acting at the macula, the staphyloma-related scleral-retinal mismatch. In such instances, an MB is necessary to provide support for the staphyloma [29, 145, 146]. Although further research and long-term follow-up studies are warranted to validate these findings, the combination of vitrectomy and MB surgery holds great potential as a comprehensive treatment option for effectively managing MTM.

4. Choroidal vascularity index

CVI has gained popularity as a convenient and noninvasive measure owing to its simplicity and calculation method [147–149]. The CVI can be derived from enhanced OCT images by using digital binarization and quantification techniques [150, 151]. Unlike choroidal thickness, the CVI provides a more comprehensive assessment of choroidal structure by capturing both vascular and stromal changes. Numerous studies have associated changes in the CVI with the development and progression of various retinal diseases [147, 152, 153]. CVI can detect specific microcirculatory alterations in the retina [154–156] and is associated with visual function after vitrectomy [157]. Given that retinal diseases often involve multiple processes affecting the choroid, such as inflammation, edema, and leakage, the CVI has been proposed as a potentially valuable biomarker for evaluating the integrity of the choroidal vascular network [152, 158]. Moreover, earlier investigations have demonstrated that the CVI remains unaffected by factors such as AXL, blood pressure, and intraocular pressure, making it a reliable measurement [159].

4.1 Methodology applied to calculate the CVI and its clinical relevance

Initially, the CVI was computed using a horizontal B-scan that passed through the fovea, and it subsequently became a widely adopted conventional method in numerous studies found in the literature. Agrawal et al. demonstrated that the scanning area, whether subfoveal, total macular, or central macular, does not influence the final CVI results in healthy individuals [160]. Therefore, a single subfoveal scan could reliably represent the posterior pole. Furthermore, the type of OCT scan, whether swept-source (SS) or spectral-domain (SD), had no impact on the CVI values [161].

The CVI values were calculated based on macular images obtained using SD-OCT. High-resolution 9-mm horizontal OCT-B images were chosen and imported into ImageJ analysis software (version 1.53, http://imagej.nih.gov/ij/). These images are initially converted into an 8-bit format and adjusted using the Niblack automatic local threshold. Next, the subfoveal choroid area was manually selected from 750 μm nasal to 750 μm temporal in the horizontal plane from the foveal center and from the RPE-Bruch membrane to the scleral border in the vertical plane. The total choroidal area (TCA) was measured using an adaptable geometric polygon tool. Subsequently, the stromal vascular tissue area was determined by counting the number of white pixels, whereas the luminal area (LA) at the enhanced choroid was calculated by applying the threshold tool and quantifying the number of dark pixels. Finally, the dark-to-light pixel ratio is expressed as a percentage and defined as CVI, as previously described by Agrawal et al. [148, 152].

CVI is derived by taking the ratio of LA to the total choroidal area (TCA), and it is expressed as a percentage [162]. This parameter offers a distinct opportunity to acquire information about choroidal perfusion, as it precisely mirrors the vascular alterations in the choroid [1]. CVI is calculated as follows: CVI – (luminal area/total choroidal area) × 100.

CVI is usually expressed as a percentage, representing the proportion of the choroid occupied by the blood vessels. The protocol study method for the binarization method is shown in **Figure 10**.

4.2 Clinical relevance and role of the CVI in assessing choroidal vascular changes in MTM

CVI has proven to be informative in determining the condition of the choroidal vasculature across various disease and treatment scenarios [163–168]. Reliable quantitative metrics, such as the CVI, have been devised to diagnose, categorize, and track retinal disorders [169]. An increase in the CVI can result from an increase in the number of blood vessels or the diameter of choroidal blood vessels in a specific area [152]. Hayreh [170] demonstrated that the submacular choroidal supply is susceptible to general chronic ischemic conditions such as AMD because of the multiple watershed zones of the short posterior ciliary arteries in the choroid. The clinical implications of the CVI could be significant and warrant further investigation in subsequent studies [170]. Conversely, a decrease in the CVI at baseline might indicate choroidal ischemia in patients with macular disorders such as AMD or diabetes. In contrast, the CVI can be used to determine an increase in choroidal vascularity in cases of posterior uveitis or central serous chorioretinopathy. Moreover, the CVI can serve as a valuable tool for monitoring the treatment response and disease resolution [152]. MTM is a progressive condition that has been classified into four stages [171, 172]: stage 1,

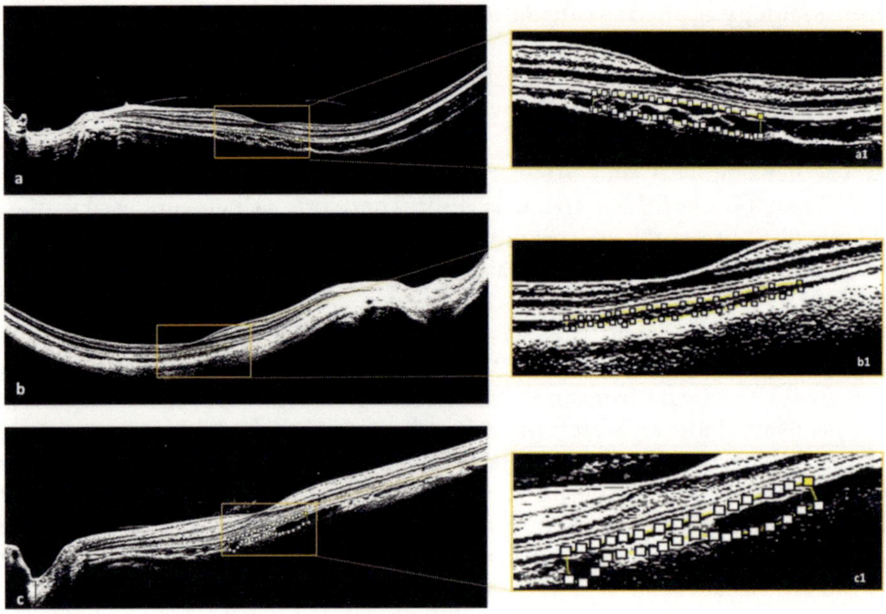

Figure 10.
Method used for quantifying the CVI in healthy myopic eyes. (a) Binarized image designed to depict the intraretinal structure and choroidal vascular layers in greater detail in a healthy, highly myopic eye with an axial length of 29.2 mm. (a1) Magnified image within the yellow square showing binarized processing of the subfoveal choroidal vascular stroma and luminal vascular visualization of the subfoveal choroidal vessels to obtain a choroidal vascularity index (CVI) of 64.2%. The selected subfoveal area of choroidal flow is clearly delineated by the white-yellow dotted line. (b) Binarized processing of choroidal flow in a healthy highly myopic eye with an axial length of 30.2 mm. (b1) Enhanced choroidal vessel visualization yielding a CVI of 62.3% inside of the magnified image within the white-yellow dotted line clearly delineating a CVI of 62.3%. (c) Binarized image corresponding to a healthy, highly myopic eye with an axial length of 29.7 mm in the control group. (c1) The white and yellow dotted lines depict the binarized choroidal flow area selected to calculate the CVI. The CVI was 63.4% inside the selected choroidal flow area in the magnified image depicting the selected area for the CVI measurements.

MF; stage 2, FRD; stage 3, myopic MHs; and stage 4, MHRD. Employing noninvasive techniques, such as CVI estimation, to monitor disease and treatment outcomes could significantly enhance the management of MTM [173]. In a case series conducted by Quiroz-Reyes et al., which included eyes with MTM, patients with more advanced disease stages tended to exhibit lower CVIs [1].

5. CVI alteration after surgery in myopic traction maculopathy

Numerous studies have established a connection between the CVI and the development and progression of various diseases, including genetic, retinal, and macular conditions [149, 152, 153]. These investigations suggest that the CVI can serve as a distinctive indicator of retinal diseases. Since retinal diseases involve multiple factors, such as inflammation, edema, and leakage, the CVI has been suggested as a potential marker because it reflects the changes that affect the integrity of the vascular network within the highly blood-supplied retinal structure known as the choroid [152, 158]. Consequently, quantifying vascular factors is believed to accurately represent the ongoing disease pathogenesis.

In a previous study [1], we investigated the CVI as a potential biomarker of myopic traction maculopathy (MTM). In this investigation, data were collected from normal eyes in the control group, one being a healthy emmetropic eye and the other a healthy highly myopic eye, with an intervention group consisting of four patients with MTM related to high myopia. The findings revealed that the CVI was significantly lower in the disease group than in the control group. This suggests that the CVI may indicate disease pathology in MTM, and a lower CVI in diseased eyes could be linked to choroidal vascular defects caused by PM or surgical procedures, potentially influencing the manifestation, progression, and functional outcomes in different stages of surgically resolved MTM. Preoperative patient characteristics were mostly similar and directly comparable, except for visual acuity, which was expected to be poor in the disease group. The study found differences in TCA and CVI between normal subjects and MTM patients; however, among the surgical groups, the CVI was similar for the surgical patients. However, the CVI proved to be a useful noninvasive biomarker, distinguishing patients in the MTM group from those in the healthy control group. It has been reported that age and the CVI are inversely related in healthy eyes, and the study showed an inverse correlation between the CVI and ILM surgical techniques, suggesting that this procedure may not favor better long-term visual recovery in patients with MTM [174]. Nevertheless, surgical intervention significantly improved visual acuity in all participants.

In conclusion, this study highlights the potential of the CVI as a biomarker for MTM and its significance in differentiating healthy eyes from eyes with MTM. Further research is needed to explore and quantify the CVI in myopic subjects to better understand its implications in high myopia.

From the surgical experience of the author, representative and complex clinical cases of highly myopic eyes in which macular surgery was performed at different stages of MTM with the corresponding long-term postoperative and enhanced binarized OCT imaging evaluation and CVI calculations are shown in **Figure 11**.

5.1 Advantages of the choroidal vascularity index

a. CVI enables the use of noninvasive imaging techniques such as OCTfor measurement, allowing patients to undergo assessments without the need for invasive procedures or contrast agents.

b. CVI shows promise in detecting early changes in ocular diseases, such as AMD and diabetic retinopathy, before significant symptoms or vision loss become apparent.

c. CVI offers a quantitative measurement, facilitating an objective and standardized evaluation of choroidal vascularity. This aspect is valuable for monitoring disease progression and gauging treatment response.

d. The CVI may aid in distinguishing between various ocular disease subtypes, leading to more precise diagnoses and personalized treatment plans.

5.2 Limitations of the choroidal vascularity index

a. Inadequate normative data: owing to its recent emergence as a biomarker, the CVI lacks sufficient normative data across diverse populations and ethnic groups.

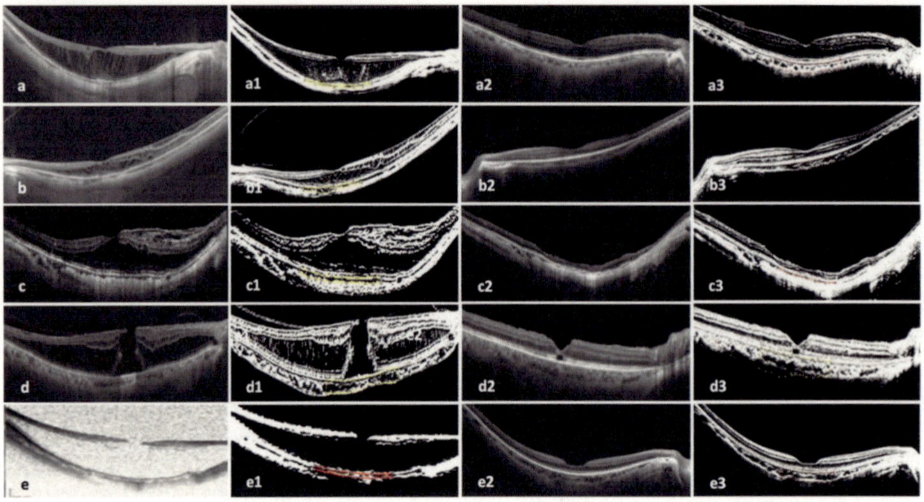

Figure 11.
Surgical cases. (a) Preoperative OCT findings consistent with myopic foveoschisis (FS) due to macular and schisis-like thickening of the inner and outer retinal layers at the macula. (a1) Binarized image of the preoperative myopic FS in a symptomatic, highly myopic patient. This is a very complex FS with outer and inner retinal layer-like thickening, tractional elongation of Henle's layer, and a very thin superficial foveal layer. This preoperative binarized image showed a CVI index of 64.6% between the normal range among the normal controls. (a2) After a 31-month follow-up, the center of the macular region appeared thinner, with a normal foveal profile and without evidence of a macular hole (MH). OCT biomarkers, such as a normal foveal contour and internal and outer neuroretinal lines with total restoration of the central subfoveal ellipsoid zone (EZ), were observed. (a3) Postoperative long-term binarized image with a CVI of 53.3% lower than the mean control value. (b) Preoperative myopic FS in a symptomatic, highly myopic patient. This FS exhibited outer retinal layer-like thickening, tractional elongation of Henle's layer, and epiretinal membrane (ERM) proliferation mainly over the temporal side of the macula. (b1) Preoperative binarized image showing a CVI index of 61.9%. (b2) Long-term postoperative horizontal B-scan with an almost normal foveal profile and diffuse thinning of the retina layers over the temporal side, no evidence of outer or inner retinal layer thickening, and final vision of 20/60. (b3) The long-term postoperative CVI calculated from the binarized image was 49.6% lower than that of healthy myopic controls. (c) Preoperative image of the right eye exhibiting chronic myopic foveoretinal detachment (FRD) with subretinal fluid, inner and outer retina layer-like thickening in a symptomatic highly myopic eye of 28.8 mm of axial length, and a very thin superficial foveal layer. (c1) Preoperative CVI was 63.2%. (c2) Corresponding long-term postoperative horizontal B-scan depicting diffuse atrophic thinning of the retinal layers and evidence of FRD flattening without ERM remnants. (c3) The CVI calculated from the binarized image was 49.6% in the last enhanced binarized image calculation. (d) Highly myopic eye with posterior staphyloma (PS) in a very symptomatic patient. Evidence of a full-thickness myopic macular hole (FTMH) with severe tractional elongation of Henle's layer and thickening of the outer layers of the macula without evidence of macular detachment. (d1) Preoperative enhanced-definition binarized image of the corresponding highly myopic patient with FTMH showed a CVI of 61.8%. (d2) Postoperative long-term structural evaluation showed a flat macula with a recovered foveal profile, external limiting membrane (ELM) line lucency defect, and a well-preserved RPE layer. (d3) The long-term perfusion evaluation showed a CVI of 47.8% lower than the mean CVI of the healthy control eyes. (e) The 9 mm high-definition horizontal b-scan depicts full-thickness macular hole (MH)-related retinal detachment (RD). (e1) Corresponding preoperative enhanced-definition image showing a preoperative CVI of 59.7% in this 28.8 mm axial length highly myopic eye with a two-week evolution of very symptomatic MHRD. (e2) Corresponding postoperative image depicting a recovered foveal profile with diffuse retinal thinning and well-defined outer retinal markers. (e3) The corresponding long-term postoperative CVI in this enhanced binarized image was calculated as 45.9%, lower than that in the healthy myopic control eyes.

This limitation poses challenges for the accurate interpretation of the CVI values and their universal application.

b. Measurement variability: the CVI measurements can be affected by various factors, including image quality, segmentation algorithms, and observer differences. These variables may have led to inconsistent results.

c. Limited disease specificity: although the CVI can be valuable in detecting changes in choroidal vascularity, it may not offer specific insights into other retinal or optic nerve abnormalities associated with certain ocular conditions.

5.3 Comparison with other biomarkers

a. Compared with CMT, the CVI focuses on evaluating choroidal vascularity instead of retinal thickness. The CVI offers additional information about the health of the choroid and may provide complementary insights beyond what CMT can reveal in the context of retinal diseases.

b. CVI and retinal nerve fiber layer (RNFL) thickness are widely used biomarkers; however, they serve different purposes. While the RNFL thickness is commonly used in glaucoma evaluation, the CVI provides valuable information about choroidal vascular changes, which are not assessed by RNFL thickness measurements. Each biomarker had its own significance within its respective area of focus.

c. When comparing CVI with visual acuity (VA), it is evident that while VA measures a person's ability to see, CVI is a quantitative biomarker that offers more detailed information about vascular changes in the choroid. By incorporating the CVI along with the VA, healthcare professionals can potentially enhance the accuracy of diagnosing and monitoring various ocular diseases.

6. Future directions

The investigation of MTM and its link to choroidal perfusion via the CVI has yielded valuable insights into the underlying mechanisms and clinical characteristics of this condition. Nonetheless, several aspects require further inquiry to advance our understanding and enhance patient care.

1. **Longitudinal investigations:** longitudinal studies to observe the progression of MTM and its relationship with changes in the CVI over time could provide crucial information about the natural history of the disease and identify potential risk factors for its progression.

2. **Genetic and environmental influences:** delving into the impact of genetic and environmental factors on the development and progression of MTM and their association with the CVI may provide insights into individual susceptibility and possible preventive measures.

3. **Advancements in imaging**: leveraging advancements in imaging technology, such as OCT-A and indocyanine green angiography (ICGA), may open new avenues for studying choroidal perfusion and its relevance to MTM. Combining various imaging modalities can yield comprehensive data on choroidal vascular changes.

4. **Therapeutic interventions:** investigating the effects of different treatment approaches, including pharmacological agents, intravitreal injections, and surgical

methods, on CVI and MTM progression may lead to the development of more effective therapeutic strategies.

5. **Collaborative large-scale studies**: collaborative efforts involving multiple centers and patient cohorts could lead to larger-scale studies, strengthen the statistical significance of findings, and improve the generalizability of results.

6. **Animal models**: developing animal models that mimic the pathophysiology of MTM and enable the assessment of choroidal perfusion may provide additional insights into the disease mechanisms and potential treatment targets.

7. **Comparison with other retinal diseases:** comparing the CVI alterations in MTM with other retinal diseases, such as AMD or diabetic retinopathy, may help identify specific patterns of choroidal perfusion unique to MTM.

8. **Functional correlations**: investigating the functional implications of the CVI alterations and their relationship with VA and other functional outcomes in patients with MTM could aid clinicians in prognostication and treatment decision making.

7. Conclusions

In conclusion, this chapter presents a comprehensive overview of MTM, emphasizing the importance of choroidal perfusion assessed through the CVI evaluation. Through discussions on various topics, including the pathophysiology of MTM, its different stages, clinical manifestations, and surgical approaches, we have gained a better understanding of this complex condition. The introduction of the CVI calculation as a noninvasive and quantitative tool for evaluating choroidal vascular changes has demonstrated promising clinical relevance and broadens the knowledge of MTM. It offers valuable information about the vascular status, potentially assisting in early diagnosis and prognostication. Moreover, alterations in the CVI have been observed after surgery, suggesting its potential role as a prognostic indicator of surgical outcomes. However, much remains to be explored in the field of MTM and choroidal perfusion. Further research is crucial to unravel the intricacies of this condition and its correlation with the CVI. Longitudinal studies, the exploration of genetic and environmental factors, advancements in imaging techniques, and comparative analyses of other retinal diseases represent promising future directions. By addressing these research gaps and continuing to investigate the relationship between MTM and CVI, we can pave the way for a more precise diagnosis, improve patient management, and enhanced treatment strategies, ultimately improving the quality of life of individuals affected by this sight-threatening condition.

Acknowledgements

We express our deep appreciation to the technical staff of the Retina Department at Oftalmologia Integral ABC (Nonprofit Medical and Surgical Organization), Mexico City, Mexico, affiliated with The Postgraduate Study Division at the National Autonomous University of Mexico.

Funding

No funding or grant support was received for this study.

Conflict of interest

The authors declare no conflicts of interest.

Acronyms and abbreviations

AMD	age-related macular degeneration
ATN	classification system for myopic maculopathy including atrophic (A), tractional (T), and neovascular (N) components
AXL	axial length
BCVA	best-corrected visual acuity
BM	Bruch's membrane
CMT	central macular thickness
CNV	choroidal neovascularization
CVI	choroidal vascularity index
DSM	dome-shaped macula
ELM	external limiting membrane
ERM	epiretinal membrane
EZ	ellipsoid zone
FSIP	foveal-sparing internal limiting membrane peeling
FRD	foveoretinal detachment
FS	foveoschisis
HM	high myopia
I-MS	inner macular schisis
ILMF	inverted internal limiting membrane flap technique
ILM	internal limiting membrane
ILMP	internal limiting membrane peeling technique
I-LMH	inner lamellar macular hole
IMH	idiopathic macular hole
I-MS	inner macular schisis
LMHEP	lamellar macular hole-related epiretinal proliferation
LCA	luminal choroidal area
LMHEP	lamellar macular hole-associated epiretinal proliferation
LogMAR	logarithm of the minimum angle of resolution
MD	macular detachment
MH	macular hole
MS	macular schisis
MS-MD	macular schisis with macular detachment
MSS	myopic traction maculopathy staging system
MHRD	macular hole-related retinal detachment
MTM	myopic traction maculopathy
OCT	optical coherence tomography
OCT-A	optical coherence tomography angiography
O-LMH	outer lamellar macular hole

O-MS	outer macular schisis
PPV	pars plana vitrectomy
PPVP	posterior precortical vitreous pocket
PM	pathologic myopia
PSR	posterior scleral reinforcement
PS	posterior staphyloma
RNFL	retinal nerve fiber layer
RPE	retinal pigment epithelium
RS	retinoschisis
RD	retinal detachment
SD-OCT	spectral-domain OCT
SO	silicon oil
SS-OCT	swept source OCT
SCA	stromal choroidal area
SRF	subretinal fluid
TCA	total choroidal area
VA	visual acuity
VMT	vitreomacular traction

Author details

Miguel A. Quiroz-Reyes[1*] and Erick A. Quiroz-Gonzalez[1,2]

1 Retina Department of Oftalmologia Integral ABC (Nonprofit Medical and Surgical Organization), Affiliated with the Postgraduate Studies Division of the National Autonomous University of Mexico, Mexico City, Mexico

2 Institute of Ophthalmology, Fundacion Conde de Valenciana (Nonprofit Organization), Affiliated with the Postgraduate Studies Division of the National Autonomous University of Mexico, Mexico City, Mexico

*Address all correspondence to: drquiroz@prodigy.net.mx

References

[1] Quiroz-Reyes MA, Quiroz-Gonzalez EA, Quiroz-Gonzalez MA, Lima-Gomez V. Association of the choroidal vascularity index with myopic traction maculopathy: A preliminary case-series report. Latin. American Journal of Ophthalmology. 2023;**6**:2

[2] Vitale S, Sperduto RD, Ferris FL. Increased prevalence of myopia in the United States between 1971-1972 and 1999-2004. Archives of Ophthalmology. 2009;**127**(12):1632-1639

[3] Ohno-Matsui K, Lai TY, Lai C-C, Cheung CMG. Updates of pathologic myopia. Progress in Retinal and Eye Research. 2016;**52**:156-187

[4] Holden BA, Fricke TR, Wilson DA, Jong M, Naidoo KS, Sankaridurg P, et al. Global prevalence of myopia and high myopia and temporal trends from 2000 through 2050. Ophthalmology. 2016;**123**(5):1036-1042

[5] Morgan IG, French AN, Ashby RS, Guo X, Ding X, He M, et al. The epidemics of myopia: Etiology and prevention. Progress in Retinal and Eye Research. 2018;**62**:134-149

[6] Iwase A, Araie M, Tomidokoro A, Yamamoto T, Shimizu H, Kitazawa Y, et al. Prevalence and causes of low vision and blindness in a Japanese adult population: The Tajimi Study. Ophthalmology. 2006;**113**(8):1354-1362 e1

[7] Wallace DK, Group PEDI. A randomized trial to evaluate 2 hours of daily patching for strabismic and anisometropic amblyopia in children. Ophthalmology. 2006;**113**(6):904-912

[8] Parolini B, Palmieri M, Finzi A, Besozzi G, Frisina R. Myopic traction maculopathy: A new perspective on classification and management. The Asia-Pacific Journal of Ophthalmology. 2021;**10**(1):49-59

[9] Phillips CI. Retinal detachment at the posterior pole. The British Journal of Ophthalmology. 1958;**42**(12):749-753

[10] Takano M, Kishi S. Foveal retinoschisis and retinal detachment in severely myopic eyes with posterior staphyloma. American Journal of Ophthalmology. 1999;**128**(4):472-476

[11] Panozzo G, Mercanti A. Optical coherence tomography findings in myopic traction maculopathy. Archives of Ophthalmology. 2004;**122**(10):1455-1460

[12] Shimada N, Ohno-Matsui K, Yoshida T, Sugamoto Y, Tokoro T, Mochizuki M. Progression from macular retinoschisis to retinal detachment in highly myopic eyes is associated with outer lamellar hole formation. British Journal of Ophthalmology. 2008;**92**(6):762-764

[13] Ruiz-Medrano J, Montero JA, Flores-Moreno I, Arias L, García-Layana A, Ruiz-Moreno JM. Myopic maculopathy: Current status and proposal for a new classification and grading system (ATN). Progress in Retinal and Eye Research. 2019;**69**:80-115

[14] Parolini B, Palmieri M, Finzi A, Besozzi G, Lucente A, Nava U, et al. The new myopic traction maculopathy staging system. European Journal of Ophthalmology. 2021;**31**(3):1299-1312

[15] Li KK, Wong DH, Li PS. Are we facing an increasing surgical demand for high myopic traction maculopathies?

A 12-year study from Hong Kong. BMC Ophthalmology. 2023;**23**(1):31

[16] Baba T, Ohno-Matsui K, Futagami S, Yoshida T, Yasuzumi K, Kojima A, et al. Prevalence and characteristics of foveal retinal detachment without macular hole in high myopia. American Journal of Ophthalmology. 2003;**135**(3):338-342

[17] Gaucher D, Haouchine B, Tadayoni R, Massin P, Erginay A, Benhamou N, et al. Long-term follow-up of high myopic foveoschisis: Natural course and surgical outcome. American Journal of Ophthalmology. 2007;**143**(3):455-462. e1

[18] Benhamou N, Massin P, Haouchine B, Erginay A, Gaudric A. Macular retinoschisis in highly myopic eyes. American Journal of Ophthalmology. 2002;**133**(6):794-800

[19] Sayanagi K, Ikuno Y, Gomi F, Tano Y. Retinal vascular microfolds in highly myopic eyes. American Journal of Ophthalmology. 2005;**139**(4):658-663

[20] Sayanagi K, Ikuno Y, Tano Y. Tractional internal limiting membrane detachment in highly myopic eyes. American Journal of Ophthalmology. 2006;**142**(5):850-852

[21] Bando H, Ikuno Y, Choi J-S, Tano Y, Yamanaka I, Ishibashi T. Ultrastructure of internal limiting membrane in myopic foveoschisis. American Journal of Ophthalmology. 2005;**139**(1):197-199

[22] Ikuno Y. Overview of the complications of high myopia. Retina. 2017;**37**(12):2347-2351

[23] Panozzo G, Mercanti A. Vitrectomy for myopic traction maculopathy. Archives of Ophthalmology. 2007;**125**(6):767-772

[24] Müller B, Joussen A. Myopic traction maculopathy-vitreoretinal traction syndrome in high myopic eyes and posterior staphyloma. Klinische Monatsblatter fur Augenheilkunde. 2011;**228**(9):771-779

[25] Ratiglia R, Osnaghi S, Bindella A, Pirondini C. Posterior traction retinal detachment in highly myopic eyes: Clinical features and surgical outcome as evaluated by optical coherence tomography. Retina. 2005;**25**(4):473-478

[26] Polito A, Lanzetta P, Del Borrello M, Bandello F. Spontaneous resolution of a shallow detachment of the macula in a highly myopic eye. American Journal of Ophthalmology. 2003;**135**(4):546-547

[27] Shimada N, Tanaka Y, Tokoro T, Ohno-Matsui K. Natural course of myopic traction maculopathy and factors associated with progression or resolution. American Journal of Ophthalmology. 2013;**156**(5):948-957. e1

[28] Zheng B, Chen Y, Zhao Z, Zhang Z, Zheng J, You Y, et al. Vitrectomy and internal limiting membrane peeling with perfluoropropane tamponade or balanced saline solution for myopic foveoschisis. Retina. 2011;**31**(4):692-701

[29] Mateo C, Burés-Jelstrup A, Navarro R, Corcóstegui B. Macular buckling for eyes with myopic foveoschisis secondary to posterior staphyloma. Retina. 2012;**32**(6):1121-1128

[30] Quiroz-Reyes MA, Quiroz-Gonzalez EA, Quiroz-Gonzalez MA, Lima-Gomez V. Postoperative choroidal vascularity index after the management of macula-off rhegmatogenous retinal detachment. International Journal of Retina and Vitreous. 2023;**9**(1):19

[31] Ouyang P-B, Duan X-C, Zhu X-H. Diagnosis and treatment

of myopic traction maculopathy. International Journal of Ophthalmology. 2012;**5**(6):754

[32] Oie Y, Ikuno Y, Fujikado T, Tano Y. Relation of posterior staphyloma in highly myopic eyes with macular hole and retinal detachment. Japanese Journal of Ophthalmology. 2005;**49**:530-532

[33] VanderBeek BL, Johnson MW. The diversity of traction mechanisms in myopic traction maculopathy. American Journal of Ophthalmology. 2012;**153**(1):93-102

[34] Byer NE. Natural history of posterior vitreous detachment with early management as the premier line of defense against retinal detachment. Ophthalmology. 1994;**101**(9):1503-1514

[35] Novak MA, Welch RB. Complications of acute symptomatic posterior vitreous detachment. American Journal of Ophthalmology. 1984;**97**(3):308-314

[36] Bond-Taylor M, Jakobsson G, Zetterberg M. Posterior vitreous detachment–prevalence of and risk factors for retinal tears. Clinical Ophthalmology. 2017;**11**:1689-1695

[37] Gishti O, van den Nieuwenhof R, Verhoekx J, van Overdam K. Symptoms related to posterior vitreous detachment and the risk of developing retinal tears: A systematic review. Acta Ophthalmologica. 2019;**97**(4):347-352

[38] Mastropasqua L, Carpineto P, Ciancaglini M, Falconio G, Gallenga PE. Treatment of retinal tears and lattice degenerations in fellow eyes in high risk patients suffering retinal detachment: A prospective study. British Journal of Ophthalmology. 1999;**83**(9):1046-1049

[39] Xue K, Muqit MM, Ezra E, Charles SJ, Yorston D, Mitra A, et al. Incidence, mechanism and outcomes of schisis retinal detachments revealed through a prospective population-based study. British Journal of Ophthalmology. 2017;**101**(8):1022-1026

[40] La Cour M, Friis J. Macular holes: Classification, epidemiology, natural history and treatment. Acta Ophthalmologica Scandinavica. 2002;**80**(6):579-587

[41] Arevalo JF, Ramirez E, Suarez E, Morales-Stopello J, Cortez R, Ramirez G, et al. Incidence of vitreoretinal pathologic conditions within 24 months after laser in situ keratomileusis. Ophthalmology. 2000;**107**(2):258-262

[42] Chan CK, Lawrence FC II. Macular hole after laser in situ keratomileusis and photorefractive keratectomy. American Journal of Ophthalmology. 2001;**131**(5):666-667

[43] Mitry D, Singh J, Yorston D, Siddiqui MR, Wright A, Fleck BW, et al. The predisposing pathology and clinical characteristics in the Scottish retinal detachment study. Ophthalmology. 2011;**118**(7):1429-1434

[44] Crim N, Esposito E, Monti R, Correa LJ, Serra HM, Urrets-Zavalia JA. Myopia as a risk factor for subsequent retinal tears in the course of a symptomatic posterior vitreous detachment. BMC Ophthalmology. 2017;**17**:1-5

[45] Curtin BJ, Jampol LM. The myopias: Basic science and clinical management. Retina. 1986;**6**(2):132

[46] Akiba J. Prevalence of posterior vitreous detachment in high myopia. Ophthalmology. 1993;**100**(9):1384-1388

[47] Itakura H, Kishi S, Li D, Nitta K, Akiyama H. Vitreous changes in high

myopia observed by swept-source optical coherence tomography. Investigative Ophthalmology & Visual Science. 2014;**55**(3):1447-1452

[48] Spaide RF, Fisher Y. Removal of adherent cortical vitreous plaques without removing the internal limiting membrane in the repair of macular detachments in highly myopic eyes. Retina. 2005;**25**(3):290-295

[49] Kwok A, Lai T, Yip W. Vitrectomy and gas tamponade without internal limiting membrane peeling for myopic foveoschisis. British Journal of Ophthalmology. 2005;**89**(9):1180-1183

[50] Yokota R, Hirakata A, Hayashi N, Hirota K, Rii T, Itoh Y, et al. Ultrastructural analyses of internal limiting membrane excised from highly myopic eyes with myopic traction maculopathy. Japanese Journal of Ophthalmology. 2018;**62**:84-91

[51] Yonemoto J, Ideta H, Sasaki K, Tanaka S, Hirose A, Oka C. The age of oneset of posterior vitreous detachment. Graefe's Archive for Clinical and Experimental Ophthalmology. 1994;**232**:67-70

[52] Morita H, Funata M, Tokoro T. A clinical study of the development of posterior vitreous detachment in high myopia. Retina. 1995;**15**(2):117-124

[53] Lim L, Cheung G, Lee S. Comparison of spectral domain and swept-source optical coherence tomography in pathological myopia. Eye. 2014;**28**(4):488-491

[54] Muqit MM, Stanga PE. Fourier-domain optical coherence tomography evaluation of retinal and optic nerve head neovascularisation in proliferative diabetic retinopathy. British Journal of Ophthalmology. 2014;**98**(1):65-72

[55] Ng D, Cheung C, Luk F, Mohamed S, Brelen M, Yam J, et al. Advances of optical coherence tomography in myopia and pathologic myopia. Eye. 2016;**30**(7):901-916

[56] Itakura H, Kishi S. Evolution of vitreomacular detachment in healthy subjects. JAMA Ophthalmology. 2013;**131**(10):1348-1352

[57] Takahashi H, Tanaka N, Shinohara K, Yokoi T, Yoshida T, Uramoto K, et al. Ultrawidefield optical coherence tomographic imaging of posterior vitreous in eyes with high myopia. American Journal of Ophthalmology. 2019;**206**:102-112

[58] Hayashi K, Sato T, Manabe S-i, Hirata A. Sex-related differences in the progression of posterior vitreous detachment with age. Ophthalmology Retina. 2019;**3**(3):237-243

[59] You QS, Peng XY, Xu L, Chen CX, Wei WB, Wang Y, et al. Macular Bruch membrane defects in highly myopic eyes: The Beijing Eye Study. Retina. 2016;**36**(3):517-523

[60] Chirco K, Sohn E, Stone E, Tucker B, Mullins R. Structural and molecular changes in the aging choroid: Implications for age-related macular degeneration. Eye. 2017;**31**(1):10-25

[61] Jonas JB, Ohno-Matsui K, Jiang WJ, Panda-Jonas S. Bruch membrane and the mechanism of myopization: A new theory. Retina. 2017;**37**(8):1428-1440

[62] Ohno-Matsui K, Jonas JB, Spaide RF. Macular Bruch membrane holes in highly myopic patchy chorioretinal atrophy. American Journal of Ophthalmology. 2016;**166**:22-28

[63] Ohno-Matsui K, Jonas JB, Spaide RF. Macular bruch membrane holes in

choroidal neovascularization–related myopic macular atrophy by swept-source optical coherence tomography. American Journal of Ophthalmology. 2016;**162**(133-9):e1

[64] Fang Y, Jonas JB, Yokoi T, Cao K, Shinohara K, Ohno-Matsui K. Macular Bruch's membrane defect and dome-shaped macula in high myopia. PLoS One. 2017;**12**(6):e0178998

[65] Meng L-H, Yuan M-Z, Zhao X-Y, Chen Y-X. Macular Bruch's membrane defects and other myopic lesions in high myopia. International Journal of Ophthalmology. 2022;**15**(3):466

[66] Xie R, Qiu B, Chhablani J, Zhang X. Evaluation of choroidal thickness using optical coherent tomography: A review. Frontiers in Medicine. 2021;**8**:783519

[67] Tan K-A, Gupta P, Agarwal A, Chhablani J, Cheng C-Y, Keane PA, et al. State of science: Choroidal thickness and systemic health. Survey of Ophthalmology. 2016;**61**(5):566-581

[68] Phillips CI. Retinal detachment at the posterior pole. The British Journal of Ophthalmology. 1958;**42**(12):749

[69] Wu P, Chen Y, Chen Y, Chen C, Shin S, Tsai C, et al. Factors associated with foveoschisis and foveal detachment without macular hole in high myopia. Eye. 2009;**23**(2):356-361

[70] Phillips C, Dobbie J. Posterior staphyloma and retinal detachment. American Journal of Ophthalmology. 1963;**55**(2):332-335

[71] Fujimoto M, Hangai M, Suda K, Yoshimura N. Features associated with foveal retinal detachment in myopic macular retinoschisis. American Journal of Ophthalmology. 2010;**150**(6):863-870. e1

[72] Sayanagi K, Morimoto Y, Ikuno Y, Tano Y. Spectral-domain optical coherence tomographic findings in myopic foveoschisis. Retina. 2010;**30**(4):623-628

[73] Ceklic L, Munk MR, Wolf-Schnurrbusch U, Gekkieva M, Wolf S. Visual acuity outcomes of ranibizumab treatment in pathologic myopic eyes with macular retinoschisis and choroidal neovascularization. Retina (Philadelphia, Pa). 2017;**37**(4):687

[74] Ikuno Y, Gomi F, Tano Y. Potent retinal arteriolar traction as a possible cause of myopic foveoschisis. American Journal of Ophthalmology. 2005;**139**(3):462-467

[75] Hoang QV, Chen C-L, Garcia-Arumi J, Sherwood PR, Chang S. Radius of curvature changes in spontaneous improvement of foveoschisis in highly myopic eyes. British Journal of Ophthalmology. 2016;**100**(2):222-226

[76] Witkin AJ, Ko TH, Fujimoto JG, Schuman JS, Baumal CR, Rogers AH, et al. Redefining lamellar holes and the vitreomacular interface: An ultrahigh-resolution optical coherence tomography study. Ophthalmology. 2006;**113**(3):388-397

[77] Reibaldi M, Parravano M, Varano M, Longo A, Avitabile T, Uva MG, et al. Foveal microstructure and functional parameters in lamellar macular hole. American Journal of Ophthalmology. 2012;**154**(6):974-980. e1

[78] Frisina R, Tessarolo F, Marchesoni I, Piccoli F, Bonomi E, Caciagli P, et al. Microscopic observation of proliferative membranes in fibrocontractive retinal disorders. Journal of Ophthalmology. 2019;**61**(2):73-82

[79] Bottoni F, Deiro AP, Giani A, Orini C, Cigada M, Staurenghi G. The natural history of lamellar macular holes: A spectral domain optical coherence tomography study. Graefe's Archive for Clinical and Experimental Ophthalmology. 2013;**251**:467-475

[80] Parolini B, Schumann RG, Cereda MG, Haritoglou C, Pertile G. Lamellar macular hole: A clinicopathologic correlation of surgically excised epiretinal membranes. Investigative Ophthalmology & Visual Science. 2011;**52**(12):9074-9083

[81] Frisina R, Pilotto E, Midena E. Lamellar macular hole: State of the art. Ophthalmic Research. 2019;**61**(2):73-82

[82] Zampedri E, Romanelli F, Semeraro F, Parolini B, Frisina R. Spectral-domain optical coherence tomography findings in idiopathic lamellar macular hole. Graefe's Archive for Clinical and Experimental Ophthalmology. 2017;**255**:699-707

[83] Lai T-T, Yang C-M. Lamellar hole-associated epiretinal proliferation in lamellar macular hole and full-thickness macular hole in high myopia. Retina. 2018;**38**(7):1316-1323

[84] Duker JS, Kaiser PK, Binder S, de Smet MD, Gaudric A, Reichel E, et al. The International Vitreomacular Traction Study Group classification of vitreomacular adhesion, traction, and macular hole. Ophthalmology. 2013;**120**(12):2611-2619

[85] Govetto A, Dacquay Y, Farajzadeh M, Platner E, Hirabayashi K, Hosseini H, et al. Lamellar macular hole: Two distinct clinical entities? American Journal of Ophthalmology. 2016;**164**:99-109

[86] Hubschman JP, Govetto A, Spaide RF, Schumann R, Steel D, Figueroa MS, et al. Optical coherence tomography-based consensus definition for lamellar macular hole. British Journal of Ophthalmology. 2020;**104**(12):1741-1747

[87] Hattori K, Kataoka K, Takeuchi J, Ito Y, Terasaki H. Predictive factors of surgical outcomes in vitrectomy for myopic traction maculopathy. Retina. 2018;**38**:S23-S30

[88] Lin C, Ho T, Yang C. The development and evolution of full thickness macular hole in highly myopic eyes. Eye. 2015;**29**(3):388-396

[89] dell'Omo R, Virgili G, Bottoni F, Parolini B, De Turris S, Di Salvatore A, et al. Lamellar macular holes in the eyes with pathological myopia. Graefe's Archive for Clinical and Experimental Ophthalmology. 2018;**256**:1281-1290

[90] Hsia Y, Ho T-C, Yang C-H, Hsieh Y-T, Lai T-T, Yang C-M. Clinical characteristics and long-term evolution of lamellar macular hole in high myopia. PLoS One. 2020;**15**(5):e0232852

[91] Rino F, Elena Z, Ivan M, Paolo B, Barbara P, Federica R. Lamellar macular hole in high myopic eyes with posterior staphyloma: Morphological and functional characteristics. Graefe's Archive for Clinical and Experimental Ophthalmology. 2016;**254**:2141-2150

[92] Frisina R, Gius I, Palmieri M, Finzi A, Tozzi L, Parolini B. Myopic traction maculopathy: Diagnostic and management strategies. Clinical Ophthalmology. 2020;**14**:3699-3708

[93] Ikuno Y, Sayanagi K, Soga K, Oshima Y, Ohji M, Tano Y. Foveal anatomical status and surgical results in vitrectomy for myopic foveoschisis. Japanese Journal of Ophthalmology. 2008;**52**:269-276

[94] Jo Y, Ikuno Y, Nishida K. Retinoschisis: A predictive factor in

vitrectomy for macular holes without retinal detachment in highly myopic eyes. British Journal of Ophthalmology. 2012;**96**(2):197-200

[95] Ohno-Matsui K, Kawasaki R, Jonas JB, Cheung CMG, Saw S-M, Verhoeven VJ, et al. International photographic classification and grading system for myopic maculopathy. American Journal of Ophthalmology. 2015;**159**(5):877-883. e7

[96] Ruiz-Medrano J, Flores-Moreno I, Ohno-Matsui K, Cheung CMG, Silva R, Ruiz-Moreno JM. Validation of the recently developed ATN classification and grading system for myopic maculopathy. Retina (Philadelphia, Pa). 2020;**40**(11):2113

[97] Zhang R-r, Yu Y, Hou Y-f, Wu C-f. Intra-and interobserver concordance of a new classification system for myopic maculopathy. BMC Ophthalmology. 2021;**21**(1):1-7

[98] Quiroz-Reyes M, Andrade B, Quiroz-Gonzalez E, Quiroz-Gonzalez M, Kim H. Long-term postoperative structural and functional evaluation in myopic foveoretinal detachment. International Journal of Ophthalmology and Clinical Research. 2021;**8**:132

[99] Borley W, Snyder A. Surgical treatment of degenerative myopia; the combined lamellar scleral resection with scleral reinforcement using donor eye. Transactions – American Academy of Ophthalmology and Otolaryngology. 1958;**62**(6):791-801

[100] Qi Y, Duan AL, You QS, Jonas JB, Wang N. Posterior scleral reinforcement and vitrectomy for myopic foveoschisis in extreme myopia. Retina. 2015;**35**(2):351-357

[101] Snyder AA, Thompson FB. A simplified technique for surgical treatment of degenerative myopia. American Journal of Ophthalmology. 1972;**74**(2):273-277

[102] Peng C, Xu J, Ding X, Lu Y, Zhang J, Wang F, et al. Effects of posterior scleral reinforcement in pathological myopia: A 3-year follow-up study. Graefe's Archive for Clinical and Experimental Ophthalmology. 2019;**257**:607-617

[103] Frisina R. A customized posterior scleral reinforcement for myopic macular hole with retinal detachment and posterior staphyloma: A case report. European Journal of Ophthalmology. 2021;**31**(5):NP88-NP92

[104] Momose A. Surgical treatment of myopia—With special references to posterior scleral support operation and radial keratotomy. Indian Journal of Ophthalmology. 1983;**31**(6):759-767

[105] Schepens CL, Okamura I, Brockhurst R. The scleral buckling procedures: 1. Surgical techniques and management. AMA. Archives of Ophthalmology. 1957;**58**(6):797-811

[106] Ripandelli G, Coppé AM, Fedeli R, Parisi V, D'Amico DJ, Stirpe M. Evaluation of primary surgical procedures for retinal detachment with macular hole in highly myopic eyes: A randomized comparison of vitrectomy versus posterior episcleral buckling surgery. Ophthalmology. 2001;**108**(12):2258-2264

[107] Theodossiadis GP, Theodossiadis PG. The macular buckling procedure in the treatment of retinal detachment in highly myopic eyes with macular hole and posterior staphyloma: Mean follow-up of 15 years. Retina. 2005;**25**(3):285-289

[108] Shinohara K, Tanaka N, Jonas JB, Shimada N, Moriyama M, Yoshida T, et al. Ultrawide-field OCT to investigate

relationships between myopic macular retinoschisis and posterior staphyloma. Ophthalmology. 2018;**125**(10):1575-1586

[109] Zheng F, Wong CW, Sabanayagam C, Cheung YB, Matsumura S, Chua J, et al. Prevalence, risk factors and impact of posterior staphyloma diagnosed from wide-field optical coherence tomography in Singapore adults with high myopia. Acta Ophthalmologica. 2021;**99**(2):e144-ee53

[110] Sasoh M, Yoshida S, Ito Y, Matsui K, Osawa S, Uji Y. Macular buckling for retinal detachment due to macular hole in highly myopic eyes with posterior staphyloma. Retina (Philadelphia, Pa). 2000;**20**(5):445-449

[111] Ward B, Tarutta E, Mayer M. The efficacy and safety of posterior pole buckles in the control of progressive high myopia. Eye. 2009;**23**(12):2169-2174

[112] Alkabes M, Mateo C. Macular buckle technique in myopic traction maculopathy: A 16-year review of the literature and a comparison with vitreous surgery. Graefe's Archive for Clinical and Experimental Ophthalmology. 2018;**256**:863-877

[113] Yeh SI, Chang WC, Chen LJ. Vitrectomy without internal limiting membrane peeling for macular retinoschisis and foveal detachment in highly myopic eyes. Acta Ophthalmologica. 2008;**86**(2):219-224

[114] Johnson MW. Myopic traction maculopathy: Pathogenic mechanisms and surgical treatment. Retina. 2012;**32**:S205-SS10

[115] Sasaki H, Shiono A, Kogo J, Yomoda R, Munemasa Y, Syoda M, et al. Inverted internal limiting membrane flap technique as a useful procedure for macular hole-associated retinal detachment in highly myopic eyes. Eye. 2017;**31**(4):545-550

[116] Kinoshita T, Onoda Y, Maeno T. Long-term surgical outcomes of the inverted internal limiting membrane flap technique in highly myopic macular hole retinal detachment. Graefe's Archive for Clinical and Experimental Ophthalmology. 2017;**255**:1101-1106

[117] Kadonosono K, Yazama F, Itoh N, Uchio E, Nakamura S, Akura J, et al. Treatment of retinal detachment resulting from myopic macular hole with internal limiting membrane removal. American Journal of Ophthalmology. 2001;**131**(2):203-207

[118] Lu L, Li Y, Cai S, Yang J. Vitreous surgery in highly myopic retinal detachment resulting from a macular hole. Clinical & Experimental Ophthalmology. 2002;**30**(4):261-265

[119] Kobayashi H, Kishi S. Vitreous surgery for highly myopic eyes with foveal detachment and retinoschisis. Ophthalmology. 2003;**110**(9):1702-1707

[120] Shimada N, Sugamoto Y, Ogawa M, Takase H, Ohno-Matsui K. Fovea-sparing internal limiting membrane peeling for myopic traction maculopathy. American Journal of Ophthalmology. 2012;**154**(4):693-701

[121] Ho T-C, Yang C-M, Huang J-S, Yang C-H, Yeh P-T, Chen T-C, et al. Long-term outcome of foveolar internal limiting membrane nonpeeling for myopic traction maculopathy. Retina. 2014;**34**(9):1833-1840

[122] Uchida A, Shinoda H, Koto T, Mochimaru H, Nagai N, Tsubota K, et al. Vitrectomy for myopic foveoschisis with internal limiting membrane peeling and no gas tamponade. Retina. 2014;**34**(3):455-460

[123] Futagami S, Inoue M, Hirakata A. Removal of internal limiting membrane for recurrent myopic traction maculopathy. Clinical & Experimental Ophthalmology. 2008;**36**(8):782-785

[124] Shin JY, Yu HG. Visual prognosis and spectral-domain optical coherence tomography findings of myopic foveoschisis surgery using 25-gauge transconjunctival sutureless vitrectomy. Retina. 2012;**32**(3):486-492

[125] Taniuchi S, Hirakata A, Itoh Y, Hirota K, Inoue M. Vitrectomy with or without internal limiting membrane peeling for each stage of myopic traction maculopathy. Retina. 2013;**33**(10):2018-2025

[126] Figueroa MS, Ruiz-Moreno JM, del Valle FG, Govetto A, De La Vega C, Plascencia RN, et al. Long-term outcomes of 23-gauge pars plana vitrectomy with internal limiting membrane peeling and gas tamponade for myopic traction maculopathy: A prospective study. Retina. 2015;**35**(9):1836-1843

[127] Kumagai K, Furukawa M, Ogino N, Larson E. Factors correlated with postoperative visual acuity after vitrectomy and internal limiting membrane peeling for myopic foveoschisis. Retina. 2010;**30**(6):874-880

[128] Gao X, Ikuno Y, Fujimoto S, Nishida K. Risk factors for development of full-thickness macular holes after pars plana vitrectomy for myopic foveoschisis. American Journal of Ophthalmology. 2013;**155**(6):1021-1027. e1

[129] Kim KS, Lee SB, Lee WK. Vitrectomy and internal limiting membrane peeling with and without gas tamponade for myopic foveoschisis. American Journal of Ophthalmology. 2012;**153**(2):320-326. e1

[130] Lim SJ, Kwon YH, Kim SH, You YS, Kwon OW. Vitrectomy and internal limiting membrane peeling without gas tamponade for myopic foveoschisis. Graefe's Archive for Clinical and Experimental Ophthalmology. 2012;**250**:1573-1577

[131] Tian T, Jin H, Zhang Q, Zhang X, Zhang H, Zhao P. Long-term surgical outcomes of multiple parfoveolar curvilinear internal limiting membrane peeling for myopic foveoschisis. Eye. 2018;**32**(11):1783-1789

[132] Ho T-C, Chen M-S, Huang J-S, Shih Y-F, Ho H, Huang Y-H. Foveola nonpeeling technique in internal limiting membrane peeling of myopic foveoschisis surgery. Retina. 2012;**32**(3):631-634

[133] Lee CL, Wu WC, Chen KJ, Chiu LY, Wu KY, Chang YC. Modified internal limiting membrane peeling technique (maculorrhexis) for myopic foveoschisis surgery. Acta Ophthalmologica. 2017;**95**(2):e128-ee31

[134] Michalewska Z, Michalewski J, Adelman RA, Nawrocki J. Inverted internal limiting membrane flap technique for large macular holes. Ophthalmology. 2010;**117**(10):2018-2025

[135] Kannan NB, Kohli P, Parida H, Adenuga O, Ramasamy K. Comparative study of inverted internal limiting membrane (ILM) flap and ILM peeling technique in large macular holes: A randomized-control trial. BMC Ophthalmology. 2018;**18**:1-6

[136] Lin J-P, Yang C-M. Combined fovea-sparing internal limiting membrane peeling with internal limiting membrane flap technique for progressive myopic traction maculopathy. Graefe's Archive for Clinical and Experimental Ophthalmology. 2022;**260**(2):1-8

[137] Kokame GT, Yamamoto I. Silicone oil versus gas tamponade. Ophthalmology. 2004;**111**(4):851-852

[138] Mester V, Kuhn F. Internal limiting membrane removal in the management of full-thickness macular holes. American Journal of Ophthalmology. 2000;**129**(6):769-777

[139] Kanda S, Uemura A, Sakamoto Y, Kita H. Vitrectomy with internal limiting membrane peeling for macular retinoschisis and retinal detachment without macular hole in highly myopic eyes. American Journal of Ophthalmology. 2003;**136**(1):177-180

[140] Mete M, Parolini B, Maggio E, Pertile G. 1000 cSt silicone oil vs heavy silicone oil as intraocular tamponade in retinal detachment associated with myopic macular hole. Graefe's Archive for Clinical and Experimental Ophthalmology. 2011;**249**:821-826

[141] Ikuno Y, Sayanagi K, Ohji M, Kamei M, Gomi F, Harino S, et al. Vitrectomy and internal limiting membrane peeling for myopic foveoschisis. American Journal of Ophthalmology. 2004;**137**(4):719-724

[142] Scholda C, Wirtitsch M, Biowski R, Stur M. Primary silicone oil tamponade without retinopexy in highly myopic eyes with central macular hole detachments. Retina. 2005;**25**(2):141-146

[143] Susvar P, Sood G. Current concepts of macular buckle in myopic traction maculopathy. Indian Journal of Ophthalmology. 2018;**66**(12):1772

[144] Wang S, Peng Q, Zhao P. SD-OCT use in myopic retinoschisis preand postvitrectomy. Optometry and Vision Science. 2012;**89**(5):678-683

[145] Baba T, Tanaka S, Maesawa A, Teramatsu T, Noda Y, Yamamoto S. Scleral buckling with macular plombe for eyes with myopic macular retinoschisis and retinal detachment without macular hole. American Journal of Ophthalmology. 2006;**142**(3):483-487

[146] Devin F, Tsui I, Morin B, Duprat J-P, Hubschman J-P. T-shaped scleral buckle for macular detachments in high myopes. Retina. 2011;**31**(1):177-180

[147] Agarwal A, Agrawal R, Khandelwal N, Invernizzi A, Aggarwal K, Sharma A, et al. Choroidal structural changes in tubercular multifocal serpiginoid choroiditis. Ocular Immunology and Inflammation. 2018;**26**(6):838-844

[148] Agrawal R, Gupta P, Tan K-A, Cheung CMG, Wong T-Y, Cheng C-Y. Choroidal vascularity index as a measure of vascular status of the choroid: Measurements in healthy eyes from a population-based study. Scientific Reports. 2016;**6**(1):21090

[149] Agrawal R, Li LKH, Nakhate V, Khandelwal N, Mahendradas P. Choroidal vascularity index in Vogt–Koyanagi–Harada disease: An EDI-OCT derived tool for monitoring disease progression. Translational Vision Science & Technology. 2016;**5**(4):7

[150] Yazdani N, Ehsaei A, Hoseini-Yazdi H, Shoeibi N, Alonso-Caneiro D, Collins MJ. Wide-field choroidal thickness and vascularity index in myopes and emmetropes. Ophthalmic and Physiological Optics. 2021;**41**(6):1308-1319

[151] Iovino C, Au A, Hilely A, Violanti S, Peiretti E, Gorin MB, et al. Evaluation of the choroid in eyes with retinitis pigmentosa and cystoid macular edema. Investigative Ophthalmology & Visual Science. 2019;**60**(15):5000-5006

[152] Agrawal R, Salman M, Tan K-A, Karampelas M, Sim DA, Keane PA, et al. Choroidal vascularity index (CVI)—A novel optical coherence tomography parameter for monitoring patients with panuveitis? PLoS One. 2016;**11**(1):e0146344

[153] Aribas YK, Hondur AM, Tezel TH. Choroidal vascularity index and choriocapillary changes in retinal vein occlusions. Graefe's Archive for Clinical and Experimental Ophthalmology. 2020;**258**:2389-2397

[154] Sakata K, Funatsu H, Harino S, Noma H, Hori S. Relationship between macular microcirculation and progression of diabetic macular edema. Ophthalmology. 2006;**113**(8):1385-1391

[155] Chin EK, Kim DY, Hunter AA, Pilli S, Wilson M, Zawadzki RJ, et al. Staging of macular telangiectasia: Power-Doppler optical coherence tomography and macular pigment optical density. Investigative Ophthalmology & Visual Science. 2013;**54**(7):4459-4470

[156] Veverka KK, AbouChehade JE, Iezzi R Jr, Pulido JS. Noninvasive grading of radiation retinopathy: The use of optical coherence tomography angiography. Retina. 2015;**35**(11):2400-2410

[157] Marques JH, Marta A, Castro C, Baptista PM, José D, Almeida D, et al. Choroidal changes and associations with visual acuity in diabetic patients. International Journal of Retina and Vitreous. 2022;**8**(1):6

[158] Kim M, Kim RY, Park Y-H. Choroidal vascularity index and choroidal thickness in human leukocyte antigen-B27-associated uveitis. Ocular Immunology and Inflammation. 2019;**27**(8):1280-1287

[159] Singh SR, Invernizzi A, Rasheed MA, Cagini C, Goud A, Vupparaboina KK, et al. Wide-field choroidal vascularity in healthy eyes. American Journal of Ophthalmology. 2018;**193**:100-105

[160] Agrawal R, Wei X, Goud A, Vupparaboina KK, Jana S, Chhablani J. Influence of scanning area on choroidal vascularity index measurement using optical coherence tomography. Acta Ophthalmologica. 2017;**95**(8):e770-e7e5

[161] Agrawal R, Seen S, Vaishnavi S, Vupparaboina KK, Goud A, Rasheed MA, et al. Choroidal vascularity index using swept-source and spectral-domain optical coherence tomography: A comparative study. Ophthalmic Surgery, Lasers and Imaging Retina. 2019;**50**(2):e26-e32

[162] Iovino C, Pellegrini M, Bernabei F, Borrelli E, Sacconi R, Govetto A, et al. Choroidal vascularity index: An in-depth analysis of this novel optical coherence tomography parameter. Journal of Clinical Medicine. 2020;**9**(2):595

[163] Chun H, Kim JY, Kwak JH, Kim RY, Kim M, Park Y-G, et al. The effect of phacoemulsification performed with vitrectomy on choroidal vascularity index in eyes with vitreomacular diseases. Scientific Reports. 2021;**11**(1):19898

[164] Bernabei F, Pellegrini M, Taroni L, Roda M, Toschi PG, Schiavi C, et al. Choroidal vascular changes after encircling scleral buckling for rhegmatogenous retinal detachment. Eye. 2021;**35**(9):2619-2623

[165] Rizzo S, Savastano A, Finocchio L, Savastano MC, Khandelwal N, Agrawal R. Choroidal vascularity index changes after vitreomacular surgery. Acta Ophthalmologica. 2018;**96**(8):e950-e9e5

[166] Dou N, Yu S, Tsui C-K, Yang B, Lin J, Lu X, et al. Choroidal vascularity index as a biomarker for visual response to antivascular endothelial growth factor treatment in diabetic macular edema. Journal of Diabetes Research. 2021;**2021**:3033219

[167] Nicolini N, Tombolini B, Barresi C, Pignatelli F, Lattanzio R, Bandello F, et al. Assessment of diabetic choroidopathy using ultrawidefield optical coherence tomography. Translational Vision, Science & Technology. 2022;**11**(3):35

[168] Foo VHX, Gupta P, Nguyen QD, Chong CCY, Agrawal R, Cheng C-Y, et al. Decrease in Choroidal Vascularity Index of Haller's layer in diabetic eyes precedes retinopathy. BMJ Open Diabetes Research and Care. 2020;**8**(1):e001295

[169] Agrawal R, Ding J, Sen P, Rousselot A, Chan A, Nivison-Smith L, et al. Exploring choroidal angioarchitecture in health and disease using choroidal vascularity index. Progress in Retinal and Eye Research. 2020;**77**:100829

[170] Hayreh SS. Segmental nature of the choroidal vasculature. British Journal of Ophthalmology. 1975;**59**(11):631-648

[171] Margolis R, Spaide RF. A pilot study of enhanced depth imaging optical coherence tomography of the choroid in normal eyes. American Journal of Ophthalmology. 2009;**147**(5):811-815

[172] Imamura Y, Fujiwara T, Margolis R, Spaide RF. Enhanced depth imaging optical coherence tomography of the choroid in central serous chorioretinopathy. Retina. 2009;**29**(10):1469-1473

[173] Fan H, Chen H-Y, Ma H-J, Chang Z, Yin H-Q, Ng DS-C, et al. Reduced macular vascular density in myopic eyes. Chinese Medical Journal. 2017;**130**(04):445-451

[174] Koçak N, Subaşı M, Yeter V. Effects of age and binarising area on choroidal vascularity index in healthy eyes: An optical coherence tomography study. International Ophthalmology. 2021;**41**:825-834

Chapter 10

Update on Retinal Displacement Following Surgical Repair of Retinal Detachment

Romana García Gil, Anselmo Feliciano Sánchez, Paula Boned-Fustel and Laura Fernández García

Abstract

Retinal displacement following surgical repair of retinal detachment is a common complication. It involves the repositioning and fixation of the retina in a non-optimal area. Associated risk factors include pars plana vitrectomy as a surgical technique, the use of gas as a tamponading agent, or a retinal detachment involving the macula. Among complementary diagnostic tests, autofluorescence plays a pivotal role, revealing the presence of retinal vessel imprints through the depiction of hyperautofluorescent lines that run parallel to the vessels. These lines represent the original vascular pattern and serve as a distinctive hallmark. Despite the surgical repair of retinal detachment, there is a high incidence of metamorphopsia and visual dissatisfaction among patients suffering from retinal displacement. Several approaches have been proposed to reduce retinal displacement, including the use of a smaller gas bubble as a tamponade, immediate placement of the patient face down in the operating room, and maintaining this position for at least 2 hours after surgery. In this chapter, we will elaborate on these aspects based on recent literature.

Keywords: retinal displacement, retinal detachment, autofluorescence, gas tamponade, pars plana vitrectomy, pneumatic retinopexy

1. Introduction

The incidence of retinal detachment (RD) ranges from 6.3 to 17.9 per 100,000 inhabitants, with a significant geographic variation [1].

In RD, there is a separation and accumulation of fluid between the retinal pigment epithelium (RPE) and the neurosensory retina due to one or more tears in the retina that allow fluid to pass between these layers. It is considered a cause of visual loss, which can be severe and even lead to permanent visual disability.

There are different types of RD depending on their etiopathogenesis (rhegmatogenous RD, exudative RD, tractional RD). Rhegmatogenous retinal detachment (RRD), caused by a full-thickness retinal tear, stands as the most prevalent form [2].

RPE cells facilitate retinal cohesion by pumping "virtual" subretinal fluid into the choriocapillaris and additionally, to a matrix of proteoglycans called the interphotoreceptor matrix (IPM), which acts as an adhesive intermediary between the neurosensory retina and the RPE, ensuring their connection [2].

The primary pathological process that gives rise to RRD is vitreous syneresis, which involves partial liquefaction of the vitreous gel. This liquefaction can be attributed to various factors, including aging, myopia, which permit the movement of vitreous gel fluid within the eye. Additionally, tractions occurring at vitreoretinal adhesion points, such as the optic disc border and retinal vessels (with stronger adhesions anterior to the equator than posterior), as well as at the vitreous base, can disrupt the cohesive forces between the neurosensory retina and RPE, thereby precipitating retinal tears. This phenomenon allows liquefied vitreous to traverse into the subretinal space in quantities exceeding the pumping capacity of the RPE, resulting in the initiation and subsequent progression of RD [2].

RD damages the neurosensory retina in a characteristic pattern of apoptosis. Photoreceptor cells undergo apoptosis lasting from 1 to 180 days, with the peak occurring at 2 days and the lowest level at 7–14 days. Anatomically, this is expressed by disruption of the outer and inner segments of photoreceptors [3]. Additionally, glial cells undergo anatomical and biochemical changes, such as retraction of synaptic terminals, hypertrophy of Müller cells, and altered expression of certain proteins like the apoptosis-inducing factor [4].

These physiological changes in primary RD sensitize photoreceptors to future apoptotic signals. In cases of recurrent RD, this prior sensitization leads to greater retinal damage compared to that in primary RD [5].

Repositioning of the retina requires surgical treatment, with possible options including scleral buckle (SB) surgery and pars plana vitrectomy (PPV). In cases of localized tears, scleral buckling or pneumatic retinopexy can be used. For cases without localized tears, those with giant tears, lesions with vitreous tractions, or proliferative vitreoretinopathy, PPV emerges as the preferred approach [6].

Scleral buckling constitutes an extraocular surgical procedure involving the application of pressure on the sclera through the placement of a sponge or band at the location of the retinal tear. This indentation effect serves to approximate the sclera to the retina, thereby mitigating vitreous traction on the retinal tissue [2, 7].

PPV, an intraocular surgical procedure, entails the utilization of small-gauge instruments to access the vitreous cavity through the pars plana. This approach facilitates the extraction of the vitreous humor and the rectification of the RD from within. This includes draining the subretinal fluid through the retinal tears, posteriorly sealing the tears using laser or cryopexy, and ocular tamponade employing diverse agents like gas or silicone oil [2, 8].

A noteworthy complication of RD surgical repair is the potential displacement of the retina followed by fixation in an anatomically suboptimal region. This phenomenon can result in structural modifications of photoreceptors and the subsequent manifestation of corresponding visual anomalies.

It has been reported that retinal displacement subsequent to surgical intervention for RD could be observed in a notable proportion of cases, reaching up to 35% as indicated by recent studies [9].

The first description of retinal displacement was presented in 2010 by Shiragami et al., who described hyperautofluorescent lines in the fundus autofluorescence of patients who underwent standard PPV for RRD. These lines ran parallel to the retinal vessels in the area where the RD had occurred [10]. These hyperautofluorescent lines were termed "imprints of retinal vessels," which perfectly encapsulate the underlying etiology [11].

This chapter provides an update on retinal displacement after retinal surgery and discusses factors to consider during surgery to minimize this complication.

2. Emerging terminology and concepts in retinal repositioning

According to the literature, in the surgical treatment of RRD, achieving complete retinal reattachment after the first surgery is considered a primary anatomical success, and achieving this complete retinal reattachment after multiple surgeries is considered a final anatomical success.

However, these concepts of surgical success only consider the reattachment of the retina in all four quadrants, without considering the quality of that reattachment. This led to the proposal of two new terms in 2020: high-integrity retinal reattachment and low-integrity retinal reattachment (**Figure 1**) [12].

High-integrity retinal reattachment is characterized by repositioning the retina as closely as possible to its original location, allowing alignment of photoreceptors as close as possible to their original positions. This achieves better functionality and reduces vertical metamorphopsia [12].

Conversely, low-integrity retinal reattachment involves repositioning the retina far from its original location, without aligning the photoreceptors to their original positions, resulting in poorer functionality.

To assess the integrity of the reattachment, fundus autofluorescence is employed. In cases of high-integrity retinal reattachment, the imprint of retinal vessels will not be observed in autofluorescence. However, in cases of low-integrity retinal reattachment, the imprint of retinal vessels will be evident in autofluorescence imaging.

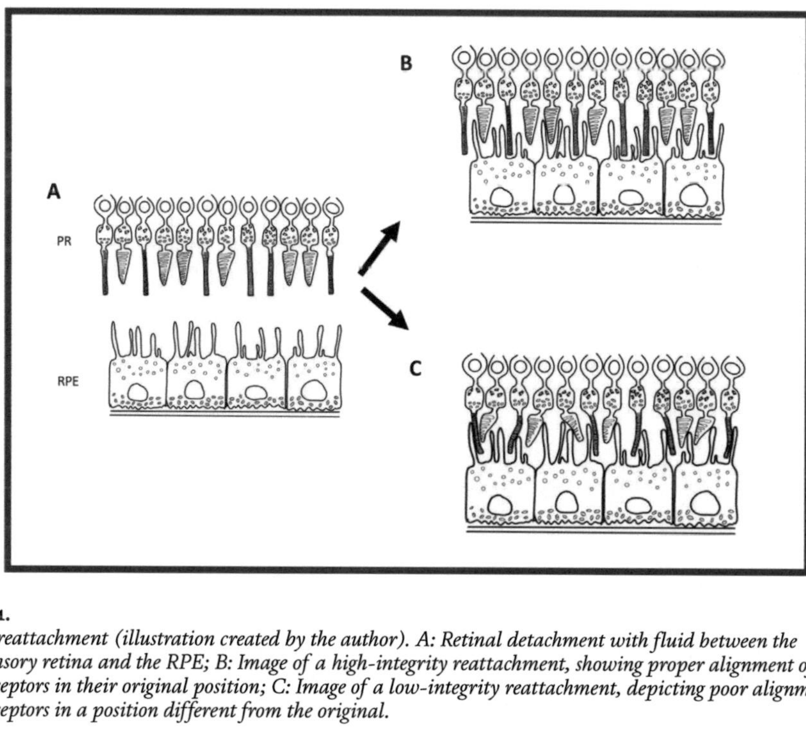

Figure 1.
Retinal reattachment (illustration created by the author). A: Retinal detachment with fluid between the neurosensory retina and the RPE; B: Image of a high-integrity reattachment, showing proper alignment of photoreceptors in their original position; C: Image of a low-integrity reattachment, depicting poor alignment of photoreceptors in a position different from the original.

3. Factors associated with retinal displacement following rhegmatogenous retinal detachment surgery

Several studies have identified factors that can influence the occurrence of retinal displacement, either predisposing to or mitigating the risk of this complication.

Consensus across all studies indicates a heightened risk of retinal displacement in surgeries employing PPV compared to scleral surgery and pneumatic retinopexy. Scleral surgery without the use of tamponade presents the lowest risk of retinal displacement, followed by pneumatic retinopexy [12].

The type of tamponade agent used during surgery also makes a difference, with an increased risk observed in cases involving gas in comparison to silicone oil [13]. Nevertheless, distinctions based on the specific type of gas employed (such as SF6 or C3F8) do not appear to be evident (**Table 1**).

An additional factor under scrutiny in cases of RRD is macular involvement. RRDs that affect the macula demonstrate an increased susceptibility to retinal displacement subsequent to surgical intervention, accompanied by more pronounced visual implications. Conversely, the initial extent of RRD without macular involvement has not been conclusively correlated with retinal displacement [14].

However, a definitive correlation between the utilization of perfluorocarbon liquids (PFCL) to achieve retinal flattening during surgery and the implementation of posterior retinotomy for subretinal fluid drainage, with the occurrence of retinal displacement, has not been firmly established [15].

4. Pathogenesis of retinal displacement

PPV has emerged as the most common approach in the surgical management of RRD due to technological advancements, refined instrumentation, enhanced visualization systems, its established safety profile, and the achievement of favorable surgical outcomes. Despite surgical efficacy, the occurrence of retinal displacement remains a potential concern.

Within the context of PPV, retinal displacement's mechanism is attributed to the persistence of a small amount of subretinal fluid immediately after surgery. The large gas bubble injected during PPV generates significant buoyant force and stretches the retina. In this scenario, during the patient's vertical positioning, the fluid prompts a downward retinal displacement and an anomalous interdigitation of photoreceptors with the retinal pigment epithelium (RPE) [10].

Flattering displacement	Less displacement	Factors not clearly related to displacement
PPV	Scleral buckling, pneumatic retinopexy	Type of gas
Tamponade gas	Tamponade silicon oil	Initial extension of the RRD
Macula Off	Immediate face-down positioning post-surgery	Use of PFCL
		Performing posterior retinotomy

PPV: pars plana vitrectomy; RRD: rhegmatogenous retinal detachment; PFCL: liquid perfluorocarbon.

Table 1.
Factors related to retinal displacement after RRD surgery.

In pneumatic retinopexy, the gas bubble introduced into the vitreous cavity during surgery is smaller than in PPV, resulting in smaller buoyancy force exerted on the retina. This enables gradual subretinal fluid reabsorption by the RPE pump. This gradual reabsorption, combined with face-down positioning followed by vertical positioning, facilitates proper photoreceptor interdigitation with the RPE and thereby contributes to a decreased incidence lower of displacement [12].

In more recent literature, the hypothesis of residual subretinal fluid, strong buoyancy force, and a thin and elastic retina has gained prominence as the mechanism leading to retinal stretching and displacement. This hypothesis aligns with the observation that displacement mainly occurs downward, influenced by gravity and head position.

Conversely, instances of upward retinal displacement have been reported in patients undergoing pneumatic retinopexy, particularly when using silicone oil as a tamponade agent. In pneumatic retinopexy, fluid can be displaced upward during the transition from supine to sitting position in the immediate postoperative period, as some patients remain seated for a few minutes before adopting a face-down position. Similarly, when silicone oil is employed as a tamponade agent, residual fluid can also be pushed upward from its posterior pole position by the pressure exerted by the silicone bubble itself.

5. Clinical presentation

Following successful anatomical restoration through surgical retinal detachment repair, there can be cases where patients remain dissatisfied, despite achieving good visual acuity outcomes.

The symptom of distorted lines in the operated eye, known as metamorphopsia, has been strongly associated to retinal displacement in up to 83% of cases [12, 16, 17]. This visual phenomenon is responsible for the visual dissatisfaction experienced by these patients.

On the other hand, several studies have considered decreased corrected visual acuity [14, 16] and alterations in binocular vision due to the perception of an object's image with different sizes in each eye, known as aniseikonia, as clinical manifestations specific to surgically repaired retinal detachment rather than being solely attributed to retinal displacement [12, 18].

In general, current evidence suggests that metamorphopsia is the only symptom clearly linked to retinal displacement.

6. Imaging tests

Retinal displacement is a complication that remains imperceptible via conventional ophthalmoscopic examination, yet can be readily detected through imaging modalities such as autofluorescence.

Autofluorescence imaging of the fundus has emerged as a prominent non-invasive technique for retinal examination in recent years. It relies on the retina's ability, as well as its natural fluorophores like lipofuscin, to emit light within the 500–750 nm range upon stimulation by short-wave light.

In the visual cycle, the RPE is responsible for renewing the outer segments of photoreceptors and degrading their constituents (lipids, proteins, fluorophores).

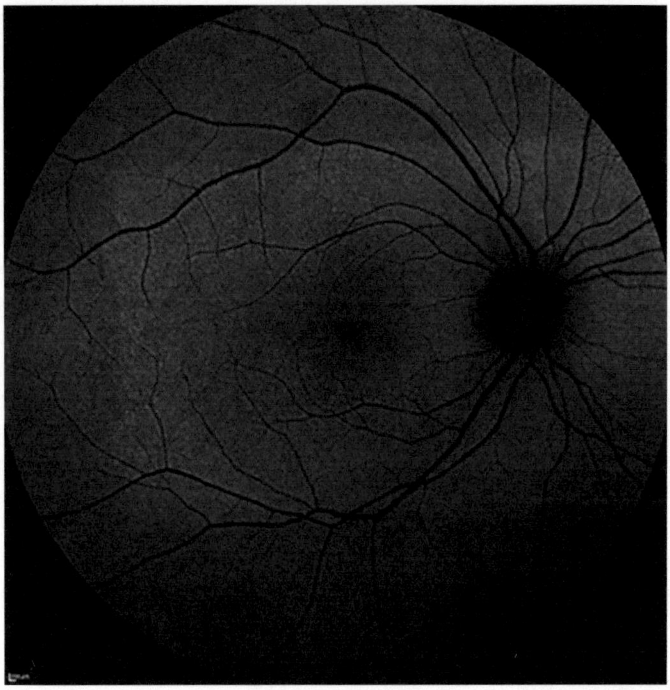

Figure 2.
Normal fundus autofluorescence image. The image depicts the normal autofluorescence of the fundus, highlighting hypoautofluorescent areas (in black), such as the optic nerve and retinal vessels.

However, a fraction of these bioproducts remains unprocessed by RPE lysosomes and accumulates at this level, forming lipofuscin aggregates responsible for the physiological autofluorescence of the retina [10, 19]. Additionally, structures devoid of RPE, such as the optic nerve and retinal vessels, appear dark or hypoautofluorescent in autofluorescence fundus images (**Figure 2**).

This imaging technique allows for the visualization of subtle alterations in retinal layers, including the detection of retinal displacement, which might not be apparent through conventional examination modalities.

In retinal displacement, fundus autofluorescence reveals itself through slightly hyperautofluorescent lines, running parallel to adjacent retinal vessels. These lines accurately reflect the caliber and orientation of these vessels. Such lines correspond to the original imprints of retinal vessels, which have shifted along with the retina following its reattachment (**Figures 3** and **4**) [13].

There are different theories concerning the genesis of these hyperautofluorescent lines. Some authors suggest that these lines might arise due to heightened metabolic activity within segments of the RPE when exposed to light following retinal displacement [10]. On the contrary, another proposition posits the presence of a distinctive composition and attributes of fluorophores within the RPE cells situated in the region of retinal vessel imprints that were concealed prior to the occurrence of retinal displacement [21].

These hyperfluorescent lines in autofluorescence become visible after RRD surgery once the gas has dissipated and the retina becomes explorable, which is typically around 10 days post-surgery. They maintain their morphological appearance, range, and brightness up to 3 months after surgery [10]. However, starting from 12 months

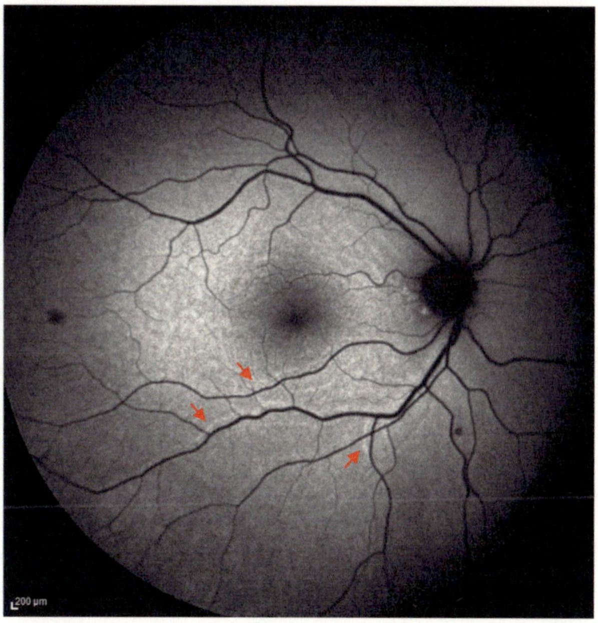

Figure 3.
Autofluorescence of retinal displacement. The image displays the hypoautofluorescence of the optic disc, retinal vessels, and the foveal avascular zone. Additionally, the impressions of retinal vessels are evident in the lower retina, attributed to downward displacement after retinal detachment repair with PPV (red arrows).

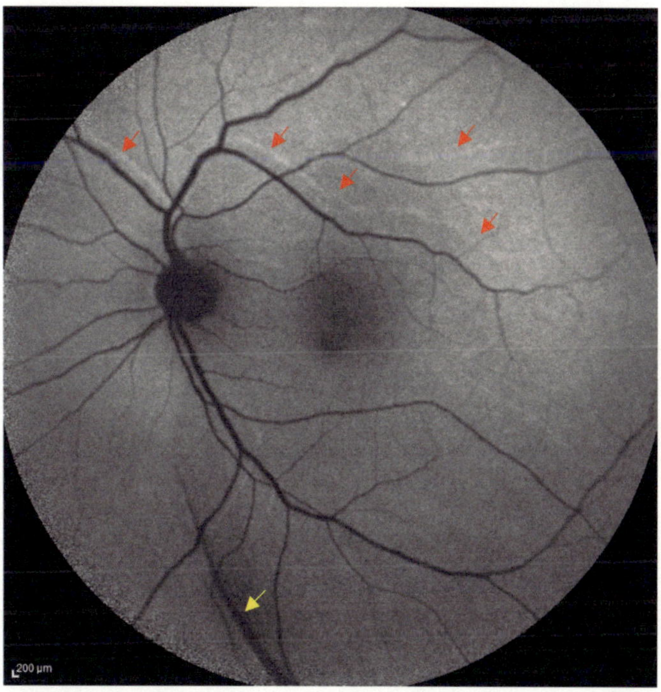

Figure 4.
Retinal displacement autofluorescence. Postoperative images of a patient who underwent upper rhegmatogenous retinal detachment repair in their left eye using PPV [20]. Impressions of retinal vessels (red arrows), inferior retinal fold (yellow arrow).

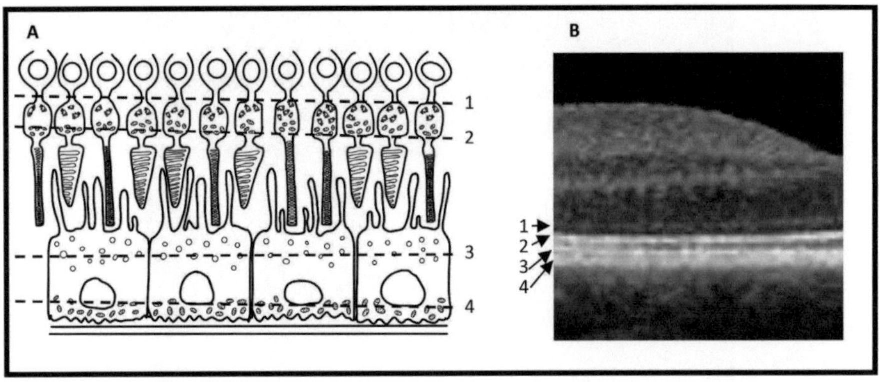

Figure 5.
Microstructure of the outer retina. A: Self-created schematic representation; B: Optical coherence tomography (OCT). 1: External limiting membrane, 2: Photoreceptor ellipsoids, 3: Phagosomes of the outer segments of photoreceptors (apical zone of the RPE), 4: Basal region of the RPE.

post-surgery, a slight repositioning toward the original vessels can be observed. Thus, the retinal alteration in fundus autofluorescence diminishes over the course of a year following RRD surgical repair [22].

While there is an observed tendency for retinal displacement to gradually resolve over time, conclusive evidence supporting complete reversion remains lacking [9].

Another complementary diagnostic test is optical coherence tomography (OCT), which enables the study of the microstructure of the outer retina in patients with retinal displacement. As previously discussed, retinal displacement leads to an abnormal

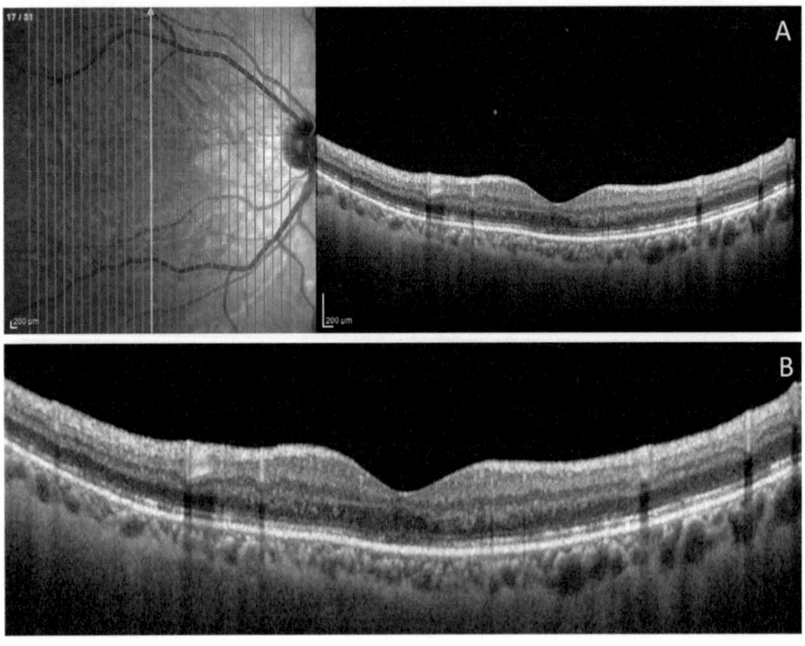

Figure 6.
Optical coherence tomography of a patient with retinal displacement. A. Infrared image en face (left), structural OCT (right). B. Structural OCT B-scan: Subfoveal outer retina anomaly.

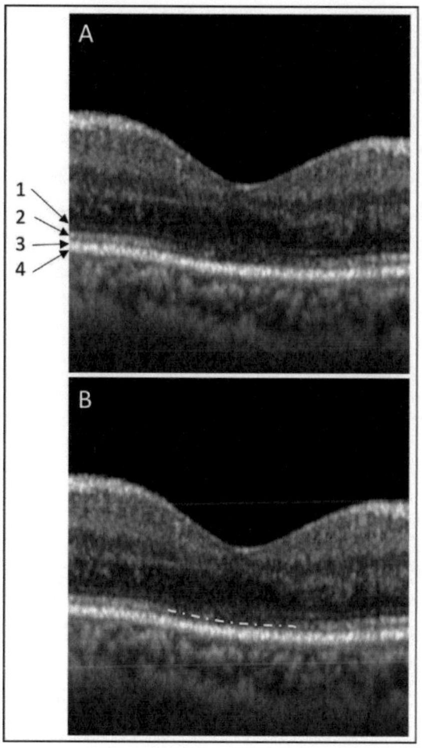

Figure 7.
Optical coherence tomography of a patient with retinal displacement. A: Outer retinal microstructure. Four hyperreflective lines. 1: External limiting membrane, 2: Photoreceptor ellipsoids, 3: Apical zone of RPE containing phagosomes of outer segments of photoreceptors, 4: Mitochondria at the base of RPE. B. Alteration of subfoveal hyperreflective lines (yellow dashed line).

arrangement of photoreceptors within the interdigitation zones of the RPE. These structural changes can be effectively visualized through OCT imaging.

In a normal OCT scan of the outer retina, four distinct hyperreflective lines are discernible. The first corresponds to the external limiting membrane, the second to the ellipsoids of the photoreceptors, the third to the apical region of the RPE containing phagosomes of the outer segment of the photoreceptors, and the fourth corresponds to mitochondria at the base of the RPE (**Figure 5**) [23].

Patients who exhibit retinal displacement with low-integrity reattachment, as evidenced by alterations in the third line (phagosomes of the outer segments of photoreceptors), experience such alterations in up to 95% of cases. This disruption is accountable for the visual dissatisfaction experienced by these patients (**Figures 6** and 7).

7. Prevention of retinal displacement

Prevention of retinal displacement can be addressed through two distinct approaches: during the surgical procedure and in the immediate postoperative phase.

During surgery, several authors propose using a smaller gas bubble as a tamponade than what is conventionally used in both pneumatic retinopexy and PPV. This could facilitate the natural reabsorption of a substantial portion of subretinal fluid, ultimately contributing to a diminished risk of retinal displacement [24, 25].

From the second perspective of the immediate postoperative period, numerous studies agree that performing PPV with gas and immediately positioning the patient in a face-down position in the operating room, maintaining this position for at least 2 hours, can effectively reduce the occurrence of retinal displacement [9].

On the contrary, positions involving a brief period of head elevation or resting supine postures in the immediate postoperative period result in higher rates of retinal displacement. Immediate face-down positioning postoperatively causes the subretinal fluid remaining in the posterior pole to distribute in all directions, not just downward. This is the reason why placing patients face-down after surgery leads to lower rates of retinal displacement. Publications have demonstrated that immediate face-down positioning post-surgery reduces the proportion of patients with retinal displacement from 63.6 to 24.0% [26].

8. Conclusions

No surgical procedure is exempt from potential complications. In the context of retinal detachment, retinal displacement stands as a frequent complication. Despite achieving anatomical success, the dissatisfaction experienced by patients can pose challenges for surgeons. Recognizing this entity can lead to implementing improvements aimed at mitigating this complication.

The utility of fundus autofluorescence lies in its straightforward, rapid, and secure nature as a diagnostic tool. The identification of retinal vessel imprints renders this technique indispensable for the monitoring of patients who have undergone retinal detachment surgery.

Furthermore, understanding the concept of low-integrity reattachment by vitreoretinal surgeons may lead to further refinements in the techniques employed during vitreoretinal surgery for primary rhegmatogenous retinal detachment repair. This, in turn, may yield improved functional outcomes for patients.

Conflict of interest

The authors declare no conflict of interest.

Nomenclature

RPE	retinal pigment epithelium
PPV	Pars plana vitrectomy
RD	retinal detachment
RRD	rhegmatogenous retinal detachment
OCT	optical coherence tomography
AF	autofluorescence
PFCL	perfluorocarbon liquid
PR	photoreceptors
SB	scleral buckling
SF6	sulfur hexafluoride
C3F8	perfluoropropane

DOI: http://dx.doi.org/10.5772/intechopen.1003007

Appendices

Autofluorescence and optical coherence tomography (OCT) images were obtained using SD-OCT (Spectralis®, Heidelberg Engineering, Heidelberg, Germany).

Author details

Romana García Gil*, Anselmo Feliciano Sánchez, Paula Boned-Fustel and Laura Fernández García
Ophthalmology Department, University and Polytechnic Hospital La Fe, Valencia, Spain

*Address all correspondence to: dra.garciagil@gmail.com

References

[1] Mitry D, Charteris DG, Fleck BW, Campbell H, Singh J. The epidemiology of rhegmatogenous retinal detachment: Geographical variation and clinical associations. The British Journal of Ophthalmology [Internet]. 2010 [citado 25 de julio de 2023];**94**(6):678-684. DOI: 10.1136/bjo.2009.157727

[2] Kuhn F, Aylward B. Rhegmatogenous retinal detachment: A reappraisal of its pathophysiology and treatment. Ophthalmic Research [Internet]. 2014 [citado 6 de agosto de 2023];**51**(1):15-31. Available from: https://www.karger.com/Article/FullText/355077

[3] Erickson PA, Fisher SK, Anderson DH, Stern WH, Borgula GA. Retinal detachment in the cat: The outer nuclear and outer plexiform layers. Investigative Ophthalmology & Visual Science [Internet]. 1983 [citado 10 de agosto de 2023];**24**(7):927-942. Available from: https://iovs.arvojournals.org/article.aspx?articleid=2159684

[4] Hisatomi T, Sakamoto T, Murata T, Yamanaka I, Oshima Y, Hata Y, et al. Relocalization of apoptosis-inducing factor in photoreceptor apoptosis induced by retinal detachment in vivo. The American Journal of Pathology [Internet]. 2001 [citado 10 de agosto de 2023];**158**(4):1271-1278. Available from: https://linkinghub.elsevier.com/retrieve/pii/S0002944010640783

[5] Arroyo JG, Yang L, Bula D, Chen DF. Photoreceptor apoptosis in human retinal detachment. American Journal of Ophthalmology [Internet]. 2005 [citado 10 de agosto de 2023];**139**(4):605-610. Available from: https://linkinghub.elsevier.com/retrieve/pii/S0002939404014096

[6] Falkner-Radler CI, Myung JS, Moussa S, Chan RVP, Smretschnig E, Kiss S, et al. Trends in primary retinal detachment surgery: Results of a Bicenter study. Retina [Internet]. 2011 [citado 6 de agosto de 2023];**31**(5):928-936. Available from: https://journals.lww.com/00006982-201105000-00016

[7] Heydinger S, Ufret-Vincenty R, Robertson ZM, He YG, Wang AL. Comparison of surgical outcomes for uncomplicated primary retinal detachment repair. Clinical Ophthalmology [Internet]. 2023 [citado 6 de agosto de 2023];**17**:907-915. Available from: https://www.dovepress.com/comparison-of-surgical-outcomes-for-uncomplicated-primary-retinal-deta-peer-reviewed-fulltext-article-OPTH

[8] Feltgen N, Walter P. Rhegmatogenous Retinal Detachment. Dtsch Ärztebl Int [Internet]. 6 de enero de 2014 [citado 6 de agosto de 2023];**111**(1-2):12-22. Available from https://www.aerzteblatt.de/10.3238/arztebl.2014.0012

[9] Mason RH, Minaker SA, Marafon SB, Figueiredo N, Hillier RJ, Muni RH. Retinal displacement following rhegmatogenous retinal detachment: A systematic review and meta-analysis. Survey of Ophthalmology [Internet]. 2022 [citado 27 de julio de 2023];**67**(4):950-964. Available from: https://linkinghub.elsevier.com/retrieve/pii/S0039625722000029

[10] Shiragami C, Shiraga F, Yamaji H, Fukuda K, Takagishi M, Morita M, et al. Unintentional displacement of the retina after standard vitrectomy for Rhegmatogenous retinal detachment. Ophthalmology [Internet]. 2010 [citado 25 de julio de 2023];**117**(1):86-92.e1. Available from:

https://linkinghub.elsevier.com/retrieve/pii/S016164200900654X

[11] Dell'Omo R, Mura M, Lesnik Oberstein SY, Bijl H, Tan HS. Early simultaneous fundus autofluorescence and optical coherence tomography features after pars plana vitrectomy for primary rhegmatogenous retinal detachment. Retina [Internet]. 2012 [citado 27 de julio de 2023];**32**(4):719-728. Available from: https://journals.lww.com/00006982-201204000-00012

[12] Brosh K, Francisconi CLM, Qian J, Sabatino F, Juncal VR, Hillier RJ, et al. Retinal displacement following pneumatic Retinopexy vs pars Plana vitrectomy for Rhegmatogenous retinal detachment. JAMA Ophthalmology [Internet]. 2020 [citado 25 de julio de 2023];**138**(6):652. Available from: https://jamanetwork.com/journals/jamaophthalmology/fullarticle/2764533

[13] dell'Omo R, Scupola A, Viggiano D, Sammarco MG, De Turris S, Romano MR, et al. Incidence and factors influencing retinal displacement in eyes treated for Rhegmatogenous retinal detachment with vitrectomy and gas or silicone oil. Investigative Ophthalmology & Visual Science [Internet]. 2017 [citado 27 de julio de 2023];**58**(6):BIO191. Available from: http://iovs.arvojournals.org/article.aspx?doi=10.1167/iovs.17-21466

[14] Mahmoudzadeh R, Salabati M, Yonekawa Y, Kuriyan AE, Khan MA, Klufas MA, et al. Retinal displacement following incisional Rhegmatogenous retinal detachment repair. Investigative Ophthalmology & Visual Science [Internet]. 2021 [citado 27 de julio de 2023];**62**(8):3084-3084. Available from: https://iovs.arvojournals.org/article.aspx?articleid=2776336

[15] Casswell EJ, Yorston D, Lee E, Heeren TFC, Harris N, Zvobgo TM, et al. Effect of face-down positioning vs support-the-break positioning after macula-involving retinal detachment repair: The PostRD randomized clinical trial. JAMA Ophthalmology [Internet]. 2020 [citado 27 de julio de 2023];**138**(6):634. Available from: https://jamanetwork.com/journals/jamaophthalmology/fullarticle/2764385

[16] Chelazzi P, Azzolini C, Bellina C, Cappelli F, Del Genovese I, Caraffa L, et al. Efficacy and safety of vitrectomy without using perfluorocarbon liquids and drainage Retinotomy associated with postoperative positioning based on residual subretinal fluid for Rhegmatogenous retinal detachment. Journal of Ophthalmology [Internet]. 2021 [citado 29 de julio de 2023];**2021**:1-9. Available from: https://www.hindawi.com/journals/joph/2021/5588479/

[17] Schawkat M, Valmaggia C, Lang C, Scholl HPN, Harsum S, Guber I, et al. Influence of postoperative posture on macular slippage after macula-off retinal detachment: A randomized controlled trial. Ophthalmology and Therapy [Internet]. 2019 [citado 6 de agosto de 2023];**8**(4):519-525. Available from: http://link.springer.com/10.1007/s40123-019-0204-8

[18] Lee E, Williamson TH, Hysi P, Shunmugam M, Dogramaci M, Wong R, et al. Macular displacement following rhegmatogenous retinal detachment repair. The British Journal of Ophthalmology [Internet]. 2013 [citado 29 de julio de 2023];**97**(10):1297-1302. Available from: https://bjo.bmj.com/lookup/doi/10.1136/bjophthalmol-2013-303637

[19] Spaide R. Autofluorescence from the outer retina and subretinal space: Hypothesis and review. Retina [Internet]. 2008 [citado 30 de julio de 2023];**28**(1):5-35. Available from: https://journals.lww.com/00006982-200801000-00002

[20] García-Gil R, Feliciano-Sánchez A, España GE. Desplazamiento retiniano tras cirugía de desprendimiento de retina. Archivos de la Sociedad Española de Oftalmología [Internet]. 2022 [citado 29 de julio de 2023];**97**(12):722. Available from: https://linkinghub.elsevier.com/retrieve/pii/S0365669122001927

[21] dell'Omo R, Cifariello F, dell'Omo E, De Lena A, Di Iorio R, Filippelli M, et al. Influence of retinal vessel printings on Metamorphopsia and retinal architectural abnormalities in eyes with idiopathic macular Epiretinal membrane. Investigative Ophthalmology & Visual Science [Internet]. 2013 [citado 27 de julio de 2023];**54**(12):7803. Available from: http://iovs.arvojournals.org/article.aspx?doi=10.1167/iovs.13-12817

[22] Guber J, Schawkat M, Scholl HPN, Guber I, Valmaggia C. Long-term outcome of macular shift after retinal detachment repair. Graefe's Archive for Clinical and Experimental Ophthalmology [Internet]. 2021 [citado 27 de julio de 2023];**259**(6):1487-1491. Available from: https://link.springer.com/10.1007/s00417-020-05019-6

[23] Pinilla I, Ruiz-Moreno JM, Cuenca N. Correlation of optical coherence tomography with retinal histology. Archivos de la Sociedad Española de Oftalmología [Internet]. 2012 [citado 30 de julio de 2023];**87**(9):275-277. Available from: https://linkinghub.elsevier.com/retrieve/pii/S2173579412001405

[24] Muni RH, Bansal A, Lee WW, Escaf LC. A method to decrease the frequency of unintentional slippage after vitrectomy for rhegmatogenous retinal detachment. Retina [Internet]. 2023 [citado 28 de julio de 2023];**17**(3):247-250. Available from: https://journals.lww.com/10.1097/ICB.0000000000001174

[25] Muni RH, Felfeli T, Figueiredo N, Marafon SB, Escaf LC, Juncal VR. Minimal gas vitrectomy technique for reducing risk of retinal displacement following rhegmatogenous retinal detachment repair. Retina [Internet]. 2022 [citado 28 de julio de 2023];**16**(6):681-684. Available from: https://journals.lww.com/10.1097/ICB.0000000000001076

[26] Shiragami C, Fukuda K, Yamaji H, Morita M, Shiraga F. A method to decrease the frequency of unintentional slippage after vitrectomy for rhegmatogenous retinal detachment. Retina [Internet]. 2015 [citado 27 de julio de 2023];**35**(4):758-763. Available from: https://journals.lww.com/00006982-201504000-00021